HANDBOOK OF THE VULNERABLE PLAQUE

Edited by

Ron Waksman MD
Professor of Medicine (Cardiology)
Georgetown University
Director, Division of Cardiology
Washington Hospital Center
Washington, DC
USA

Patrick W Serruys MD PhD
Professor of Interventional Cardiology
Erasmus University
Thoraxcenter
Rotterdam
The Netherlands

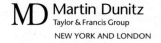

MD Martin Dunitz
Taylor & Francis Group
NEW YORK AND LONDON

© 2004 Taylor & Francis, an imprint of the Taylor & Francis Group plc

First published in the United Kingdom in 2004
by Taylor & Francis, an imprint of the Taylor & Francis Group plc, 11 New Fetter Lane,
London EC4P 4EE

Tel: +44 (0)20 7583 9855
Fax: +44 (0)20 7842 2298
E-mail: info@dunitz.co.uk
Website: http://www.dunitz.co.uk

Although every effort has been made to ensure that all owners of copyright material have
been acknowledged in this publication, we would be glad to acknowledge in subsequent
reprints or editions any omissions brought to our attention.

A CIP record for this book is available from the British Library.

Library of Congress Cataloging-in-Publication Data.

Data available on application.

ISBN 1 84184 323 7

Distributed in North and South America by

Taylor & Francis
2000 NW Corporate Blvd
Boca Raton, FL 33431, USA

Within Continental USA
Tel: 800 272 7737; Fax: 800 374 3401
Outside Continental USA
Tel: 561 994 0555; Fax: 561 361 6018
E-mail: orders@crcpress.com

Distributed in the rest of the world by
Thomson Publishing Services
Cheriton House, North Way
Andover, Hampshire SP10 5BE, UK
Tel: +44 (0)1264 332424
E-mail: salesorder.tandf@thomsonpublishingservices.co.uk

Composition by Creative P&D

Printed and bound in Spain by Grafos, SA

CONTENTS

To my wife who went through a vulnerable period. . . during the gestation of this handbook

Patrick W Serruys

To my wife Tali and my children Ori, Yarden, Jonathan and Daniel

Ron Waksman

LIST OF CONTRIBUTORS

John A Ambrose MD
Comprehensive Cardiovascular Center
Department of Medicine
St. Vincent's Hospital and Medical Center
New York, NY 10011-8202
USA

Chourmouzios A Arampatzis MD
Department of Cardiology
Thoraxcenter
Erasmus Medical Center
NL-3015 GD Rotterdam
The Netherlands

Juan J Badimon PhD
Professor of Medicine
Director, The Zena & Michael A Wiener
    Cardiovascular Institute
Mount Sinai School of Medicine
New York, NY 10029
USA

Antonio Bayes-Genis MD
Minneapolis Heart Institute Foundation
Minnesota Cardiovascular Research
    Institute
Minneapolis, MN 55407
USA

Christoph R Becker MD
Department of Clinical Radiology
University of Munich
Grosshadern
Germany

Brett Bouma PhD
Massachusetts General Hospital
Boston, MA 02114
USA

Vincent J Burgess
Volcano Therapeutics
2870 Kilgore Road
Rancho Cordova, CA 95670
USA

Allen Burke MD
Department of Cardiovascular Pathology
Armed Forces Institute of Pathology
Washington, DC
USA

Fhilippo Cademartiri MD
Department of Radiology
Erasmus Medical Center
NL-3015 GD Rotterdam
The Netherlands

Andrew J Carter DO
Medical Director, Cardiovascular Research
Providence Heart Institute
Portland, OR 97225
USA

S Ward Casscells MD
Professor and Associate Director Of
    Cardiology Research
Texas Heart Institute
6431 Fannin Street
Houston, TX 77030
USA

Robin P Choudhury DM MRCP
Department of Cardiovascular Medicine
University of Oxford Medical School
John Radcliffe Hospital
Oxford OX3 9DU
UK

Cheryl A Conover PhD
Minneapolis Heart Institute Foundation
Minnesota Cardiovascular Research
    Institute
Minneapolis, MN 55407
USA

Brian K Courtney
Division of Cardiovascular Medicine
Center for Research in CV Interventions
Stanford University Medical Center,
    H3554
300 Pasteur Drive
Stanford, CA 94305
USA

David D'Agate DO
Comprehensive Cardiovascular Center
Department of Medicine
St. Vincent's Hospital and Medical Center
New York, NY 10011-8202
USA

Pim J de Feyter MD PhD
Department of Cardiology and Radiology
Thoraxcenter
Erasmus Medical Center
NL-3015 GD Rotterdam
The Netherlands

Chris L de Korte MD
Clinical Physics Laboratory, CUKZ 435
University Medical Center St Radboud
PO Box 9101
6500 HB, Nijmen
The Netherlands

Andrew Farb MD
Department of Cardiovascular Pathology
Armed Forces Institute of Pathology
Washington, DC
USA

Zahi A Fayad PhD
ACC Lecturer, Assistant Professor of
    Radiology
Departments of Radiology and Medicine
    (Cardiology)
The Zena & Michael A Wiener
    Cardiovascular Institute
The Mount Sinai School of Medicine
New York, NY 10029
USA

Aloke V Finn MD
Cardiac Unit
Department of Internal Medicine
Massachusetts General Hospital
Bigelow 800
Boston, MA 02114
USA

Peter J Fitzgerald MD
Assistant Professor of Medicine
Division of Cardiovascular Medicine
Center for Research in CV Interventions
Stanford University Medical Center
300 Pasteur Drive
Stanford, CA 94305
USA

Valentin Fuster MD PhD
Professor of Medicine
Director, The Zena & Michael A Wiener
    Cardiovascular Institute
Mount Sinai School of Medicine
New York, NY 10029
USA

Frank J Gijsen PhD
Erasmus MC Rotterdam
Hemodynamics Laboratory
PO Box 1738, Room 23.11
NL-3000 Rotterdam
The Netherlands

Herman K Gold MD
Cardiac Unit
Department of Internal Medicine
Massachusetts General Hospital
Bigelow 800
Boston, MA 02114
USA

Timothy D Henry MD
Minneapolis Heart Institute Foundation
Minnesota Cardiovascular Research
    Institute
Minneapolis, MN 55407
USA

W Craig Hooper PhD
Hematologic Disease Branch
Centers for Disease Control and
    Prevention
1600 Clifton Road
Atlanta, GA 30333
USA

Angela Hoye MB MRCP
Department of Cardiology
Thoraxcenter
Erasmus Medical Center
NL-3015 GD Rotterdam
The Netherlands

Ik-Kyung Jang MD PhD
Cardiology Division
Massachusetts General Hospital
Bulfinch Building, 55 Fruit Street
Boston, MA 02114
USA

Tanya Khan PhD
Department of Surgery
University of Massachusetts Medical
    School
Worcester, MA
USA

Jon D Klingensmith PhD
Department of Biomedical Engineering
Mail Stop ND20
The Cleveland Clinic Foundation
9500 Eucclid Avenue
Cleveland, OH 44195
USA

Frank D Kolodgie PhD
Department of Cardiovascular Pathology
Armed Forces Institute of Pathology
Washington, DC
USA

Rob Krams MD
Department of Cardiology
Thoraxcenter
Erasmus Medical Center
NL-3015 GD Rotterdam
The Netherlands

Barry D Kuban
Department of Biomedical Engineering
Mail Stop ND20
The Cleveland Clinic Foundation
9500 Eucclid Avenue
Cleveland, OH 44195
USA

Richard E Kuntz MD
Chief, Division of Clinical Biometrics
Brigham & Women's Hospital
900 Commonwealth Avenue
Boston, MA 02215
USA

John R Lesser MD
Minneapolis Heart Institute Foundation
Minnesota Cardiovascular Research
    Institute
Minneapolis, MN 55407
USA

Silvio Litovsky MD
Senior Research Scientist
Texas Heart Institute
Assistant Professor
Department of Pathology, School of
     Medicine
University of Texas Health Science Center
6770 Bertner Avenue
Houston, TX 77030
USA

Mohammad Madjid MD
Assistant Professor of Medicine
Department of Internal Medicine
Division of Cardiology, School of
     Medicine
University of Texas Health Science Center
Texas Heart Institute
6431 Fannin Street
Houston, TX 77030
USA

Paul Magnin PhD
President and CEO
LightLab Imaging Inc
133 Littleton Road
Westford, MA 01886
USA

Willibald Maier MD
Department of Cardiology
University Hospital
CH-8097 Zürich
Switzerland

M Pauliina Margolis MD PhD
Volcano Therapeutics
2870 Kilgore Road
Rancho Cordova, CA 95670
USA

Barbara J Marshik PhD
Infraredx Inc
125 Cambridge Park Drive
Cambridge, MA 02140
USA

Frits Mastik
Experimental Echocardiography
Ee23.02, Erasmus MC
PO Box 1735
NL-3000 DR Rotterdam
The Netherlands

Bernard Meier MD FACC FESC
Professor and Head of Cardiology
Swiss Cardiovascular Center Bern
University Hospital
CH-3010 Bern
Switzerland

Nico Mollet MD
Department of Cardiology
Thoraxcenter
Erasmus Medical Center
NL-3015 GD Rotterdam
The Netherlands

Eric Mont
Department of Cardiovascular Pathology
Armed Forces Institute of Pathology
14th & Alaska, NW
Washington, DC 20306-6000
USA

Pedro R Moreno MD
Assistant Professor of Medicine
University of Kentucky
Rose Street
Lexington, KY 40536
USA

James E Muller MD
Director of Clinical Research
Co-Director of CIMIT Vulnerable Plaque
    Program
Massachusetts General Hospital
Harvard Medical School
Boston, MA 02114
USA

Elizabeth G Nabel MD
Scientific Director, Clinical Research
National Heart, Lung and Blood Institute
10 Center Drive
Bethesda, MD 20892
USA

Morteza Naghavi MD
Director
American Institute of Cardiovascular
    Science and Technology
2472 Boslover, No 439
Houston, TX 77005
USA

Anuja Nair PhD
Department of Biomedical Engineering
Mail Stop ND20
The Cleveland Clinic Foundation
9500 Eucclid Avenue
Cleveland, OH 44195
USA

Karen Nieman MD
Department of Cardiology
Thoraxcenter
Erasmus Medical Center
NL-3015 GD Rotterdam
The Netherlands

Konstantin Nikolaou MD
Imaging Science Laboratories
The Zena & Michael A Wiener
    Cardiovascular Institute
Mount Sinai School of Medicine
New York, NY 10029
USA
and
Department of Clinical Radiology
University of Munich
Grosshadern
Germany

Peter Pattynama MD PhD
Department of Radiology
Erasmus Medical Center
NL-3015 GD Rotterdam
The Netherlands

Evelyn Regar MD PhD
Department of Cardiology
Thoraxcenter
Erasmus Medical Center
NL-3015 GD Rotterdam
The Netherlands

Campbell Rogers MD
Cardiovascular Division
Brigham and Women's Hospital
Harvard Medical School
75 Francis Street
Boston, MA 02115
USA

Francesco Saia MD
Department of Cardiology
Thoraxcenter
Erasmus Medical Center
NL-3015 GD Rotterdam
The Netherlands

Giuseppe Sangiorgi MD
Minneapolis Heart Institute Foundation
Minnesota Cardiovascular Research
    Institute
Minneapolis, MN 55407
USA

Johannes A Schaar MD
Experimental Echocardiography
Ee23.02, Erasmus MC
PO Box 1735
NL-3000 DR Rotterdam
The Netherlands

Robert S Schwartz MD FACC
Minneapolis Heart Institute Foundation
Minnesota Cardiovascular Research
    Institute
Minneapolis, MN 55407
USA

Patrick W Serruys MD PhD
Professor of Interventional Cardiology
Erasmus University
Thoraxcenter
Dr. Molewaterplein 40
3015 GD, Rotterdam
The Netherlands

Cornelis J Slager PhD
Hemodynamics Laboratory
Erasmus MC
PO Box 1738, Room 23.11
NL-3000 DR Rotterdam
The Netherlands

Babs Soller PhD
Department of Surgery
University of Massachusetts Medical
    School
Worcester, MA 01655
USA

Masamichi Takano
Cardiology Division
Massachusetts General Hospital
Boston, MA 02114
USA

Guillermo J Tearney MD PhD
Cardiology Division
Massachusetts General Hospital
Boston, MA 02114
USA

Arturo G Touchard MD
Minneapolis Heart Institute Foundation
Minnesota Cardiovascular Research
    Institute
Minneapolis, MN 55407
USA

Anton FW van der Steen PhD
Head, Department of Experimental
    Echocardiography
Erasmus MC
PO Box 1735
NL-3000 DR Rotterdam
The Netherlands

Glenn van Langenhove MD PhD
Department of Interventional Cardiology
Middelheim Hospital
Antwerp
Belgium

Stefan Verheye MD
Department of Cardiology
Middelheim Hospital
Antwerp
Belgium

Juan F Viles-Gonzalez MD
Instructor of Medicine
Cardiovascular Biology Research
    Laboratory
The Zena & Michael A Wiener
    Cardiovascular Institute
Mount Sinai School of Medicine
New York, NY 10029
USA

D Geoffrey Vince PhD
Department of Biomedical Engineering
Mail Stop ND20
The Cleveland Clinic Foundation
9500 Eucclid Avenue
Cleveland, OH 44195
USA

Renu Virmani MD
Chair, Department of Cardiovascular
    Pathology
Armed Forces Institute of Pathology
14th & Alaska, NW
Washington, DC 20306-6000
USA

Marco Wainstein MD DSc
Hospital de Clinicas de Porto Alegre
Federal University of Rio Grande do Sul
Porto Alegre
Brazil

Ron Waksman MD
Professor of Medicine (Cardiology)
Georgetown University
Director, Division of Cardiology
Washington Hospital Center
Washington, DC 20010
USA

Wei Wei MD
Providence Heart Institute
Providence St Vincent Hospital and
    Medical Center
Portland, OR 97201
USA

Jolanda J Wentzel PhD
Hemodynamics Laboratory
Erasmus MC
PO Box 1738, Room 23.11
NL-3000 DR Rotterdam
The Netherlands

James T Willerson MD FACC
Medical Director
Texas Heart Institute
6770 Bertner Avenue
Houston, TX 77030
USA

Andreas Zeiher MD PhD
Head of Internal Medicine
Johann Wolfgang Goethe University
60054 Frankfurt am Main
Germany

PREFACE

Atherosclerotic cardiovascular disease continues to be a major contributor to coronary heart disease, and more specifically to acute myocardial infarction and death. The recognition of 'vulnerable plaques' and the role they play in vulnerable patients has been previously described and defined both pathologically and clinically. As a result, a new field evolved, which provided new opportunities to better define and understand the biology of vulnerable plaques, and helped develop diagnostic modalities and strategies for its prevention and treatment.

We are pleased to present the first handbook dedicated to the vulnerable plaque, an ever evolving concept facing the new frontier of interventional cardiology. Today, the interventionalist faces the daunting task of translating the ideas of the vulnerable plaque into clinical practice.

The *Handbook of the Vulnerable Plaque* provides interventionalists insight into the world of the vulnerable plaque with introductory chapters that describe the epidemiology, genetic determinants, biology and pathology of vulnerable plaques, while subsequent chapters on detection and diagnosis include biomarkers, MRI, intravascular thermography, intravascular ultrasound, and optical coherence tomography. Possible treatment options are presented in chapters describing drug therapy, photodynamic therapy, and drug-eluting stents, and the handbook's final chapters are devoted to industry representation and device selection.

It is our hope that the *Handbook of the Vulnerable Plaque* will prove useful to the medical community in its effort to serve as a comprehensive guide to understanding the many complexities of the vulnerable plaque and its role in interventional cardiology. As an instructional tool, the *Handbook* will help to enhance diagnostic capabilities and prevention and treatment strategies in our collective efforts to reduce the incidence of acute coronary syndrome, acute myocardial infarction, and sudden cardiac death in our patients.

Many thanks to all of our contributors, recognized and respected worldwide for their work with vulnerable plaque. We would also like to acknowledge the dedication of Alan Burgess of Martin Dunitz for his tremendous efforts in the collection, coordination, and subsequent production of this handbook.

Ron Waksman
Patrick W Serruys

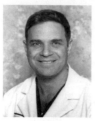

Dr Ron Waksman is the Director of the Division of Cardiology, Washington Hospital Center and the Director of Experimental Angioplasty and Vascular Brachytherapy for the Cardiovascular Research Institute at Washington Hospital Center, Washington, DC. He is also a clinical professor of medicine (cardiology) at Georgetown University. Dr Waksman

Dr Ron Waksman

is an interventional cardiologist currently involved in exploring modalities to treat vascular atherosclerotic disease with the utilization of photodynamic therapy. In addition, he is engaged in the research and development of bio-absorbable stents. He serves as a national and international principal investigator of leading studies in the field of interventional cardiology and vascular brachytherapy. Dr Waksman is also the editor-in-chief of the Cardiovascular Radiation Medicine Journal. He is an editor of three books in the field and has more than 210 peer-reviewed manuscripts published in professional journals.

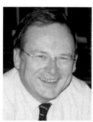

Patrick W Serruys MD PhD FACC FESC is Professor of Interventional Cardiology, Erasmus University, and Head, Department of Interventional Cardiology, Thoraxcenter, Erasmus Medical Center, The Netherlands. Co-Director of EuroPCR and Guest Faculty Member of most interventional cardiology meetings (TCT, JIM, ACC and AHA), author of at

Prof Patrick W Serruys

least 800 peer-reviewed papers and editor of over 30 books, Professor Serruys is one of the world's leading pioneers and experts in interventional cardiology and is Principal Investigator of many international randomized clinical trials. His current interests are the drug eluting stents and the vulnerable plaque.

1. DEFINITION OF THE VULNERABLE PLAQUE

James E Muller and Pedro R Moreno

The title of this handbook uses the term 'vulnerable plaque', which most would agree refers to a topic of great importance. However, there is considerable disagreement over the precise meaning of this term, and the related terms 'high-risk plaque' and 'thrombosis-prone plaque'. We propose that all three terms – high-risk plaque, vulnerable plaque and thrombosis-prone plaque – be used as synonyms to refer to a plaque at increased risk of causing thrombosis and lesion progression. We will provide support for this proposal in the discussion below, and also offer suggestions for the use of the terms 'thin-cap fibroatheroma', 'unstable plaque' and 'disrupted plaque', which are also the source of considerable confusion. If common usage of these terms was developed and widely accepted, it would facilitate communication among basic scientists, clinical researchers and clinicians working to prevent and treat acute cardiovascular disease.

History of recognition of plaque vulnerability

Plaque rupture

In 1966, Dr Paris Constantinides provided the first convincing evidence that plaque rupture was the cause of onset of most acute cardiovascular disease.[1] Prior to his work, several authors had proposed that coronary thrombosis was caused by breaks in the atheroma surface, but data supporting such a mechanism were limited.[2–4]

Dr Constantinides examined the coronary arteries of 22 patients with coronary artery disease, 17 of whom had acute coronary thrombosis. In order to avoid missing a site of rupture, he studied a total of more than 40 000 histologic sections, covering the entire segment of each artery containing a thrombus. All 17 of the acute thrombi were found to originate over cracks in the intimal surface of the plaque, confirming the hypothesis he had formulated based on the pre-existing literature, and his prior animal studies. This observation has been confirmed by many investigators, and is the basis of modern understanding of the atherosclerotic substrate causing thrombus formation in the arterial circulation.

Consequences of plaque rupture

In 1984 (and in a series of subsequent studies) Willerson et al advanced the concept that conversion of chronic to acute coronary disease occurs when such an anatomically altered plaque becomes a stimulus for platelet adhesion, aggregation and mediator accumulation.[5] Studies have now documented that thromboxane A_2, serotonin and other mediators are generated, which may cause subsequent thrombosis and vasoconstriction.[6–8] The animal model of cyclic coronary artery flow reductions developed by Folts has been particularly useful in studying such mediators and their inhibitors.[9] These outcomes of rupture of vulnerable/high-risk plaques lead to a decrease in coronary blood flow which, in turn, causes the clinical events.

Definitions of plaque vulnerability

A functional definition

By 1994, there was widespread recognition of the importance of plaque rupture, thrombosis and mediator generation in the onset of cardiovascular disease. On the basis of this knowledge, our studies on triggering of disease onset led us to propose that the term 'vulnerable' be used to describe a plaque that by becoming disrupted had a high likelihood of starting the adverse cascade.[10] This was an uncomplicated functional definition that did not (i) depend on the histologic features of the plaque and (ii) did not indicate how such a plaque might be identified prospectively, or stabilized before it caused the onset of disease.

Following the introduction of this functional definition of plaque vulnerability, evidence continued to accumulate suggesting, but not proving, that plaques with a large lipid core, thin cap and increased macrophage content were vulnerable plaques. Such plaques can be described as inflamed thin-cap fibroatheromas[11–12] (TCFAs). While inflamed TCFAs are strongly suspected to represent vulnerable plaques, there are, as yet, no prospective studies proving that they are at increased risk of leading to thrombosis and lesion progression. Also, there appear to be plaques without these histologic features that may be associated with arterial thrombosis and therefore should be considered vulnerable.[13] Hence, at the present time, for the sake of scientific rigor, it is important to describe a vulnerable plaque as a functional concept and avoid the histologic definition.

A histologic definition

Since the classic studies of Constantinides, many pathologic studies have suggested that inflamed TCFAs frequently cause coronary events.[14–24] All such studies are limited by their retrospective nature. However, just as an examination of the wreckage can yield information about an airplane's malfunction prior to a crash, these pathologic studies have made it possible to describe the likely histologic features of the plaque prior to disruption. They strongly suggest that an inflamed

TCFA is likely to be a vulnerable plaque, but proof is not yet available. In legal terms, an inflamed TCFA is indicted, but not yet convicted.

There are additional types of plaque suspected to be vulnerable. Recent pathologic studies have revealed that a number of plaques causing thrombosis – and hence proved to have been vulnerable – were not TCFAs. Farb et al analyzed plaque characteristics in 50 subjects with sudden cardiac death due to coronary thrombosis.[20] In 22 of the cases (44%) the thrombosis occurred at a site with erosion which did not occur over a thin cap and lipid pool. The plaque appeared to have an increased proteoglycan content. Hence, a plaque rich in proteoglycans might be a second histologic type of vulnerable or high-risk plaque. Furthermore, Virmani and her group have also identified a calcified nodule as a potentially vulnerable plaque.

Specificity of a TCFA for vulnerability is also limited because it is known that plaques with a large lipid pool, thin cap and increased macrophage content, which are not disrupted, can be found at autopsy.[22,24] In some cases, such plaques may cause stable angina only, although their histologic features suggest they could produce an acute coronary syndrome.

A prospective definition

The most useful definition of a vulnerable plaque is one that can be applied prospectively to individual lesions. While routine coronary angiograms are often used to make inferences about plaque vulnerability, as recently noted by Little and Applegate, 'The shadows leave a doubt'.[25] In a 1998 review, Kullo et al stated that no method reliably identifies plaques prone to rupture.[26] However, there is reason to believe that one, or more, of a broad array of new technologies will make it possible to identify vulnerable plaques prospectively in the coronary arteries of living patients.

In a study that has received much less attention than it deserves, Uchida and colleagues demonstrated that angioscopy could identify vulnerable plaques prospectively in living patients.[27] A prospective angioscopic survey was done of all three coronary arteries of 157 patients with angina. Thirteen of these patients had a glistening yellow plaque, shown in a separate autopsy series to represent a lipid pool with a very thin cap. During a 1-year follow-up, 68% of the patients with the vulnerable glistening yellow plaque experienced an acute coronary syndrome; only 4% of those without such a plaque experienced an event.

This study, when replicated in a larger group, is likely to permit a vulnerable plaque to be defined prospectively as a glistening yellow plaque identified by angioscopy. While such an achievement is valuable for research purposes, it is unlikely to have clinical utility. Angioscopy requires coronary artery occlusion, the identification of a 'glistening yellow' appearance is subjective, and angioscopy would not be expected to identify the vulnerable plaques discussed above, that are not associated with a lipid pool and a thin fibrous cap.

While non-invasive detection of vulnerable coronary plaques must be the ultimate goal, such approaches face formidable obstacles of coronary artery motion, small size and central location. Promising results have been obtained with MRI (magnetic resonance imaging) detection of presumably vulnerable plaques in the aorta and carotid arteries, which are larger and less mobile than the coronary arteries.[28–29]

It is likely that the initial prospective identification of vulnerable coronary plaques will first be achieved by one of several competing intracoronary technologies applied to patients already undergoing an intervention. In addition to angioscopy, diffuse reflectance near-infrared spectroscopy, Raman near-infrared spectroscopy, optical coherence tomography, thermography, intracoronary MRI, intracoronary ultrasound and quantitative angiography are all being advocated for vulnerable plaque detection.[30–38] Prospective clinical trials will identify the optimal intracoronary method that will aid the subsequent development of non-invasive means of detection of vulnerable coronary plaques.

For each technique (invasive, and subsequently non-invasive) to be evaluated, prospective identification should start with mapping of the three main coronary arteries for the features the technique can detect. A group of approximately 1000 patients followed prospectively for 1 year would produce a number of coronary events (unstable angina, myocardial infarction and sudden cardiac death) in which the plaque proved to be vulnerable could be localized by angiography or autopsy examination. Repeat angiography at 1 year in all patients could also identify plaques that showed major progression, but did not cause an event. Such rapid increases in stenosis have been shown to result from plaque rupture and thrombosis.

A combination of criteria for vulnerability that included clinical events and angiographic progression may provide sufficient statistical power for prospective analysis. If such a study validated the hypothesis that a certain signature of a plaque predicted a negative outcome, a great advance in the diagnostic capability of the catheterization laboratory would be achieved. By examining the baseline characteristics of coronary plaques that met the criteria for vulnerability, cardiologists would be able to identify vulnerable plaques in advance, a major challenge for contemporary medicine. It is likely that varying signatures would be associated with varying degrees of risk, i.e. plaques with a higher temperature, or more extreme spectroscopic score would be more vulnerable.

From such a study, the following prospective definition of a vulnerable plaque could then be formulated: a plaque, identified prospectively (by the technology tested), is documented to have a high likelihood of forming a thrombogenic focus. The thrombus could produce immediate disease onset, or rapid, asymptomatic, angiographic progression. On the other hand, a plaque with a low likelihood of causing such an outcome would be termed 'non-vulnerable'.

Nonetheless, as discussed above, at the present time three histologic subtypes of plaque suspected to be vulnerable have been identified: (i) a thin-capped fibroatheroma, (ii) plaques with increased proteoglycan content or inflammation leading to erosion and thrombosis, and (iii) a plaque with a calcified nodule. Prospective studies are needed to confirm these hypotheses.

Treatment of vulnerable plaques

The ability to measure plaque vulnerability would open a vast field of study of plaque stabilization therapy.[39] Systemic pharmacologic approaches that have been advocated include intense lipid lowering, matrix metalloproteinase inhibitors, ACAT (acyl-CoA: cholesterol acyltransferase) inhibitors, ACE (angiotensin converting enzyme) inhibitors, anti-inflammatory agents, antibiotics, anti-oxidants and angiogenesis inhibitors.[40–47] Local, intracoronary therapies that might stabilize vulnerable plaques include stenting of lesions with less than critical stenosis, radiation therapy, gene therapy and angioplasty or coronary stenting to induce fibrosis.[48–52]

Disrupted plaques

The term 'disrupted' has been used in some cases to refer to a plaque that causes some degree of thrombosis, but in other cases to describe the nature of the lesion. As is clear from the prior discussion, in some cases thrombosis may result from rupture of a thin cap covering a lipid pool, while in others it may be caused by erosion of the surface of a plaque rich in proteoglycans, inflammatory cells, or one having a less distinctive histologic appearance. In any case, the plaque proved itself to have been vulnerable by its transformation into a 'thrombosed plaque'.

It seems best to avoid the use of the word 'disrupted' and refer instead to 'thrombosed plaques', the meaning of which is less ambiguous. The transition would then be from a vulnerable/high-risk/thrombosis-prone plaque to a 'thrombosed plaque'. Since plaques that have recently ruptured and thrombosed are suspected to be at high risk for growth of thrombus (in the absence of anti-thrombotic therapy), a thrombosed plaque could also be considered to be yet another form of 'vulnerable' plaque.

Unstable plaques

The term 'unstable' has received highly variable usage. In some cases, it has been used to describe vulnerable plaques, and in others to refer to disrupted plaques, as defined above. A symposium has been dedicated to the topic of 'potentially unstable plaques'. Because the term also has well-accepted clinical usage to describe unstable angina pectoris, confusion between the clinical syndrome and the plaque under discussion is inevitable.

Given the difficulties with the term, and the adequacy of the terms 'vulnerable' and 'thrombosed plaque', we propose that the term 'unstable' be reserved for the clinical syndrome and not applied to the plaque.

Relation to the AHA classification of atherosclerotic lesions

The usage of the terms 'vulnerable/high-risk plaque', and 'thrombosed plaque' proposed above complements the AHA (American Heart Association) classification of atherosclerotic lesions.[53–54] The AHA classification, which is based on histologic features rather than functional significance, divides plaques into six types with increasing complexity: type I (initial changes); type II (fatty streak); type III (pre-atheroma); type IV (atheroma); type V (fibroatheroma); and type VI (complicated plaque).

The relation of thrombosed plaques with this classification is quite simple – all thrombosed lesions would be included in type VI as complicated lesions. Differences between functional and histologic definitions are more marked for the vulnerable/high-risk plaque, because, as noted by the AHA committee, thrombosis may result from any of the six histologic types. In the extreme case, thrombosis may even occur due to endothelial dysfunction at a site with no detectable histologic abnormality. However, most vulnerable/high-risk plaques will exhibit a type IV (atheroma) or type V (fibroatheroma) histologic appearance. The advent of a prospective means of quantitating vulnerability will make it possible to assign vulnerability scores to the different AHA classification types.

Virmani et al have noted several deficiencies of the AHA histologic classification and proposed alternative categories.[55] Alteration of histologic categories would not affect the usage of 'vulnerable/high-risk plaque' and 'thrombosed plaque' proposed above.

Frequency of suspected vulnerable/high-risk plaques in individual patients

There are several obstacles to answering the seemingly simple question of the frequency of vulnerable plaques in individual patients. While clinical events indicate how many vulnerable plaques might cause symptoms in a given group of patients, for instance, a 5% annual rate of cardiac events in a population of post-myocardial infarction patients would signify that, at the least, 5% of the patients had one vulnerable plaque; not all thrombosis caused by a vulnerable plaque leads to symptoms. Some patients may have collateral vessels that can provide an alternative source of blood flow. In other patients, the thrombosis may not be occlusive, and the residual flow may be sufficient to meet the needs of the myocardium downstream.

An additional obstacle to determining frequency of vulnerable plaques, or even thrombosed plaques, has been the lack of a method to easily identify either type of plaque in patients.

Finally, since, as stated earlier, there are no prospective studies clearly establishing that any particular histologic type of plaque is indeed a vulnerable plaque, it is not possible, without the use of simplifying assumptions, to identify the frequency of vulnerable plaque. Efforts therefore shift to detection of an inflamed thin-cap fibroatheroma, which is a suspected, but not proven, vulnerable plaque.

While autopsy-based studies have a certain selection bias, the best evidence about the frequency of various histologic types of plaques comes from post-mortem specimens. It is, of course, easier to determine the incidence of thrombosed plaques, than vulnerable plaques. Falk identified 103 ruptured plaques in 47 patients dying from coronary atherosclerosis preceded by chest pain.[56] Forty of these were associated with occlusive thrombosis. The remaining 63 ruptured sites were associated with grossly discernible intimal hemorrhage without occlusive thrombosis but with a tiny mural thrombus sealing the ruptured site.[56] Davies and Thomas identified 115 thrombotic segments in 74 patients dying from sudden cardiac death. Of note, intraluminal thrombus was also found in eight out of 79 control patients dying from non-cardiac causes.[57] In addition, Frink identified 211 ruptured plaques in 83 patients dying from acute coronary events.[58] This number included many sites of chronic rupture, which no longer demonstrated any sign of intraluminal thrombosis. This supports the concept of atherosclerosis as a multifocal process in which multiple vulnerable plaques can develop and thrombose, with only a subset of thromboses leading to clinical events.[58]

Although the visualization of ruptured plaques in patients is not an easy task, intravascular ultrasound (IVUS) has provided some information about their frequency in patients with acute coronary events. Rioufol et al reported on IVUS evidence of ruptured plaques obtained in 24 patients with acute coronary events.[59] Many ruptured plaques (41/50) were identified at sites other than the site responsible for the clinical event. These additional ruptured lesions were less stenotic and less calcified than the culprit lesions.[59]

Angioscopy, which is more difficult to perform than IVUS but provides better information about endoluminal structures, has also been used to identify thrombosed plaques. Asakura et al performed three-vessel coronary angioscopy in 20 patients 1 month after acute myocardial infarction. The incidence of coronary thrombosis, as might be expected, was 81% on lesions responsible for the event.[60] In addition, 2% of lesions not associated with the clinical event also showed evidence of thrombosis.[60] This occurred despite the likelihood that such post-myocardial infarction patients were receiving anti-thrombotic therapy.

The deficiencies in information about the number of thrombosed plaques are minor compared to problems of identifying the number of vulnerable/high-risk plaques for the reasons stated above. If the assumption is made that an inflamed TCFA is a vulnerable plaque, some information is available.

Post-mortem studies were performed by Burke et al in 113 individuals who died suddenly of severe coronary artery disease.[61] They identified an average of 1.2 TCFA per patient. TCFAs were more frequently found in white, hypercholesterolemic men and correlated directly with levels of blood cholesterol. Similar findings were found in women by the same group of investigators.[62]

Precise quantitation of the frequency of TCFAs in living patients is difficult due to limitations of the technology that is currently available. For instance, few instruments have the capability of determining that a cap is less than 65 μm in thickness. However, yellow appearance of a plaque has been taken as presumptive evidence of a thin cap covering a lipid pool. Asakura et al identified yellow plaques as a rather common angioscopic finding in living patients after acute myocardial infarction.[60] Yellow plaques were equally prevalent in the infarct-related and non-infarct-related coronary arteries (3.7 ± 1.6 and 3.4 ± 1.8 plaques/artery, respectively). However, detailed pathologic studies have found that yellow plaques often have a fibrous cap thickness greater than 65 μm and hence would not qualify as TCFAs.[17]

In the study cited earlier,[27] Uchida et al have reported that *glistening* yellow plaques have an average fibrous cap thickness of only 10 μm and hence could be considered to be TCFAs. Uchida identified 118 white and 39 yellow plaques in 186 consecutive patients with stable angina who underwent three-vessel angioscopy. Of the 39 yellow plaques identified, 13 were glistening and 26 non-glistening. Hence in this carefully studied group of patients with stable angina pectoris, there were 13 (7%) presumed TCFAs.

In the following chapters, many techniques are described that will provide improved characterization of plaques in living patients. Studies conducted with these new instruments will provide much better information about the incidence of vulnerable and thrombosed plaques than is currently available.

Summary

A simplified terminology is proposed for the types of plaque causing acute coronary disease. Vulnerable/high-risk/thrombosis-prone plaques are those defined prospectively to have a high likelihood of causing thrombosis which in turn may lead to asymptomatic lesion progression and/or a clinical event. These terms are proposed for use as concepts. The histologic features of such plaques are not yet clearly identified. TCFA, proteoglycan-rich areas and calcified nodules are suspected to be three types of vulnerable plaque, but confirmatory evidence is needed. Thrombosed plaques are those complicated by any degree of thrombosis. The term 'unstable' is reserved for the clinical syndrome.

In the chapters that follow, the reader will encounter variable use of these terms. The individual chapters have not been tailored to conform to the definitions given above, nor is such usage universal in the current literature. However, it is hoped that the proposed terminology will facilitate understanding of the underlying message despite variable usage.

In his classic 1966 publication, Dr Constantinides noted that 'it would appear rewarding to search not only for changes in the blood favouring coagulation, but also for factors increasing the fragility – or provoking the fracture – of atheroma surfaces in human victims of coronary thrombosis'.[1] A standardized nomenclature will assist this search, and lead to rewarding efforts to diagnose and treat dangerous plaques before they cause their catastrophic consequences.

References

1. Constantinides P. Plaque fissures in human coronary thrombosis. *J Atheroscler Res* 1966; **6**:1–17.

2. Koch LKaW. Uber die Formen des Coronarrerschlusses, die Anderungen im Coronarkreislauf und die Beziehungen zur Angina Pectoris. *Alleg Pathol* 1932; **90**:21–84.

3. Drury R. The role of initmal haemorrhage in coronary occlusion. *J Pathol Bacteriol* 1954; **67**:207–15.

4. Leary T. Atherosclerosis; special consideration of aortic lesions. *Arch Pathol* 1936; **21**:419–52.

5. Willerson JT, Campbell WB, Winniford MD et al. Conversion from chronic to acute coronary artery disease: speculation regarding mechanisms. *Am J Cardiol* 1984; **54**:1349–54.

6. Willerson JT, Hillis LD, Winniford M, Buja LM. Speculation regarding mechanisms responsible for acute ischemic heart disease syndromes. *J Am Coll Cardiol* 1986; **8**:245–50.

7. Willerson JT, Golino P, Eidt J, Campbell WB, Buja LM. Specific platelet mediators and unstable coronary artery lesions. Experimental evidence and potential clinical implications. *Circulation* 1989; **80**:198–205.

8. Willerson JT. Stable angina pectoris: recent advances in predicting prognosis and treatment. *Adv Intern Med* 1998; **43**:175–202.

9. Maalej N, Folts JD. Increased shear stress overcomes the antithrombotic platelet inhibitory effect of aspirin in stenosed dog coronary arteries. *Circulation* 1996; **93**:1201–5.

10. Muller JE, Abela GS, Nesto RW, Tofler GH. Triggers, acute risk factors and vulnerable plaques: the lexicon of a new frontier. *J Am Coll Cardiol* 1994; **23**:809–13.

11. Kolodgie FD, Burke AP, Farb A et al. The thin-cap fibroatheroma: a type of vulnerable plaque: the major precursor lesion to acute coronary syndromes. *Curr Opin Cardiol* 2001; **16**:285–92.

12. Virmani R, Burke AP, Kolodgie FD, Farb A. Pathology of the thin-cap fibroatheroma: a type of vulnerable plaque. *J Interv Cardiol* 2003; **16**:267–72.

13. Farb A, Tang AL, Burke AP et al. Sudden coronary death. Frequency of active coronary lesions, inactive coronary lesions, and myocardial infarction. *Circulation* 1995; **92**:1701–9

14. Davies MJ. Detecting vulnerable coronary plaques. *Lancet* 1996; **347**:1422–3.

15. Moreno PR, Falk E, Palacios IF et al. Macrophage infiltration in acute coronary syndromes. Implications for plaque rupture. *Circulation* 1994; **90**:775–8.

16. Falk E, Shah PK, Fuster V. Coronary plaque disruption. *Circulation* 1995; **92**:657–71.

17. Libby P. Molecular bases of the acute coronary syndromes. *Circulation* 1995; **91**:2844–50.

18. Davies MJ. Acute coronary thrombosis – the role of plaque disruption and its initiation and prevention. *Eur Heart J* 1995; **16 (Suppl L)**:3–7.

19. Moreno PR, Bernardi VH, Lopez-Cuellar J et al. Macrophages, smooth muscle cells, and tissue factor in unstable angina. Implications for cell-mediated thrombogenicity in acute coronary syndromes. *Circulation* 1996; **94**:3090–7.

20. Farb A, Burke AP, Tang AL et al. Coronary plaque erosion without rupture into a lipid core. A frequent cause of coronary thrombosis in sudden coronary death. *Circulation* 1996; **93**:1354–63.

21. Burke AP, Farb A, Malcom GT et al. Plaque rupture and sudden death related to exertion in men with coronary artery disease. *JAMA* 1999; **281**:921–6.

22. Pasterkamp G, Schoneveld AH, van der Wal AC et al. Inflammation of the atherosclerotic cap and shoulder of the plaque is a common and locally observed feature in unruptured plaques of femoral and coronary arteries. *Arterioscler Thromb Vasc Biol* 1999; **19**:54–8.

23. Shah PK, Falk E, Badimon JJ et al. Human monocyte-derived macrophages induce collagen breakdown in fibrous caps of atherosclerotic plaques. Potential role of matrix-degrading metalloproteinases and implications for plaque rupture. *Circulation* 1995; **92**:1565–9.

24. van der Wal AC, Becker AE, Koch KT et al. Clinically stable angina pectoris is not necessarily associated with histologically stable atherosclerotic plaques. *Heart* 1996; **76**:312–16.

25. Little WC, Applegate RJ. The shadows leave a doubt – the angiographic recognition of vulnerable coronary artery plaques. *J Am Coll Cardiol* 1999; **33**:1362–4.

26. Kullo IJ, Edwards WD, Schwartz RS. Vulnerable plaque: pathobiology and clinical implications. *Ann Intern Med* 1998; **129**:1050–60.

27. Uchida Y, Nakamura F, Tomaru T et al. Prediction of acute coronary syndromes by percutaneous coronary angioscopy in patients with stable angina. *Am Heart J* 1995; **130**:195–203.

28. Fuster V. Mechanisms of arterial thrombosis: foundation for therapy. *Am Heart J* 1998; **135**:S361–6.

29. Toussaint JF, Pachot-Clouard M, Bridal SL, Gouya H, Berger G. Non-invasive imaging of atherosclerosis by MRI and ultrasonography. *Arch Mal Coeur Vaiss* 1999; **92**:349–54.

30. Cassis LA, Lodder RA. Near-IR imaging of atheromas in living arterial tissue. *Anal Chem* 1993; **65**:1247–56.

31. Dempsey RJ, Cassis LA, Davis DG, Lodder RA. Near-infrared imaging and spectroscopy in stroke research: lipoprotein distribution and disease. *Ann NY Acad Sci* 1997; **820**:149–69.

32. Moreno PR, Lodder RA, Purushothaman KR et al. Detection of lipid pool, thin fibrous cap and inflammatory cell infiltration in human aortic atherosclerotic plaques by near infrared spectroscopy. *Circulation* 2002; **105**:923–7.

33. Moreno PR, Lodder R, O'Connor WN et al. Characterization of vulnerable plaques by near-infrared spectroscopy in an atherosclerotic rabbit model. *J Am Coll Cardiol* 1999; **33**:66A.

34. Moreno PR, Eric Ryan S, Hopkins D et al. Identification of lipid-rich plaques in human coronary artery autopsy specimens by near-infrared spectroscopy. *J Am Coll Cardiol* 2001; **37**:1219–90.

35. Brennan JF III, Romer TJ, Lees RS et al. Determination of human coronary artery composition by Raman spectroscopy. *Circulation* 1997; **96**:99–105.

36. Brezinski ME, Tearney GJ, Weissman NJ et al. Assessing atherosclerotic plaque morphology: comparison of optical coherence tomography and high frequency intravascular ultrasound. *Heart* 1997; **77**:397–403.

37. Casscells W, Hathorn B, David M et al. Thermal detection of cellular infiltrates in living atherosclerotic plaques: possible implications for plaque rupture and thrombosis. *Lancet* 1996; **347**:1447–51.

38. Stefanadis C, Diamantopoulos L, Vlachopoulos C et al. Thermal heterogeneity within human atherosclerotic coronary arteries detected in vivo: a new method of detection by application of a special thermography catheter. *Circulation* 1999; **99**:1965–71.

39. Moreno PR, Shah PK, Falk E. Triggering of acute coronary syndromes – implications for prevention. In: *Determinants of Rupture of Atherosclerotic Coronary Lesions*. The Netherlands: Kluwer Academic Publishers, 1996:268–83.

40. Bocan TM, Mueller SB, Brown EQ et al. HMG-CoA reductase and ACAT inhibitors act synergistically to lower plasma cholesterol and limit atherosclerotic lesion development in the cholesterol-fed rabbit. *Atherosclerosis* 1998; 139:21–30.

41. MacIsaac AI, Thomas JD, Topol EJ. Toward the quiescent coronary plaque. *J Am Coll Cardiol* 1993; **22**:1228–41.

42. Cheng JW, Ngo MN. Current perspective on the use of angiotensin-converting enzyme inhibitors in the management of coronary (atherosclerotic) artery disease. *Ann Pharmacother* 1997; **31**:1499–506.

43. Gurfinkel E, Bozovich G, Daroca A, Beck E, Mautner B. Randomised trial of roxithromycin in non-Q-wave coronary syndromes: ROXIS Pilot Study. ROXIS Study Group. *Lancet* 1997; **350**:404–7.

44. Gupta S, Leatham EW, Carrington D et al. Elevated *Chlamydia pneumoniae* antibodies, cardiovascular events, and azithromycin in male survivors of myocardial infarction. *Circulation* 1997; **96**:404–7.

45. Anderson JL, Muhlestein JB, Carlquist J et al. Randomized secondary prevention trial of azithromycin in patients with coronary artery disease and serological evidence for *Chlamydia pneumoniae* infection: The Azithromycin in Coronary Artery Disease: Elimination of Myocardial Infection with *Chlamydia* study. *Circulation* 1999; **99**:1540–7.

46. Stein O, Dabach Y, Hollander G et al. Dexamethasone impairs cholesterol egress from a localized lipoprotein depot in vivo. *Atherosclerosis* 1998; **137**:303–10.

47. Stephens NG, Parsons A, Schofield PM et al. Randomised controlled trial of vitamin E in patients with coronary disease: Cambridge Heart Antioxidant Study (CHAOS). *Lancet* 1996; **347**:781–6.

48. Isner JM, Walsh K, Symes J et al. Arterial gene therapy for therapeutic angiogenesis in patients with peripheral artery disease. *Circulation* 1995; **91**:2687–92.

49. Teirstein PS, Massullo V, Jani S et al. Catheter-based radiotherapy to inhibit restenosis after coronary stenting. *N Engl J Med* 1997; **336**:1697–703.

50. Condado JA, Waksman R, Gurdiel O et al. Long-term angiographic and clinical outcome after percutaneous transluminal coronary angioplasty and intracoronary radiation therapy in humans. *Circulation* 1997; **96**:727–32.

51. Lafont A, Libby P. The smooth muscle cell: sinner or saint in restenosis and the acute coronary syndromes? *J Am Coll Cardiol* 1998; **32**:283–5.

52. Moreno PR, Kilpatrick D, Purushothaman KR, Coleman L, O'Connor WN. Stenting vulnerable plaques improves fibrous cap thickness and reduces lipid content: understanding alternatives for plaque stabilization. *Am J Cardiol* 2002: **90**:50H

53. Stary HC, Chandler AB, Dinsmore RE et al. A definition of advanced types of atherosclerotic lesions and a histological classification of atherosclerosis. A report from the Committee on Vascular Lesions of the Council on Arteriosclerosis, American Heart Association. *Circulation* 1995; **92**:1355–74.

54. Stary HC, Chandler AB, Glagov S et al. A definition of initial, fatty streak, and intermediate lesions of atherosclerosis. A report from the Committee on Vascular Lesions of the Council on Arteriosclerosis, American Heart Association. *Arterioscler Thromb* 1994; **14**:840–56.

55. Virmani R, Farb A, Burke AP. Risk factors in the pathogenesis of coronary artery disease. *Compr Ther* 1998; **24**:519–29.

56. Falk E. Plaque rupture with severe pre-existing stenosis precipitating coronary thrombosis. Characteristics of coronary atherosclerotic plaques underlying fatal occlusive thrombi. *Br Heart J* 1983; **50**:127–34.

57. Davies MJ, Thomas A. Thrombosis and acute coronary-artery lesions in sudden cardiac ischemic death. *N Engl J Med* 1984; **310**:1137–40.

58. Frink RJ. Chronic ulcerated plaques: new insights into the pathogenesis of acute coronary disease. *J Invasive Cardiol* 1994; **6**:173–85.

59. Rioufol G, Finet G, Ginon I et al. Multiple atherosclerotic plaque rupture in acute coronary syndrome: a three-vessel intravascular ultrasound study. *Circulation* 2002; **106**:804.

60. Asakura M, Ueda Y, Yamaguchi O et al. Extensive development of vulnerable plaques as a pan-coronary process in patients with myocardial infarction: an angioscopic study. *J Am Coll Cardiol* 2001; **37**:1284–8.

61. Burke AP, Farb A, Malcom GT et al. Coronary risk factors and plaque morphology in men with coronary disease who died suddenly. *N Engl J Med* 1997; **336**:1276–82.

62. Burke AP, Farb A, Malcom GT et al. Effect of risk factors on the mechanism of acute thrombosis and sudden coronary death in women. *Circulation* 1998; **97**:2110–6.

2. PLATELETS AND THE VULNERABLE PLAQUE

Juan F Viles-Gonzalez, Valentin Fuster and
Juan J Badimon

Introduction

Arterial thrombosis is the acute complication that develops on disrupted atherosclerotic lesions and causes unstable angina, myocardial infarction, sudden cardiovascular death and stroke, the most common causes of morbidity and mortality in the Western world today. Platelets and fibrin are prominent components of the thrombi that occlude arteries, but may also participate in the development and progression of the atherosclerotic plaque. Thus, platelets are central to the process of atherothrombosis, a term that describes the combination of acute thrombotic event and a chronic disease that begins early in childhood (atherosclerosis) and affects different vascular beds.

The function of platelets, however, is to arrest bleeding from wounds, which requires adhesion to injured vascular surfaces and rapid cellular activation with the ensuing accumulation of additional platelets and fibrin into a growing thrombus. An intact and healthy endothelium (Figure 2.1) possesses antiatherogenic activity and normally prevents platelet activation, but the intimal injury associated with endothelial denudation and plaque rupture exposes subendothelial collagen and von Willebrand factor (vWF), which support prompt platelet adhesion and activation. Circulating platelets can adhere either directly to collagen or indirectly, via the binding of vWF, to the glycoprotein (GP) Ib/IX complex. The present consensus is that in high-shear rate conditions, both platelet GP Ib and GP IIb/IIIa appear to be involved in the events of platelet adhesion, whereas GP IIb/IIIa may be involved predominantly in platelet–platelet interaction. Local platelet activation promotes thrombus formation and additional platelet recruitment by supporting cell surface thrombin formation and releasing potent platelet agonists, perpetuating the thrombotic process. The central role of platelet activation in acute coronary syndromes (ACS) is supported by increased platelet-derived thromboxane and prostaglandin metabolites detected in patients with ACS and the clear clinical benefit of treatment with aspirin for prevention of acute coronary events.[1]

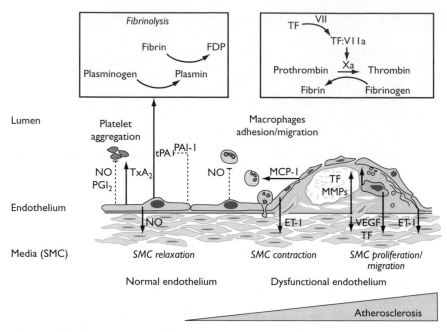

Figure 2.1 *The role of endothelium in plaque development. Endothelial dysfunction and inflammatory processes are crucial in the initiation and progression of atherosclerotic lesions. The major goal of endothelial activity is to maintain constant hemostatic and hemorheologic conditions through a balanced production of several vasoactive and thrombotic / antithrombotic substances. Arrow, promotion; -----, inhibition; ET, endothelin; FDP, fibrin degrading products; MCP-1, monocyte chemoattractant protein-1; M-CSF, macrophage colony-stimulating factor; MMP, matrix metalloproteinase; NO, nitric oxide; PAI-1, plasminogen activator inhibitor-1; PGI$_2$, prostaglandin; SMC, smooth muscle cell; TF, tissue factor; tPA, tissue plasminogen activator; TXA$_2$, thromboxane A$_2$; VEGF, vascular endothelial growth factor.*

Atherothrombosis and vulnerable plaque

Atherosclerosis is a systemic disease involving the intima of large and medium arteries, including the aorta and the carotid, coronary, and peripheral arteries. Normal endothelium plays a pivotal role in vascular homeostasis (through the balanced production of potent vasodilators such as nitric oxide (NO) and vasoconstrictors such as endothelin-1 (ET-1) and limits the development of atherosclerosis (see Figure 2.1). Endothelial dysfunction is considered the earliest pathologic signal of atherosclerosis. Cardiovascular risk factors impair endothelial function and may trigger atherosclerosis without the need for physical endothelial injury.[2] These risk factors have been recognized to induce endothelial dysfunction by reducing the bioavailability of NO, increasing tissue ET-1 content,[3] and

16

activating proinflammatory signaling pathways such as nuclear factor κB.[4] The nuclear factor κB signaling transduction pathway is an essential regulator of the transcription of a number of proinflammatory genes, such as those that lead to the expression of many cytokines, enzymes and adhesion molecules (i.e. intercellular adhesion molecule 1 (ICAM-1); vascular-cell adhesion molecule 1 (VCAM-1); E-selectin.[5] In hypercholesterolemia, for example, endothelium-dependent relaxation is impaired, while contraction and adhesion of monocytes and platelets are enhanced. A recent study has demonstrated that treatment with recombinant HDL (high-density lipoprotein) restores normal endothelial function in hypercholesterolemic patients, explaining the protective effect of HDL in ACS, reducing the occurrence and pointing out the potential role of the endothelium as a therapeutic target.[6]

Atherosclerosis is characterized by intimal thickening due to cellular and lipid accumulation that is due to an imbalance in lipid influx and efflux.[7,8] Secondary changes may occur in the underlying media and adventitia, particularly in advanced disease stages. Fatty streaks have been found in the intima of infants.[9] These progress to fibroatheroma by developing a cap of smooth muscle cells and collagen. The early atherosclerotic lesions can progress without compromising the lumen because of compensatory vascular enlargement (remodeling).[10] Importantly, the culprit lesions leading to ACS are often mildly stenotic and therefore not detected by angiography.[11] These rupture-prone lesions usually have a large lipid core, a thin fibrous cap and a high density of inflammatory cells, particularly at the shoulder region, where disruptions most often occur.[12] Monocytes and macrophages are key to the development of vulnerable plaques. Macrophages produce growth, mitogenic, proinflammatory and lytic factors that enhance the progression of atherosclerotic lesions.[13] Vulnerable plaques (type IV and Va), which are commonly composed of an abundant lipid core separated from the lumen by a thin fibrotic cap, are particularly soft and prone to disruption (Figure 2.2).[8,11] Platelets and inflammatory cells may be a source and targets for inflammatory mediators.[13]

Three major factors determine the vulnerability of the fibrous cap: circumferential wall stress or cap 'fatigue,' lesion characteristics (location, size and consistency) and blood flow characteristics.[14] Pathologic evidence suggests that a plaque must be considered vulnerable when the lipid core accounts for more than 40% of the whole. This may explain the effects of lipid-lowering therapy in reducing coronary events.[8]

Plaque disruption, however, is not a purely mechanical process. Inflammation is also important.[15,16] Activated inflammatory cells have been detected in the disrupted areas of atherectomy specimens from patients with ACS.[17] These cells are capable of degrading extracellular matrix by secreting proteolytic enzymes, such as matrix metalloproteinases.[15] In addition, T cells isolated from rupture-prone sites can stimulate macrophages to produce metalloproteinases and may

17

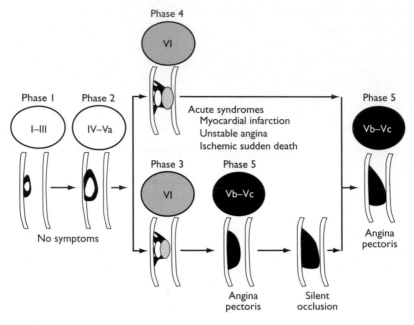

Figure 2.2 *Lesion morphology and phases of progression of coronary atherothrombosis.*

predispose disruption of lesions by weakening their fibrous cap.[18] Matrix metalloproteinases and their co-secreted tissue inhibitors affect vascular remodeling[15] and migration of smooth muscle cells (SMCs) across the basement membrane.[7,19]

Lesion thrombogenicity correlates with its tissue factor (TF) content; furthermore, local TF inhibition reduces lesion thrombogenicity.[20] Cell apoptosis has been linked to inflammation and thrombosis via increased TF expression.[21,22] TF activity in the acellular lipid core was found mainly on apoptotic microparticles of monocytic and lymphocytic origin.[22] Recent studies have demonstrated an increased TF expression in the coronary arteries and in the plasma of patients with unstable angina or myocardial infarction compared with patients with stable angina.[22] More recently, observations obtained from pathologic analysis of human coronary and carotid artery specimens showed that TF is often co-localized in macrophage apoptotic death and released microparticles rather than in biologically active macrophages. Specific inhibition of vascular TF by TF pathway inhibitor (TFPI) was associated with a significant reduction of acute thrombus formation in lipid-rich plaques.[20] Interestingly, in the pig model of arterial injury, TFPI administration during percutaneous coronary angioplasty prevented acute thrombus formation without increasing the bleeding complications, and it reduced intimal hyperplasia without affecting SMC growth.[23]

Plaque disruption and subsequent thrombus formation is responsible for the onset of ACS, the severity of which is modulated by the magnitude or stability of the thrombus.[21] In addition, successive events of plaque disruption and asymptomatic thrombus formation may be responsible for the progression of lesions.[24]

Once the plaque is disrupted, the highly thrombogenic lipid-rich core, abundant in macrophages and TF, is exposed to the bloodstream triggering the formation of a superimposed thrombus that leads to an acute coronary event. The disruption of lipid-rich plaques facilitates the interaction between TF and flowing blood, triggering activation of the coagulation cascade, thrombin generation and platelet-rich thrombus formation.[25,26] The high level of thromboxane A_2 detected in patients with coronary artery disease supports the role of platelets in atherothrombosis. An increase in platelet reactivity can be detected in coronary artery blood in the immediate vicinity of a disrupted plaque.[27] In addition, treatment with antiplatelet agents is beneficial in patients with ACS.[1,28]

One-third of ACS, particularly sudden death, occur without plaque disruption but just superficial erosion of a markedly stenotic and fibrotic plaque.[21] Under such conditions, thrombus formation depends on the hyperthrombogenic state triggered by systemic factors. Indeed, systemic factors including elevated low-density lipoprotein (LDL) and decreased HDL cholesterol levels, cigarette smoking, diabetes and hemostasis are associated with increased thrombotic complications.[24] High levels of circulating TF have been reported in patients with hyperlipidemia, diabetes and ACS. Thus TF is postulated as the agent responsible for the 'thrombogenic state'. Our group has reported increased thrombogenicity associated with hyperlipemia as well as diabetes[29,30] that can be normalized with risk factor management.[30,31] Aside from apoptotic macrophages and microparticles from atherosclerotic plaques, activated monocytes in the circulating blood seem to be the source of TF microparticles and may represent the result of activation by the previously mentioned risk factors and others, thus contributing to thrombotic events. These observations emphasize the importance of not only the 'vulnerable' or 'high risk' atherothrombotic lesions but also the relevance of 'hyperreactive' (vulnerable?) blood.

Platelets in atherogenesis

The pathogenesis of atherosclerosis is multifactorial (Figure 2.3), but the two aspects considered to be of greatest relevance are (i) the deposition of lipids that are then metabolized abnormally and oxidized in the vascular wall and (ii) the local infiltration of leukocytes.[2] This creates an inflammatory environment[32] in which the function of endothelial cells is also affected, and one of the

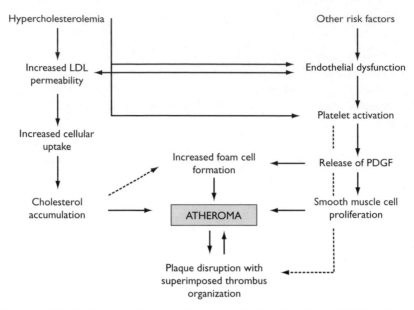

Figure 2.3 *Multifactorial theory of the origin of atherothrombosis. LDL, low-density lipoprotein; PDGF, platelet-derived growth factor.*

manifestations of this alteration is an increase in the potential for interaction with other cells including platelets.[33] A growing body of evidence highlights the interaction between platelets and endothelial cells as a cornerstone in the initiation of atherogenesis.[34] P-selectin is considered pivotal in this interplay. If P-selectin is absent, fatty streak formation is delayed in mice lacking LDL receptors and fed a cholesterol-rich diet.[35] P-selectin also seems to play a role in the advanced lesions that develop in ApoE-knockout mice. In this model, absence of P-selectin results in smaller lesions with less macrophage recruitment and smooth muscle infiltrate.[36] Both endothelial and platelet P-selectin may be involved in macrophage recruitment.[37] The recruitment and adhesion of platelets to the endothelium of atherothrombosis-prone sites was recently demonstrated in two different animal models.[38–40] Interestingly, Tailor et al established that hypercholesterolemia promotes platelet–endothelial cell interaction in the postcapillary venules of mice fed on cholesterol-rich diet.[41]

Understanding how platelets respond to alterations of the vessel wall that elicit hemostasis may explain the modalities of interaction with developing atherosclerotic plaques, where endothelial cell dysfunction may create the conditions for platelet adhesion. Enhanced secretion of vWF in response to inflammatory stimuli can lead to the local recruitment of platelets, and this process may be favored in hypercholesterolemia.[40,42] This may be one of the reasons why deficiency of vWF affords some level of protection from atherosclerosis.[42] Not all adhesion receptor–ligand pairs known to be important in thrombus formation may be equally relevant in mediating platelet interactions with developing atherosclerotic lesions, as shown by the fact that deficiency of integrin-αIIbβ3 is not associated with protection from atherosclerosis.[43]

Activated platelets attached to an atherosclerotic lesion may influence plaque progression in different ways. Platelets may provide the reactive surface for the recruitment of monocytes and lymphocytes by releasing the content of their granules, increasing the expression of adhesive ligands (such as P-selectin) or binding molecules from the plasma milieu (such as fibrinogen). These interactions may support the adhesion of leukocytes to the vessel wall even in conditions of high flow that would otherwise not permit this. Platelets also release growth factors; the involvement of platelet-derived growth factor (PDGF) in cellular proliferation has long been recognized (Figure 2.4).[44] Recent data emphasize the possible influence of platelets on the cellular metabolism of LDLs, indicating a more direct involvement in the early changes characteristic of the atherosclerotic lesion.[45] Along the same lines, processing of β-amyloid precursor protein derived

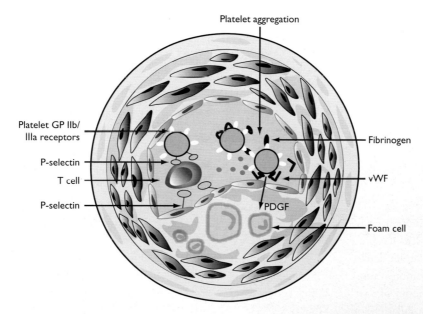

Figure 2.4 *Role of platelets in atherogenesis. Adhesive substrates (von Willebrand factor (vWF) and P-selectin) are exposed in the dysfunctional endothelium, promoting the adhesion of platelets. Adherent platelets facilitate the adhesion of leukocytes that also interact with the endothelial cells that express P-selectin. Adherent platelets release platelet-derived growth factor (PDGF), which stimulates plaque growth and increases the formation of foam cells.*

21

from engulfed platelets contributes to macrophage activation in an atherosclerotic plaque.[46] These findings support the idea that platelets adherent to the vessel wall contribute directly to the development of the chronic lesions that precede, typically by many years, the acute onset of arterial thrombosis.

Evidence suggests that plaque rupture, subsequent thrombosis and fibrous thrombus organization are also important in the progression of atherosclerosis in both asymptomatic patients and those with stable angina. Plaque disruption with subsequent change in plaque geometry and thrombosis results in a complicated lesion. Such a rapid change in atherosclerotic plaque geometry may result in acute occlusion or subocclusion with clinical manifestations of unstable angina or other ACS. More frequently, however, the rapid changes seem to result in a mural thrombus without evident clinical symptoms. This type of platelet-rich thrombus may be a main contributor to the rapid progression of atherosclerosis. A number of local and systemic circulating factors may influence the degree and duration of thrombus deposition at the time of disruption of the coronary plaque.[24]

Inflammatory role of platelets

Early evidence pointed to the involvement of inflammatory and immune-mediated mechanisms in the pathogenesis of atheroma.[32] In this context, the role of platelets goes beyond thrombosis. In fact, platelets became a critical factor linking atherosclerosis, thrombosis and inflammation. Patients with ACS not only have increased platelet interaction but also increased interaction between platelets and leukocytes (heterotypic aggregates) detectable in blood. These aggregates form when activated platelets undergo degranulation, after which they adhere to circulating leukocytes. Early work suggested that these heterotypic aggregates form in inflammatory states.[47] Platelets bind via P-selectin (CD62P) expressed on the surface of activated platelets to the leukocyte receptor, P-selectin glycoprotein ligand-1 (PSGL-1).[48] This initial association leads to increased expression of the integrin CD11b/CD18 (Mac-1) on leukocytes,[49] which itself supports interactions with platelets (perhaps because bivalent fibrinogen links this integrin with its platelet surface counterpart GP IIb/IIIa).[50] The importance of platelet–leukocyte aggregates in vascular disease is supported by a recent study demonstrating that the infusion of recombinant human PSGL-1 in an animal model of vascular injury reduced myocardial reperfusion injury and preserved vascular endothelial function.[51]

Measurement of platelet–leukocyte aggregates might be a better reflection of plaque instability and ongoing vascular thrombosis and inflammation. Platelet–leukocyte aggregates also may be a more sensitive marker of platelet activation than surface P-selectin expression because degranulated platelets rapidly lose surface P-selectin in vivo but continue to be detected in circulation. This observation was recently reported by Michelson et al,[52] who demonstrated that after acute myocardial infarction, circulating monocyte–platelet aggregates are a more sensitive marker of in vivo platelet activation than platelet surface P-selectin. In addition, two recent publications[53,54] showed that the number of circulating monocyte–platelet aggregates in ACS patients was increased compared with subjects with non-cardiac chest pain.

The binding of platelets and monocytes in ACS highlights, once again, the interaction between inflammation and thrombosis in cardiovascular disease. Plaque rupture promotes activation of the inflammatory response, and increased expression of TF initiates extrinsic coagulation. The expression of TF on both endothelial cells and monocytes is partially regulated by proinflammatory cytokines, including tumor necrosis factor (TNF) and interleukin (IL)-1.[55] In addition to initiating coagulation, TF interacts with P-selectin, accelerating fibrin formation and deposition.[55] Platelet surface P-selectin also induces the expression of TF on monocytes, enhances monocyte cytokine expression and promotes CD11b/CD18 expression.[49]

T lymphocytes in human plaque were known to stain positively for CD40L. The role of CD40L in lesion progression and thrombosis was established through gene-targeting studies utilizing murine knockout models. In an LDL deficient knockout, treatment with an anti-CD40L monoclonal antibody significantly reduced atherosclerotic lesion size and macrophage, T lymphocyte and lipid content.[56] Furthermore, Schonbeck et al utilizing the same murine model in a temporally longer, randomized study not only demonstrated that anti-CD40L monoclonal antibody limited atherosclerotic disease evolution, but also conferred stable plaque characteristics.[57] Moreover, CD40L deficiency was shown to protect against microvascular thrombus formation, while recombinant soluble CD40L (sCD40L) restored normal thrombosis.[58] Recently, much attention has been focused on CD40L's cryptic existence in platelets and its potential role in mediating platelet-dependent inflammatory response associated with the atherothrombotic state. Pioneering work has shown platelet-associated CD40L to elicit an inflammatory response from endothelial cells[59] and induce human monocytic,[60] endothelial[61,62] and vascular smooth muscle[63] TF expression in a CD40/CD40L-dependent manner. Furthermore, Henn et al have demonstrated that upon platelet stimulation, CD40L is expressed on the surface and then subsequently cleaved to generate a soluble, trimeric fragment, sCD40L.[64] Although no definitive data identify platelets as the sole source of sCD40L found in the circulation[64,65] platelet counts[66] and platelet activation[67] have been shown to correlate with sCD40L. Additionally, sCD40L is able to ligate platelet GP IIb/IIIa complex conferring a thrombogenic proclivity, and through this mechanism may play a role in high-shear-dependent platelet aggregation.[58]

CD40L and sCD40L both consist of homologous, multifunctional structural domains. They both bind CD40 by way of their TNF homology domain[68–70] to induce cellular signaling. Moreover, they both bind the platelet GP IIb/IIIa receptor through their KGD peptide sequence and may stabilize arterial thrombi in this manner.[58] GP IIb/IIIa receptor antagonists at clinically relevant doses inhibit platelet release of sCD40L in vitro.[71] On the other hand, subtherapeutic dosing of these potent antiplatelet agents increases the release of the sCD40L, explaining a potential mechanism by which suboptimal doses of GP IIb/IIIa antagonists may not only be non-protective and prothrombotic, but also proinflammatory.[71] Interestingly, both GP IIb/IIIa-dependent platelet adhesion to endothelium and GP IIb/IIIa engagement upregulate platelet-associated CD40L.[72] These data define a significant role for the GP IIb/IIIa receptor in modulating the platelet-CD40L system.

C-reactive protein (CRP) is a protein of the acute-phase response and a sensitive marker of low-grade inflammation. Increased levels of CRP have been reported to predict acute coronary events,[73,74] and it seems to be a useful marker in the prediction of thrombotic events. Whether CRP reflects the inflammatory component of atherosclerotic plaques or of the circulating blood, and whether it is a surrogate marker or a biologically active element in plaque development of thrombus formation at the site of the atherosclerotic vessel, are not known. However, recent studies support the hypothesis that CRP is an activator of blood monocyte and vessel-wall endothelial cells.[75]

Platelets, depression and acute coronary syndromes

Since established cardiovascular risk factors do not account for all patients who develop ACS events, the search for 'non-traditional' risk factors has emerged. Many of the immune-inflammatory factors playing a role in plaque instability have been associated with psychological factors. Elevation of plasma proinflammatory cytokines (e.g. IL-1) and decrease in anti-inflammatory cytokines (e.g. IL-4) have been associated with depression.[76] Depression is associated with enhanced activation of platelets and with enhanced release of Betathromboglobulin (BTG).[77] Depression is also associated with elevated IL-6, which as mentioned above, can activate platelets as well. In a recent study, it was demonstrated that 5-HT-mediated platelet reactivity is significantly increased in depressed patients compared with non-depressed matched controls.[78] To note, a non-5-HT agonist, adenosin diphosphate (ADP), did not differentiate depressed patients from their controls, as has been previously reported by other investigators.[79]

The etiologic theory of atherothrombosis has now been widened, to include the behavioral sciences in the equation that analyzes the factors determining the onset of ACS (plaque instability, plaque rupture and thrombosis). These processes can be explained by linking events taking place at the level of the central nervous system (e.g. brain secretion of norepinephrine), systemic immune and neuroendocrine level (e.g. recruitment of T cells), at the molecular and cellular level of the coronary plaque (e.g. macrophage release of mastrix metaloproteinases), and at blood level (e.g. exaggerated platelet aggregation in depression) all contributing to the development of an ACS.

Clinical implications

The clinical manifestations of atherosclerotic plaques depend on several factors including the degree and speed of blood flow obstruction, the duration of decreased myocardial perfusion and the myocardial oxygen demand at the time of obstruction (Figure 2.5). The thrombotic response at the time of disruption is also a major determinant. If the resulting thrombus is small (found in up to 8% of patients dying of non-cardiovascular causes), plaque rupture probably proceeds unnoticed. If however, the thrombus is large enough to compromise blood flow to the myocardium the individual may experience an acute ischemic syndrome.

Following mild injury to the vessel wall, it is likely that the thrombogenic stimulus is relatively limited and the resulting thrombotic occlusion transient, as occurs in unstable angina. The relative lack of therapeutic response to fibrinolysis suggests that therapeutic agents do not access this fibrin within a platelet-rich mixture, although anti-platelet agents may be able to influence events on the thrombus surface. Deep vessel injury secondary to plaque rupture and ulceration results in exposure of collagen, lipids and other elements of the vessel media leading to relatively persistent thrombotic occlusion and myocardial infarction.

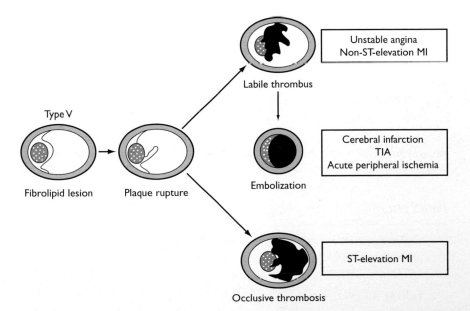

Figure 2.5 *Clinical manifestations of atherothrombosis. MI, myocardial infarction; TIA, transient ischemic attack.*

25

In patients with stable coronary artery disease, angina commonly results from increases in myocardial oxygen demand beyond the ability of stenosed arteries. In contrast, unstable angina, non-ST-elevation and ST-elevation myocardial infarction represent a continuum and are usually characterized by an abrupt cessation in coronary blood flow. In unstable angina, plaque disruption may lead to acute changes in plaque morphology and reduction in coronary blood flow. In addition to plaque disruption other mechanisms also contribute to reduce coronary blood flow. Platelets attach to the damaged endothelium and exposed media and release vasoactive substances including TXA2 and serotonin leading to further platelet aggregation and vasoconstriction. In non-ST-elevation myocardial infarction, the angiographic morphology of the culprit lesion is similar to that seen in unstable angina suggesting that plaque disruption is similar in both syndromes. Approximately one-fourth of patients with non-ST-elevation infarction have a completely occluded infarct-related vessel at early angiography with the distal territory usually supplied by collaterals. In ST-elevation infarction, plaque rupture is frequently associated with deep arterial injury or ulceration resulting in the formation of a fixed and persistent thrombus with abrupt cessation of myocardial perfusion and subsequent necrosis. The coronary lesion responsible for the infarction is usually only mildly stenotic suggesting that plaque rupture with superimposed thrombosis is the primary determinant of acute occlusion rather than lesion severity.[7]

Conclusion

The discussion in this chapter emphasizes the role of endothelial dysfunction, platelet reactivity and TF activity in acute arterial thrombosis after atherosclerotic plaque disruption (atherothrombosis). Recent evidence points toward TF as a key trigger on platelet-rich thrombus formation upon plaque rupture, hence highlights the role of this molecule as a novel therapeutic target. The progress in understanding the mechanism of these factors in the pathogenesis of atherothrombosis, may lead to the development of more effective therapy in the prevention of ACS.

References

1. Collaborative meta-analysis of randomised trials of antiplatelet therapy for prevention of death, myocardial infarction, and stroke in high risk patients. *BMJ* 2002; **324**:71–86.

2. Lusis AJ. Atherosclerosis. *Nature* 2000; **407**:233–41.

3. Ruschitzka F, Moehrlen U, Quaschning T et al. Tissue endothelin-converting enzyme activity correlates with cardiovascular risk factors in coronary artery disease. *Circulation* 2000; **102**:1086–92.

4. Kinlay S, Libby P, Ganz P. Endothelial function and coronary artery disease. *Curr Opin Lipidol* 2001; **12**:383–9.

5. Barnes PJ, Karin M. Nuclear factor-kappaB: a pivotal transcription factor in chronic inflammatory diseases. *N Engl J Med* 1997; **336**:1066–71.

6. Spieker LE, Sudano I, Hurlimann D et al. High-density lipoprotein restores endothelial function in hypercholesterolemic men. *Circulation* 2002; **105**:1399–402.

7. Fuster V, Fayad ZA, Badimon JJ. Acute coronary syndromes: biology. *Lancet* 1999; **353 (Suppl 2)**:SII5–9

8. Libby P. Current concepts of the pathogenesis of the acute coronary syndromes. *Circulation* 2001; **104**:365–72.

9. Stary HC, Chandler AB, Glagov S et al. A definition of initial, fatty streak, and intermediate lesions of atherosclerosis. A report from the Committee on Vascular Lesions of the Council on Arteriosclerosis, American Heart Association. *Arterioscler Thromb* 1994; **14**:840–56.

10. Ambrose JA, Weinrauch M. Thrombosis in ischemic heart disease. *Arch Intern Med* 1996; **156**:1382–94.

11. Falk E, Shah PK, Fuster V. Coronary plaque disruption. *Circulation* 1995; **92**:657–71.

12. Moreno PR, Bernardi VH, Lopez-Cuellar J et al. Macrophage infiltration predicts restenosis after coronary intervention in patients with unstable angina. *Circulation* 1996; **94**:3098–102.

13. Libby P, Simon DI. Inflammation and thrombosis: the clot thickens. *Circulation* 2001; **103**:1718–20.

14. Sata M, Saiura A, Kunisato A et al. Hematopoietic stem cells differentiate into vascular cells that participate in the pathogenesis of atherosclerosis. *Nat Med* 2002; **8**:403–9.

15. Galis ZS, Johnson C, Godin D et al. Targeted disruption of the matrix metalloproteinase-9 gene impairs smooth muscle cell migration and geometrical arterial remodeling. *Circ Res* 2002; **91**:852–9.

16. Scott J. ATVB in focus: lipoproteins, inflammation, and atherosclerosis. *Arterioscler Thromb Vasc Biol* 2003; **23**:528.

17. Moreno PR, Falk E, Palacios IF et al. Macrophage infiltration in acute coronary syndromes. Implications for plaque rupture. *Circulation* 1994; **90**:775–8.

18. Uzui H, Harpf A, Liu M et al. Increased expression of membrane type 3-matrix metalloproteinase in human atherosclerotic plaque: role of activated macrophages and inflammatory cytokines. *Circulation* 2002; **106**:3024–30.

19. Toschi V, Gallo R, Lettino M et al. Tissue factor modulates the thrombogenicity of human atherosclerotic plaques. *Circulation* 1997; **95**:594–9.

20. Badimon JJ, Lettino M, Toschi V et al. Local inhibition of tissue factor reduces the thrombogenicity of disrupted human atherosclerotic plaques: effects of tissue factor pathway inhibitor on plaque thrombogenicity under flow conditions. *Circulation* 1999; **99**:1780–7.

21. Virmani R, Kolodgie FD, Burke AP, Farb A, Schwartz SM. Lessons from sudden coronary death: a comprehensive morphological classification scheme for atherosclerotic lesions. *Arterioscler Thromb Vasc Biol* 2000; **20**:1262–75.

22. Mallat Z, Tedgui A. Current perspective on the role of apoptosis in atherothrombotic disease. *Circ Res* 2001; **88**:998–1003.

23. Roque M, Reis ED, Fuster V et al. Inhibition of tissue factor reduces thrombus formation and intimal hyperplasia after porcine coronary angioplasty. *J Am Coll Cardiol* 2000; **36**:2303–10.

24. Burke AP, Kolodgie FD, Farb A et al. Healed plaque ruptures and sudden coronary death: evidence that subclinical rupture has a role in plaque progression. *Circulation* 2001; **103**:934–40.

25. Fuster V, Fallon JT, Nemerson Y. Coronary thrombosis. *Lancet* 1996; **348(Suppl 1)**:S7–S10.

26. Sambola A, Osende J, Hathcock J et al. Role of risk factors in the modulation of tissue factor activity and blood thrombogenicity. *Circulation* 2003; **107**:973–7.

27. Kabbani SS, Watkins MW, Holoch PA et al. Platelet reactivity in coronary ostial blood: a reflection of the thrombotic state accompanying plaque rupture and of the adequacy of anti-thrombotic therapy. *J Thromb Thrombolysis* 2001; **12**:171–6.

28. Patrono C, Coller B, Dalen JE et al. Platelet-active drugs: the relationships among dose, effectiveness, and side effects. *Chest* 2001; **119**:39S–63S.

29. Osende JI, Badimon JJ, Fuster V et al. Blood thrombogenicity in type 2 diabetes mellitus patients is associated with glycemic control. *J Am Coll Cardiol* 2001; **38**:1307–12.

30. Rauch U, Crandall J, Osende JI et al. Increased thrombus formation relates to ambient blood glucose and leukocyte count in diabetes mellitus type 2. *Am J Cardiol* 2000; **86**:246–9.

31. Corti R, Badimon JJ. Value or desirability of hemorheological-hemostatic parameter changes as endpoints in blood lipid-regulating trials. *Curr Opin Lipidol* 2001; **12**:629–37.

32. Ross R. Atherosclerosis is an inflammatory disease. *Am Heart J* 1999; **138**:S419–20.

33. Sachais BS. Platelet–endothelial interactions in atherosclerosis. *Curr Atheroscler Rep* 2001; **3**:412–16.

34. Huo Y, Schober A, Forlow SB et al. Circulating activated platelets exacerbate atherosclerosis in mice deficient in apolipoprotein E. *Nat Med* 2003; **9**:61–7.

35. Johnson RC, Chapman SM, Dong ZM et al. Absence of P-selectin delays fatty streak formation in mice. *J Clin Invest* 1997; **99**:1037–43.

36. Dong ZM, Brown AA, Wagner DD. Prominent role of P-selectin in the development of advanced atherosclerosis in ApoE-deficient mice. *Circulation* 2000; **101**:2290–5.

37. Burger PE, Coetzee S, McKeehan WL et al. Fibroblast growth factor receptor-1 is expressed by endothelial progenitor cells. *Blood* 2002; **100**:3527–35.

38. Massberg S, Brand K, Gruner S et al. A critical role of platelet adhesion in the initiation of atherosclerotic lesion formation. *J Exp Med* 2002; **196**:887–96.

39. Massberg S, Gawaz M, Gruner S et al. A crucial role of glycoprotein VI for platelet recruitment to the injured arterial wall in vivo. *J Exp Med* 2003; **197**:41–9.

40. Theilmeier G, Michiels C, Spaepen E et al. Endothelial von Willebrand factor recruits platelets to atherosclerosis-prone sites in response to hypercholesterolemia. *Blood* 2002; **99**:4486–93.

41. Tailor A, Granger DN. Hypercholesterolemia promotes p-selectin-dependent platelet-endothelial cell adhesion in postcapillary venules. *Arterioscler Thromb Vasc Biol* 2003; **23**:675–80.

42. Methia N, Andre P, Denis CV, Economopoulos M, Wagner DD. Localized reduction of atherosclerosis in von Willebrand factor-deficient mice. *Blood* 2001; **98**:1424–8.

43. Shpilberg O, Rabi I, Schiller K et al. Patients with Glanzmann thrombasthenia lacking platelet glycoprotein alpha(IIb)beta(3) (GPIIb/IIIa) and alpha(v)beta(3) receptors are not protected from atherosclerosis. *Circulation* 2002; **105**:1044–8.

44. Ross R. The pathogenesis of atherosclerosis: a perspective for the 1990s. *Nature* 1993; **362**:801–9.

45. Sachais BS, Kuo A, Nassar T et al. Platelet factor 4 binds to low-density lipoprotein receptors and disrupts the endocytic machinery, resulting in retention of low-density lipoprotein on the cell surface. *Blood* 2002; **99**:3613–22.

46. De Meyer GR, De Cleen DM, Cooper S et al. Platelet phagocytosis and processing of beta-amyloid precursor protein as a mechanism of macrophage activation in atherosclerosis. *Circ Res* 2002; **90**:1197–204.

47. Arber N, Berliner S, Rotenberg Z et al. Detection of aggregated leukocytes in the circulating pool during stress-demargination is not necessarily a result of decreased leukocyte adhesiveness. *Acta Haematol* 1991; **86**:20–4.

48. Rinder HM, Bonan JL, Rinder CS, Ault KA, Smith BR. Dynamics of leukocyte-platelet adhesion in whole blood. *Blood* 1991; **78**:1730–7.

49. Neumann FJ, Zohlnhofer D, Fakhoury L, Ott I et al. Effect of glycoprotein IIb/IIIa receptor blockade on platelet–leukocyte interaction and surface expression of the leukocyte integrin Mac-1 in acute myocardial infarction. *J Am Coll Cardiol* 1999; **34**:1420–6.

50. Simon DI, Ezratty AM, Francis SA, Rennke H, Loscalzo J. Fibrin(ogen) is internalized and degraded by activated human monocytoid cells via Mac-1 (CD11b/CD18): a nonplasmin fibrinolytic pathway. *Blood* 1993; **82**:2414–22.

51. Hayward R, Campbell B, Shin YK, Scalia R, Lefer AM. Recombinant soluble P-selectin glycoprotein ligand-1 protects against myocardial ischemic reperfusion injury in cats. *Cardiovasc Res* 1999; **41**:65–76.

52. Michelson AD, Barnard MR, Krueger LA, Valeri CR, Furman MI. Circulating monocyte-platelet aggregates are a more sensitive marker of in vivo platelet activation than platelet surface P-selectin: studies in baboons, human coronary intervention, and human acute myocardial infarction. *Circulation* 2001; **104**: 1533–7.

53. Sarma J, Laan CA, Alam S et al. Increased platelet binding to circulating monocytes in acute coronary syndromes. *Circulation* 2002; **105**:2166–71.

54. Furman MI, Barnard MR, Krueger LA et al. Circulating monocyte-platelet aggregates are an early marker of acute myocardial infarction. *J Am Coll Cardiol* 2001; **38**:1002–6.

55. Shebuski RJ, Kilgore KS. Role of inflammatory mediators in thrombogenesis. *J Pharmacol Exp Ther* 2002; **300**:729–35.

56. Mach F, Schonbeck U, Sukhova GK, Atkinson E, Libby P. Reduction of atherosclerosis in mice by inhibition of CD40 signalling. *Nature* 1998; **394**:200–3.

57. Schonbeck U, Sukhova GK, Shimizu K, Mach F, Libby P. Inhibition of CD40 signaling limits evolution of established atherosclerosis in mice. *Proc Natl Acad Sci USA* 2000; **97**:7458–63.

58. Andre P, Prasad KS, Denis CV et al. CD40L stabilizes arterial thrombi by a beta3 integrin-dependent mechanism. *Nat Med* 2002; **8**:247–52.

59. Henn V, Slupsky JR, Grafe M et al. CD40 ligand on activated platelets triggers an inflammatory reaction of endothelial cells. *Nature* 1998; **391**:591–4.

60. Lindmark E, Tenno T, Siegbahn A. Role of platelet P-selectin and CD40 ligand in the induction of monocytic tissue factor expression. *Arterioscler Thromb Vasc Biol* 2000; **20**:2322–8.

61. Slupsky JR, Kalbas M, Willuweit A et al. Activated platelets induce tissue factor expression on human umbilical vein endothelial cells by ligation of CD40. *Thromb Haemost* 1998; **80**:1008–14.

62. Bavendiek U, Libby P, Kilbride M et al. Induction of tissue factor expression in human endothelial cells by CD40 ligand is mediated via activator protein 1, nuclear factor kappa B, and Egr-1. *J Biol Chem* 2002; **277**:25032–9.

63. Schonbeck U, Mach F, Sukhova GK et al. CD40 ligation induces tissue factor expression in human vascular smooth muscle cells. *Am J Pathol* 2000; **156**:7–14.

64. Henn V, Steinbach S, Buchner K, Presek P, Kroczek RA. The inflammatory action of CD40 ligand (CD154) expressed on activated human platelets is temporally limited by coexpressed CD40. *Blood* 2001; **98**:1047–54.

65. Aukrust P, Muller F, Ueland T et al. Enhanced levels of soluble and membrane-bound CD40 ligand in patients with unstable angina. Possible reflection of T lymphocyte and platelet involvement in the pathogenesis of acute coronary syndromes. *Circulation* 1999; **100**:614–20.

66. Viallard JF, Solanilla A, Gauthier B et al. Increased soluble and platelet-associated CD40 ligand in essential thrombocythemia and reactive thrombocytosis. *Blood* 2002; **99**:2612–4.

67. Heeschen C, Dimmeler S, Hamm CW et al. Soluble CD40 ligand in acute coronary syndromes. *N Engl J Med* 2003; **348**:1104–11.

68. Bajorath J, Aruffo A. Construction and analysis of a detailed three-dimensional model of the ligand binding domain of the human B cell receptor CD40. *Proteins* 1997; **27**:59–70.

69. van Kooten C, Banchereau J. CD40-CD40 ligand. *J Leukoc Biol* 2000; **67**:2–17.

70. Mazzei GJ, Edgerton MD, Losberger C et al. Recombinant soluble trimeric CD40 ligand is biologically active. *J Biol Chem* 1995; **270**:7025–8.

71. Nannizzi-Alaimo L, Alves VL, Phillips DR. Inhibitory effects of glycoprotein IIb/IIIa antagonists and aspirin on the release of soluble CD40 ligand during platelet stimulation. *Circulation* 2003; **107**:1123–8.

72. May AE, Kalsch T, Massberg S et al. Engagement of glycoprotein IIb/IIIa (alpha(IIb)beta3) on platelets upregulates CD40L and triggers CD40L-dependent matrix degradation by endothelial cells. *Circulation* 2002; **106**:2111–17.

73. Ridker PM, Buring JE, Cook NR, Rifai N. C-reactive protein, the metabolic syndrome, and risk of incident cardiovascular events: an 8-year follow-up of 14 719 initially healthy American women. *Circulation* 2003; **107**:391–7.

74. Ridker PM, Rifai N, Rose L, Buring JE, Cook NR. Comparison of C-reactive protein and low-density lipoprotein cholesterol levels in the prediction of first cardiovascular events. *N Engl J Med* 2002; **347**:1557–65.

75. Pasceri V, Cheng JS, Willerson JT, Yeh ET, Chang J. Modulation of C-reactive protein-mediated monocyte chemoattractant protein-1 induction in human endothelial cells by anti-atherosclerosis drugs. *Circulation* 2001; **103**:2531–4.

76. Kronfol Z, Remick DG. Cytokines and the brain: implications for clinical psychiatry. *Am J Psychiatry* 2000; **157**:683–94.

77. Laghrissi-Thode F, Wagner WR, Pollock BG, Johnson PC, Finkel MS. Elevated platelet factor 4 and beta-thromboglobulin plasma levels in depressed patients with ischemic heart disease. *Biol Psychiatry* 1997; **42**:290–5.

78. Shimbo D, Child J, Davidson K et al. Exaggerated serotonin-mediated platelet reactivity as a possible link in depression and acute coronary syndromes. *Am J Cardiol* 2002; **89**:331–3.

79. Musselman DL, Marzec UM, Manatunga A et al. Platelet reactivity in depressed patients treated with paroxetine: preliminary findings. *Arch Gen Psychiatry* 2000; **57**:875–82.

3. PATHOLOGY OF THE VULNERABLE PLAQUE

Renu Virmani, Allen Burke, Andrew Farb,
Frank D Kolodgie, Aloke V Finn and Herman Gold

Introduction

Coronary artery disease is by far the largest killer not only in the Western world but also, increasingly, in the developing world.[1] It is likely to impose a huge economic burden on society in this century. Therefore, it is imperative that there be a better understanding of the disease in order to reduce its devastating effect on the world population. Atherosclerosis is now established as an inflammatory disease that occurs preferentially in individuals with acquired risk factors and a genetic predisposition,[2] and waxes and wanes with concurrent infections. It is believed that atherosclerosis affects all populations in varying degrees. Because 70% of the morbidity and mortality from coronary disease is the result of plaque rupture, it is important to establish definitions of terminologies that are used to describe the progression of atherosclerotic lesions from the early stages through to advanced, unstable, thrombosis-prone plaques.

Composition of atherosclerotic plaque

The cellular and acellular structures that participate in the establishment of atherosclerosis include elements found in the normal arterial wall, such as smooth muscle cells, collagen and proteoglycan matrix, and endothelial cells that line the lumen. Other cells are derived from the circulation and include monocyte-derived macrophages, T and B lymphocytes, mast cells, neutrophils, red blood cells and platelets. The blood coagulation factors contribute through the devastating effects of thrombosis. Analogous to tumors, the atherosclerotic plaque requires its own vascular supply to grow and develop; the role of angiogenesis in plaque progression and thrombosis is currently under intensive study.[3,4]

The various stages of atherosclerosis have been divided into six phases by the American Heart Association. Stary et al separated the stages into early (stages I–III)[5] and late (stages IV–VI)[6] (Table 3.1). The early stages consist of adaptive intimal thickening, fatty streak, and pathologic intimal thickening; the late stages include the fibroatheroma, multilayered fibrotic and calcified fibroatheroma, and surface disruption hemorrhage and thrombosis. We have modified this

Table 3.1 Classifications of atherosclerotic plaque

Traditional classification	Stary et al[5,6]	Virmani et al[7] Initial	Progression
Early plaques	Type I: microscopic detection of lipid droplets in intima and small groups of macrophage foam cells	Intimal thickening	None
Fatty streak	Type II: fatty streaks visible on gross inspection, layers of foam cells, occasional lymphocytes and mast cells	Intimal xanthoma	None
	Type III (intermediate): extracellular lipid pools present among layers of smooth muscle cells	Pathologic intimal thickening	Thrombus (erosion)
Intermediate plaque Atheroma	Type IV: well defined lipid core; may develop surface disruption (fissure)	Fibrous cap atheroma	Thrombus (erosion)[¶]
Late lesions		Thin fibrous cap atheroma	Thrombus (rupture); hemorrhage/fibrin[§]
	Type Va: new fibrous tissue overlying lipid core (multilayered fibroatheroma)[*]	Healed plaque rupture; erosion	Repeated rupture or erosion with or without total occlusion
	Type Vb: calcification[†]	Fibrocalcific plaque (with or without necrotic core)	

Table 3.1 Classifications of atherosclerotic plaque (cont.)

	Fibrous plaque	Type Vc: fibrotic lesion with minimal lipid (could be result of organized thrombi)		
Miscellaneous/ complicated features	Complicated/ advanced plaques	Type VIa: surface disruption		
			Type VIb: intraplaque hemorrhage	
			Type VIc: thrombosis	
			Calcified nodule	Thrombus (usually non-occlusive)

*May overlap with healed plaque ruptures.
†Occasionally referred to as type VII lesion.
¶May progress further with healing (healed erosion).
§May progress further with healing (healed rupture).

classification because of new knowledge regarding the lesions substrates that lead to coronary thrombosis.[7] The early stages in both classifications are similar, although the term fatty streak has been renamed intimal xanthoma because the lesions mimic xanthomas that occur outside the cardiovascular system.

The late stages include fibrous cap atheroma, thin-cap atheroma (a type of vulnerable plaque), healed plaque rupture or erosion, fibrocalcific plaque with or without a necrotic core and calcified nodule. There are some lesions that are almost purely fibrous and should be called fibrous plaques, as they possess no lipid or calcium and have a rich collagenous matrix with or without proteoglycans.

There is much confusion in the literature and poor understanding in the community at large as to the difference between lipid pool and necrotic core. *Lipid pool* is a collection of lipid interspersed in proteoglycan/collagen matrix that is devoid of smooth muscle cells and macrophages.[5,7] The absence of smooth muscle cells is likely due to cell death, as lipid pools commonly show speckled calcification indicative of smooth muscle cell calcification with use of special stains that identify calcium (e.g. von Kossa). Furthermore, electron microscopy and PAS (periodic acid Schiff) stains demonstrate empty areas devoid of intact smooth muscle cells, but heavy staining of smooth muscle cell basement membranes and surrounding vesicular bodies with or without calcification.[8,9] Macrophages may be present in these lesions, but are located away from the lipid pools, usually towards the lumen, interspersed among smooth muscle cells. The lipid pool may have cholesterol clefts but these are usually few.

Necrotic cores are regions of the fibroatheroma that are largely devoid of viable cells and consist of cellular debris and cholesterol clefts (free cholesterol). In contrast to lipid pool, the necrotic core contains cell membranes derived from macrophages, as evidenced by CD68-positive immunohistochemical staining; the periphery of the necrotic core is infiltrated by various numbers of presumably viable foamy macrophages. We have further classified necrotic core lesions into 'early' and 'late' by staining fibroatheromas with Sirius red stain for collagen, which shows collagen matrix in the *early* necrotic core, an absence of collagen in the *late* necrotic core and a sharp demarcation of the late core from the surrounding collagen matrix.

Calcification may be present at all stages of plaque development, but its character changes as the lesion enlarges. In lipid pools and early cores, it is limited to dying smooth muscle cells and occurs as microcalcifications of matrix vesicles. With plaque enlargement, large calcific areas involving fibrous tissue occur as sheets of calcium plates. When late, macrophage-rich necrotic cores calcify, these are more feathery in appearance in decalcified sections, and the calcific areas are irregular. These calcification patterns have been described as absent, speckled, fragmented, and diffuse on radiologic and ultrasonographic examination.[10]

Fibrous cap is the region of the plaque that separates the necrotic core from the lumen. The fibrous cap is rich in type I collagen, and is of variable thickness. When less than 65 μm, it has been described as a 'vulnerable' or the thin-cap variant of fibroatheroma.[11]

Lesions that lead to acute coronary syndromes

Until recently, it was thought that all coronary thrombi occur from plaque rupture. However, it has been shown in both sudden death and acute myocardial infarction that although the most common form of thrombotic plaque disruption occurs as a result of rupture of a thin fibrous cap, other mechanisms are potentially responsible. Although at least 65–70% of atherothrombi are caused by plaque rupture, 25–30% of thrombi occur from plaque erosion and 2–5% of atherothrombi occur as a result of calcified nodules that protrude into the lumen (Figure 3.1).[7]

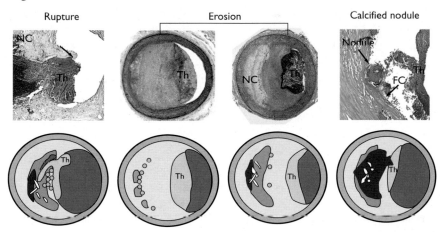

Figure 3.1 *Lesions with thrombi.* Ruptured plaques *are thin fibrous cap atheromas with luminal thrombi (Th). These lesions usually have an extensive necrotic core containing large numbers of cholesterol crystals, and a thin fibrous cap (<65 μm) infiltrated by foamy macrophages and a paucity of T lymphocytes. The fibrous cap is thinnest at the site of rupture and consists of a few collagen bundles and rarely smooth muscle cells. The luminal thrombus is in communication with the lipid-rich necrotic core.* Erosions *occur over lesions rich in smooth muscle cells and proteoglycans. Luminal thrombi overlie areas lacking surface endothelium. The deep intima of the eroded plaque often shows extracellular lipid pools, but necrotic cores are uncommon; when present, the necrotic core does not communicate with the luminal thrombus. Inflammatory infiltrate is usually absent but if present, is sparse and consists of macrophages and lymphocytes.* Calcified nodules *are plaques with luminal thrombi showing calcific nodules protruding into the lumen through a disrupted thin fibrous cap (FC). There is absence of endothelium at the site of the thrombus and inflammatory cells (macrophages, T lymphocytes) are absent. (Reproduced with permission from R Virmani et al.* Arterioscler Thromb Vasc Biol *2000; 20:1262–75.[7])*

Plaque rupture

Plaque rupture is defined as a necrotic core with a thin fibrous cap that is disrupted or ruptured, allowing the flowing blood to come in contact with the necrotic core. This exposure of tissue factor (TF) in the lipid-rich core to the circulating blood results in luminal thrombosis.[12–16] The disrupted fibrous cap is essentially devoid of smooth muscle cells and is made up of type I collagen. The cap is usually heavily infiltrated by activated macrophages and T lymphocytes, which show HLA-DR positivity.[17] T cells liberate proinflammatory cytokines such as γ-interferon, which inhibits collagen synthesis by the smooth muscle cells.[18] Interstitial collagen fibrils, especially the triple helical collagen fibril, are susceptible to degradation by proteolytic enzymes. It is believed that the macrophages in the fibrous cap release MMPs (matrix metalloproteinases),[19] of which at least 23 have been described, which weaken the fibrous cap and result in rupture. Libby and colleagues (see Sukhova et al[18]) have demonstrated overexpression of all three important interstitial collagenases in atherosclerotic plaques (MMP-1, -8, and -13) that may be responsible for the breakdown of the fibrous cap. Rupture of the fibrous cap usually occurs in the shoulder regions, the weakest portion where the stress is highest and MMP expression increased.[21] The vasa vasorum are also markedly increased within the plaque and are especially prominent in patients dying during exertion rather than those dying at rest with plaque rupture.[22]

The frequency of acute plaque rupture in series of sudden coronary death varies widely, and is dependent on the population studied and definition of the lesion. Davies,[23] Davies and Thomas[24,25] and Falk[26] believe this lesion is present in over 85% of patients dying suddenly. In our experience, however, this lesion accounts for only 30% of cases of all sudden deaths, because cases of organized thrombi with total coronary occlusion of one or more arteries are also significant substrates of terminal arrhythmias. Calcification is present in 80% of plaques that rupture but is usually either speckled or fragmented and infrequently diffuse. The coronary plaques in plaque rupture are equally concentric or eccentric and are more frequent in men and postmenopausal women.[27]

Plaque erosion

Plaque erosion is defined as a lesion with luminal thrombus with a base rich in smooth muscle cells and proteoglycan matrix.[28] At the site of thrombosis, there is absence of an endothelial layer. The underlying plaque in 50% of cases shows layering of the fibrin with interspersed smooth muscle cells and proteoglycans. The underlying plaque shows either pathologic intimal thickening or fibroatheroma with a thick fibrous cap that is rich in proteoglycans,[7] especially hyaluronan and versican along with type III collagen.[29] These lesions are usually not calcified, and when calcified the calcification is speckled.[30] Inflammatory cells are infrequently observed in the plaque underneath the thrombus. The majority of plaque erosions are eccentric, and occur most frequently in young men and women <50 years of age and are associated with smoking, especially in premenopausal women.[31]

Calcified nodule

The third type of lesion is an infrequent cause of thrombosis in patients dying a sudden coronary death and its incidence in stable or unstable angina and acute myocardial infarction is unknown. The term refers to a lesion with fibrous cap disruption, absence of endothelium and thrombus associated with eruptive, dense calcified nodule with bone formation. The origin of this lesion is unknown, but appears to be associated with healed plaque ruptures. Over one-half of these lesions are seen in the mid right coronary artery, where coronary torsion stress is maximum. The underlying plaque is associated with calcified plates and it is proposed that the breakdown of the calcified plate results in release of certain growth factors that likely induce ossification and the fibrous cap wears down from physical forces exerted by the nodules themselves or from proteases released from the surrounding cellular infiltrates. This lesion is usually seen in elderly male patients with heavily calcified and tortuous arteries.[7]

Thin-cap fibroatheroma

'Vulnerable plaque',[32] a term coined by Muller and colleagues[33,34] and Little,[35] refers to a lesion prone to thrombosis. Libby further defined the morphology of the 'vulnerable' plaque as a 'lesion composed of a lipid-rich core in an eccentric plaque'.[36] The central core contains 'many lipid-laden macrophage foam cells derived from blood monocytes' with a 'thin, friable fibrous cap'.[36]

Our laboratory has defined plaque vulnerability based on the actual cap thickness of fixed autopsy specimens (Table 3.2). The 'vulnerable' plaque, or thin-cap fibroatheroma (TCFA) was defined as a lesion with a fibrous cap <65 μm thick and infiltrated by macrophages (>25 cells per 0.3 mm diameter field).[11] A thickness of 65 μm was chosen as a criterion of instability because in rupture, the mean cap thickness was 23 ± 19 μm; 95% of caps measured less than 64 μm within a limit of only 2 standard deviations. The plaque may or may not be eccentric and the necrotic core is well developed, although there is no correlation between the thickness of the fibrous cap and size of the necrotic core. However, the fibrous cap thickness correlates with macrophage infiltration: the thinner the cap the greater the macrophage infiltration (Figure 3.2).

A detailed morphometric comparison of plaque variables between rupture and TCFA is shown in Table 3.2. This analysis of culprit lesions[38] showed that the

Table 3.2 Morphologic characteristics of plaque rupture and thin-cap fibroatheroma

Plaque type	Necrotic core (%)	Fibrous cap thickness (μm)	Macrophage density (%)	Smooth muscle cells (%)	T lymphocytes per mm² × 1000	Calcification score
Rupture	34±17	23±19	26±20	0.002±0.004	4.9±4.3	1.53±1.03
Thin cap fibroatheroma	23±17	<65	14±10	6.6±10.4	6.6±10.4	0.97±1.1
P value	NS		0.005	NS	NS	0.014

(Reproduced with permission from FD Kolodgie et al. *Curr Opin Cardiol* 2001; **16**:285–92.[35])

NS, not significant.

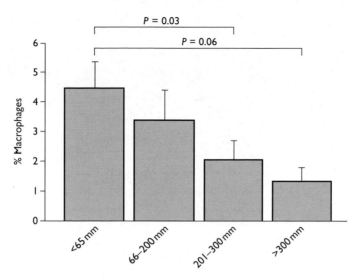

Figure 3.2 *Correlation between fibrous cap thickness and macrophage density within the fibrous cap. As the thickness increases, the density of macrophages decreases. Data are derived from post-mortem analysis of epicardial coronary artery sections from men and women dying suddenly from coronary artery disease.*

underlying necrotic core as a percent of plaque area was greatest in ruptured plaques (34±17%) but this was not significantly different (23±17%) from TCFAs. In addition, we found that ruptures had a greater concentration of macrophages in the fibrous cap than TCFAs (26±20% versus 14±10%, P = 0.005) and a significant reduction of smooth muscle cells at the rupture site compared to TCFAs. No differences were noted in the number of T lymphocytes in areas of cap thinning.

The morphologic variants of the TCFA are detailed in Figure 3.3. These include lesions with insignificant plaque burden, large eccentric or concentric lipid cores, or previous healed ruptures. In a large series of 142 cases only 11% of acute ruptures show rupture of a virgin plaque without evidence of prior rupture.[39]

Roberts and Jones have shown that at the site of rupture the necrotic core was the largest as compared to plaques with intact fibroatheromas, supporting the concept that a large necrotic core is associated with plaque vulnerability.[40] We have corroborated these data in coronary arteries from patients dying suddenly, showing that mean necrotic core size, independent of cross-sectional area luminal narrowing was greatest in plaque ruptures, followed by thin-cap atheromas and fibrous cap atheromas.[38] Ninety percent of ruptured plaques contain necrotic cores greater than 10% of plaque area; furthermore, 65% of plaque ruptures have >25% of plaque occupied by necrotic core. In contrast, only 75% of TCFAs have

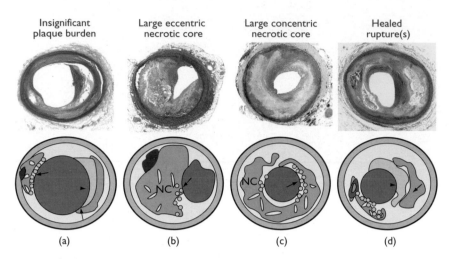

Figure 3.3 *Morphologic variants of the thin-cap fibroatheroma. Thin caps may emerge in fibroatheromas with insignificant plaque burden and insignificant luminal narrowing, in fibroatheromas with large cores that are eccentric or eccentric, and frequently in plaques with evidence of prior rupture. (a) In this plaque with insignificant plaque burden, there is an area of proteoglycan-rich smooth muscle cells (arrowhead) suggestive of a prior rupture, and multiple areas of thin caps (arrows). (b) The necrotic core (NC) is large, with an area of thinned cap (arrow). (c) The necrotic core (NC) is concentric with an extensive area of cap thinning (arrow). (d) There may be a healed rupture (arrow) with a proteoglycan-rich smooth muscle cell reparative layer (arrowhead).*

>10% of plaque area occupied by a core and only 35% of TCFAs have >25% of plaque occupied by the lipid core.[38,41] The length of the necrotic core in ruptures and TCFAs is similar, varying from 2 mm to 22 mm with a mean of 8 mm and 9 mm, respectively (Table 3.3). The mean percent cross-sectional area narrowing of TCFAs is 60% as compared to 73% for plaque ruptures. Thus TCFAs are predominantly seen in arteries with <50% diameter stenosis. Over 50% of the plaque ruptures, healed plaque ruptures and TCFAs occur in the proximal portions of the major coronary arteries, left anterior descending, right, left circumflex, and another third in the mid-portion of these arteries while the rest are distributed in the distal segments.[37]

Incidence of thin-cap atheroma in acute coronary syndromes

By far the highest incidence of TCFAs occur in patients dying with acute myocardial infarction (AMI) (3.1±2.4 TCFAs per patient), less in sudden coronary death (1.8±1.9) and least in incidental death (0.50±1.1) or plaque

Table 3.3 Approximate sizes of necrotic core, in fibroatheroma, thin-cap atheroma and acute rupture

Dimension	Plaque type		
	Fibrous cap atheroma	Thin cap atheroma	Acute plaque rupture
Length (mm: mean (range))	6 (1–18)	8 (2–17)	9 (2.5–22)
Necrotic core area (mm²)	1.2±2.2	1.7±1.1	3.8±5.5
Necrotic core area (%)	15±20	23±17	34±17

(Reproduced with permission from R Virmani et al. *J Interv Cardiol* 2002; **15**:439–46.[39])

erosion (0.50±1.0).[38] The incidence of TCFAs is greater in men than women (AMI 3.1 vs 1.7; SD 1.8 vs 1.3, respectively). We have also observed in sudden coronary death that the highest incidence of TCFA occurs in patients dying with acute rupture (1.3±1.4 per heart) than patients dying from stable plaque (1.1±1.3 per heart).[38] Similarly the incidence of TCFA was higher in healed plaque ruptures than non-healed plaque ruptures when stable plaques were separated (1.4±1.4 vs 0.5±0.8, respectively). TCFAs have not been characterized in patients dying with stable and unstable angina as these patients usually do not die during the acute phase of the disease.

Role of calcification in the detection of a thin-cap atheroma

Coronary calcification correlates with plaque burden and cardiovascular morbidity and mortality. As age advances, the mean percent calcified area increases both for plaques with moderate (≥50% and <75% area luminal narrowing) and severe (≥75% area luminal narrowing) coronary narrowing.[42,43] However, total occlusion may have less calcification and is duration dependent. It has been shown that Framingham risk factor analysis only predicts up to 50% of coronary artery disease (CAD) mortality.[44,45] Kondos et al, using electron beam tomography (EBT) to image coronary arteries in self-referred men and women who did not have prior events and were followed for 37±13 months, have shown that knowledge of coronary artery calcification provided incremental information beyond that defined by conventional CAD risk factor assessment.[46] However, pathologic analysis of coronary arteries of patients dying from sudden coronary death have shown that maximum calcification area is seen in healed plaque ruptures, followed by fibroatheroma, thin-cap atheroma, plaque hemorrhage, fibrous plaque, plaque rupture, total occlusion and plaque erosion.[9] This morphologic data suggest that calcification is not associated with plaque instability. In fact plaque ruptures and erosions showed little calcification.

We have studied post-mortem coronary radiographs and correlated the radiographs with histologic assessment of the type of atherosclerotic plaque. The radiographic calcification was typed according to Friedrich et al.[10] as absent, speckled, fragmented (linear or wide, single focus of calcium >2 mm in diameter) or diffuse (>5 mm-segment of continuous) calcification. We classified plaques histologically as plaque rupture, plaque erosion, thin-cap atheroma and healed plaque rupture. Plaque erosions had either no calcification or speckled calcification. Plaque ruptures showed speckled calcification in 70%, and the remaining 30% had a diffuse or fragmented calcification pattern. Fifty percent of TCFAs had absent or speckled calcification, and the remainder had a diffuse or fragmented calcification pattern. In contrast, 40% of healed plaque ruptures had diffuse calcification, 20% had a fragmented calcification pattern, and the remainder had predominantly speckled calcification (Figure 3.4).[30]

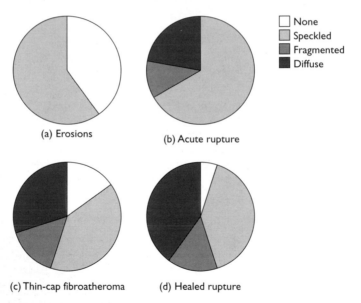

(a) Erosions   (b) Acute rupture

☐ None
▨ Speckled
▨ Fragmented
■ Diffuse

(c) Thin-cap fibroatheroma   (d) Healed rupture

Figure 3.4 *Relationship between plaque morphology and radiographic calcification. Plaque erosions (a) were exclusively present in areas with stippled or no calcification. Plaque ruptures (b) were most frequently seen in areas of speckled calcification, but were also present in blocked or diffuse calcification. Curiously, there were no ruptures in segments devoid of any calcification. Thin capped atheroma were most frequently present in areas of speckled calcification (c), but were also seen in heavily calcified or uncalcified areas, suggesting that calcification pattern is not helpful in diagnosing these lesions. Healed ruptures are almost always seen in areas of calcification, and most frequently in diffusely calcified areas (d). (Reproduced with permission from AP Burke et al. Herz 2001; 26:239–44.[8])*

Healed plaque ruptures

Not all plaque ruptures result in symptoms; therefore, there should be morphologic hallmarks that could be recognized within plaques that are representative of a previous site of thrombus. Healed ruptures in the coronary vascular bed are readily detected microscopically by the identification of the breaks in the fibrous cap, which is rich in type I collagen and an overlying repaired lesion which is richer in type III collagen. The healed lesion can be more easily recognized by Movat stain (healed site identified by the brilliant blue-green color of the proteoglycan rich matrix) and confirmed by picrosirius red staining and polarized microscopy. When viewed under polarized light, this stain highlights the breaks in the fibrous cap, which is rich in type I collagen, as yellow-red birefringence with an underlying necrotic core. The plaque overlying the fibrous cap in healed plaque rupture consists of smooth muscle cells in a proteoglycan matrix which is rich in type III collagen and has green birefringence under polarized light (Sirius red collagen stain).[40]

We and others believe that healing of a disrupted plaque is the main stimulus for plaque progression and is a major factor in causing chronic high-grade coronary stenosis once a late atherosclerotic necrotic core with a thin fibrous cap has formed.[47] This mechanism would explain the phasic rather than linear progression of coronary disease observed in angiograms taken annually of patients with chronic ischemic heart disease.[14] However, these are speculations that need to be proved in man and are only possible if we can prospectively recognize the sites of vulnerability and with follow-up show that such lesions heal and result in progressive narrowing of plaques.

In summary, there are various causes of coronary thrombosis. The major cause is plaque rupture. The precursor lesion of plaque rupture in the past has been called as the vulnerable plaque but this terminology is inaccurate as coronary thrombosis also occurs from plaque erosion and calcified nodule, and the underlying plaque morphologies are different in these two as compared to plaque rupture. Our primary goal is to identify patients who are vulnerable to developing acute coronary syndromes and the plaque morphology that underlies each of the three types of thrombosis should be descriptive. The lesion that most resembles plaque rupture is the TCFA, a lesion usually occurring at sites of mild to moderate coronary narrowing, in patients with acute myocardial infarction, in the proximal or middle regions of the three main coronary arteries.

References

1. Murray CJ, Lopez AD. Global mortality, disability, and the contribution of risk factors: Global Burden of Disease Study. *Lancet* 1997; **349**:1436–1442.

2. Libby P. Inflammation in atherosclerosis. *Nature* 2002; **420**:868–74.

3. O'Brien ER, Garvin MR, Dev R et al. Angiogenesis in human coronary atherosclerotic plaques. *Am J Pathol* 1994; **145**:883–94.

4. Depre C, Havaux X, Wijns W. Neovascularization in human coronary atherosclerotic lesions. *Cathet Cardiovasc Diagn* 1996; **39**:215–20.

5. Stary HC, Chandler AB, Glagov S et al. A definition of initial, fatty streak, and intermediate lesions of atherosclerosis. A report from the Committee on Vascular Lesions of the Council on Arteriosclerosis, American Heart Association. *Arterioscler Thromb* 1994; **14**:840–56.

6. Stary HC, Chandler AB, Dinsmore RE et al. A definition of advanced types of atherosclerotic lesions and a histological classification of atherosclerosis. A report from the Committee on Vascular Lesions of the Council on Arteriosclerosis, American Heart Association. *Arterioscler Thromb Vasc Biol* 1995; **15**:1512–31.

7. Virmani R, Kolodgie FD, Burke AP, Farb A, Schwartz SM. Lessons from sudden coronary death: a comprehensive morphological classification scheme for atherosclerotic lesions. *Arterioscler Thromb Vasc Biol* 2000; **20**:1262–75.

8. Burke AP, Weber DK, Kolodgie FD et al. Pathophysiology of calcium deposition in coronary arteries. *Herz* 2001; **26**:239–44.

9. Burke AP, Weber D, Farb A et al. Coronary calcification: insights from sudden coronary death victims. *Z Kardiol* 1999; **89**,SII:49–53.

10. Friedrich GJ, Moes NY, Muhlberger VA et al. Detection of intralesional calcium by intracoronary ultrasound depends on the histologic pattern. *Am Heart J* 1994; **128**:435–41.

11. Burke AP, Farb A, Malcom GT et al. Coronary risk factors and plaque morphology in men with coronary disease who died suddenly. *N Engl J Med* 1997; **336**:1276–82.

12. Libby P, Geng YJ, Aikawa M et al. Macrophages and atherosclerotic plaque stability. *Curr Opin Lipidol* 1996; **7**:330–5.

13. Zaman AG, Helft G, Worthley SG, Badimon JJ. The role of plaque rupture and thrombosis in coronary artery disease. *Atherosclerosis* 2000; **149**:251–66.

14. Falk E, Shah PK, Fuster V. Coronary plaque disruption. *Circulation* 1995; **92**:657–71.

15. Falk E, Fernandez-Ortiz A. Role of thrombosis in atherosclerosis and its complications. *Am J Cardiol* 1995; **75**:3B–11B.

16. Davies MJ. Acute coronary thrombosis – the role of plaque disruption and its initiation and prevention. *Eur Heart J* 1995; **16 (Suppl L)**:3–7.

17. Virmani R, Kolodgie F, Burke AP et al. Inflammation and coronary artery disease. In: Feuerstein GZ, Libby P, Mann DL, eds. *Inflammation and Cardiac Diseases*. Basel: Birkhäuser Verlag 2003:21–53.

18. Schonbeck U, Mach F, Sukhova GK et al. Regulation of matrix metalloproteinase expression in human vascular smooth muscle cells by T lymphocytes: a role for CD40 signaling in plaque rupture? *Circ Res* 1997; **81**:448–54.

19. Galis ZS, Sukhova GK, Kranzhofer R, Clark S, Libby P. Macrophage foam cells from experimental atheroma constitutively produce matrix-degrading proteinases. *Proc Natl Acad Sci USA* 1995; **92**:402–6.

20. Sukhova GK, Schonbeck U, Rabkin E et al. Evidence for increased collagenolysis by interstitial collagenases-1 and -3 in vulnerable human atheromatous plaques. *Circulation* 1999; **99**:2503–9.

21. Galis ZS, Sukhova GK, Lark MW, Libby P. Increased expression of matrix metalloproteinases and matrix degrading activity in vulnerable regions of human atherosclerotic plaques. *J Clin Invest* 1994; **94**:2493–503.

22. Burke AP, Farb A, Malcom GT et al. Plaque rupture and sudden death related to exertion in men with coronary artery disease. *JAMA* 1999; **281**:921–6.

23. Davies MJ. Pathological view of sudden cardiac death. *Br Heart J* 1981; **45**:88–96.

24. Davies MJ, Thomas A. Thrombosis and acute coronary-artery lesions in sudden cardiac ischemic death. *N Engl J Med* 1984; **310**:1137–40.

25. Davies MJ, Thomas AC. Plaque fissuring – the cause of acute myocardial infarction, sudden ischaemic death, and crescendo angina. *Br Heart J* 1985; **53**:363–73.

26. Falk E. Morphologic features of unstable atherothrombotic plaques underlying acute coronary syndromes. *Am J Cardiol* 1989; **63**:114E–120E.

27. Burke AP, Farb A, Malcom G, Virmani R. Effect of menopause on plaque morphologic characteristics in coronary atherosclerosis. *Am Heart J* 2001; **141**:S58–62.

28. Farb A, Burke A, Tang A et al. Coronary plaque erosion without rupture into a lipid core: a frequent cause of coronary thrombosis in sudden coronary death. *Circulation* 1996; **93**:1354–63.

29. Kolodgie FD, Burke AP, Farb A et al. Differential accumulation of proteoglycans and hyaluronan in culprit lesions: insights into plaque erosion. *Arterioscler Thromb Vasc Biol* 2002; **22**:1642–8.

30. Burke AP, Taylor A, Farb A, Malcom GT, Virmani R. Coronary calcification: insights from sudden coronary death victims. *Z Kardiol* 2000; **89**:49–53.

31. Burke AP, Farb A, Malcom GT et al. Effect of risk factors on the mechanism of acute thrombosis and sudden coronary death in women. *Circulation* 1998; **97**:2110–16.

32. Schroeder AP, Falk E. Vulnerable and dangerous coronary plaques. *Atherosclerosis* 1995; **118(Suppl)**:S141–S149.

33. Muller JE, Tofler GH, Stone PH. Circadian variation and triggers of onset of acute cardiovascular disease. *Circulation* 1989; **79**:733–43.

34. Muller JE, Tofler GH. Triggering and hourly variation of onset of arterial thrombosis. *Ann Epidemiol* 1992; **2**:393–405.

35. Little WC. Angiographic assessment of the culprit coronary artery lesion before acute myocardial infarction. *Am J Cardiol* 1990; **66**:44G–47G.

36. Libby P. Coronary artery injury and the biology of atherosclerosis: inflammation, thrombosis, and stabilization. *Am J Cardiol* 2000; **86**:3J–8J; discussion 8J–9J.

37. Kolodgie FD, Burke AP, Farb A et al. The thin-cap fibroatheroma: a type of vulnerable plaque: the major precursor lesion to acute coronary syndromes. *Curr Opin Cardiol* 2001; **16**:285–92.

38. Burke AP, Virmani R, Galis Z, Haudenschild CC, Muller JE. 34th Bethesda Conference: Task force #2 – What is the pathologic basis for new atherosclerosis imaging techniques? *J Am Coll Cardiol* 2003; **41**:1874–86.

39. Burke AP, Kolodgie FD, Farb A et al. Healed plaque ruptures and sudden coronary death: evidence that subclinical rupture has a role in plaque progression. *Circulation* 2001; **103**:934–40.

40. Roberts WC, Jones AA. Quantitation of coronary arterial narrowing at necropsy in sudden coronary death: analysis of 31 patients and comparison with 25 control subjects. *Am J Cardiol* 1979; **44**:39–45.

41. Virmani R, Burke AP, Kolodgie F, Farb A. The pathology of unstable coronary lesions. *J Interv Cardiol* 2002; **15**:439–46.

42. Kragel AH, Reddy SG, Wittes JT, Roberts WC. Morphometric analysis of the composition of atherosclerotic plaques in the four major epicardial coronary arteries in acute myocardial infarction and in sudden coronary death. *Circulation* 1989; **80**:1747–56.

43. Kragel AH, Reddy SG, Wittes JT, Roberts WC. Morphometric analysis of the composition of coronary arterial plaques in isolated unstable angina pectoris with pain at rest. *Am J Cardiol* 1990; **66**:562–7.

44. Wilson PW, D'Agostino RB, Levy D et al. Prediction of coronary heart disease using risk factor categories. *Circulation* 1998; **97**:1837–47.

45. Executive Summary of The Third Report of The National Cholesterol Education Program (NCEP) Expert Panel on Detection, Evaluation, And Treatment of High Blood Cholesterol In Adults (Adult Treatment Panel III). *JAMA* 2001; **285**:2486–97.

46. Kondos GT, Hoff JA, Sevrukov A et al. Electron-beam tomography coronary artery calcium and cardiac events: a 37-month follow-up of 5635 initially asymptomatic low- to intermediate-risk adults. *Circulation* 2003; **107**:2571–6.

47. Mann J, Davies MJ. Mechanisms of progression in native coronary artery disease: role of healed plaque disruption. *Heart* 1999; **82**:265–8.

4. GENETIC DETERMINANTS OF THE VULNERABLE PLAQUE

W Craig Hooper

Myocardial infarction (MI), which represents a complex multifactorial, pathologic event that evolves over time, is the clinical endpoint of coronary artery disease (CAD). During the evolution of CAD to MI, the dynamics of atherosclerotic plaque progression are constantly changing and being redefined by both clinical and pathologic parameters. The pathogenesis of CAD begins with atherosclerotic plaque formation and progression at the site of endothelial dysfunction. Pathologic analysis has demonstrated that plaque formation and progression are not uniform within an individual and consequently significant plaque variation with respect to stage and composition exists throughout the coronary tree.[1–3] The atherosclerotic plaque can trigger ischemic events either through direct luminal stenosis or by the formation of an occlusive thrombotic clot at the site of plaque rupture.[2] In recent years, the lesions found in coronary arteries with direct luminal stenosis have been referred to as stable plaque, while those with a superimposed thrombus are commonly called unstable and/or vulnerable plaque. The unstable plaque, which is the underlying cause and hallmark of the acute coronary syndromes (ACS), is thought to be responsible for up to 70% of acute MI and is clinically characterized by unstable angina, acute myocardial infarction and sudden death.[1,4] The lethality of the unstable plaque is a consequence of a sudden thrombotic-associated occlusion at the site of plaque rupture which can occur in the absence of a clinically relevant stenotic lesion.[1,4] Based largely on the increased recognition on the role of inflammation as a pivotal player in plaque dynamics, the term 'the vulnerable plaque' has emerged as possible precursor of the unstable plaque. Since there are currently no clinical or angiographic means to detect the vulnerable plaque, it is essential to develop novel non-invasive and invasive approaches for the identification of such plaques. One such approach would be the incorporation of genomics as a component of the diagnostic evaluation for either primary or secondary prevention and/or intervention. The inclusion of genomics could be used not only to identify high-risk patients and optimize therapeutic modalities, but also to individualize therapy.

Genetics of coronary artery disease/myocardial infarction: an overview

Genetic variations are commonly referred to as mutations, polymorphisms and single nucleotide polymorphisms (SNPs) (Box 4.1). Classically, mutations have been defined as disease-linked sequences present in less than 1% of individuals, while polymorphisms were referred to as DNA variations present in at least 1% of individuals with no apparent disease association. However, this view is changing in that genetic polymorphisms are now being linked to disease and the terms mutations and polymorphisms are frequently used interchangeably. As a consequence of the human genome project, the term SNP(s) is now often encountered and is defined as a genetic variation that involves only one base-pair change. It has been estimated that approximately 2–3 million SNPs are present in the human genome and account for about 90% of the genomic diversity. After SNPs, the most common genetic basis of mutations and polymorphisms are DNA changes that involve more than one base-pair such as multiple base-pair substitutions, insertions, deletions, and repeats (Box 4.1). All these DNA changes – which may have functional or physiological effects – occur in the regulatory

---

Box 4.1 Genetic definitions

Mutation: A DNA sequence which is present in less than 1% of the individuals in a population; refers to a DNA sequence that is linked to disease

Polymorphism: A DNA sequence present in at least 1% of individuals; initially believed to be neither beneficial nor harmful, this view however is changing

Single nucleotide polymorphism: A DNA sequence change that only involves one base-pair change; has been estimated to account for up to 90% of the variations present in the human genome

Substitution: The replacement of one or more nucleotides

Deletion: One or more nucleotides are deleted from a sequence

Insertion: The insertion of one or more nucleotides into a sequence

Silent substitution: The creation of new codon that codes for the original amino acid; no change in gene function

Nonsense mutation: A stop codon replaces an amino acid specifying codon; is generally associated with reduced function

Missense mutation: A different amino acid is specified by the altered codon, may or may not significantly alter function

Repeat: Identical nucleotide sequences present within the genome

---

elements, coding and non-coding regions. However in many cases, a gene variant may have no apparent functional significance despite an association with a disease phenotype. In this case, the finding still may have importance in that the variant may be in linkage disequilibrium or linked to another genetic variant which does have a functional effect and thus itself may be the disease causing or susceptible gene.

Since family studies have shown that classic risk factors do not have a significant role in the familial aggregation of cardiovascular disease, it was inferred that heredity must have an important role in the development of CAD and MI. The inference about genetics was supported by the observations of significant increases in the incidence of CAD/MI in first-degree relatives of individuals who had an MI prior to the age of 60 years.[5-7] Perhaps the best documented specific genetic determinant of CAD/MI is hyperlipidemia in which several genetic variants have been associated with lipid metabolism.[6 8] This genetic association has been underscored by clinical studies which indicated that while hyperlipidemia had a significant pathologic influence in young MI survivors, it had little effect after the age of 60 years.[6] Similar to the early family studies, these observations strongly suggested that a genetic influence was most profound in the young and less pronounced in the elderly.[6] The translation of an individual's family history into clinically relevant genetic-based risk determinants and in the formulation of individualized therapeutic modalities represents major challenges and opportunities in the new millennium.[6] Just as importantly, it will also be essential to discern DNA-based risk factors in the absence of family history.

The pathogenesis of CAD and MI can be divided into three major overlapping components: initiation, progression and expression. Throughout this disease continuum, dynamic gene–environment and gene–gene interactions along with behavioral factors are the predominant determinants that underlie atherosclerosis. These determinants may not only be interactive and operational throughout the continuum, but may also be limited to any one component (i.e. initiation versus expression). Genetic diversity within a human population not only significantly impacts the development and progression of this continuum with respect to an individual, but also affects how the genotype of the individual interacts with environmental determinants. Contributing further to the evolution of MI from CAD, are comorbid conditions that have their own set of genetic and environmental determinants such as hypertension and diabetes. The complexity of these factors are further confounded by race/ethnicity and sex. As a consequence of these parameters and the heterogeneity of atherosclerosis, defining the genetics of CAD/MI with respect to cause and effect has been difficult.

In the past decade, studies in cardiovascular genetics have predominately been centered around genetic variations within any one physiologically relevant gene, namely the candidate gene approach or as called by some, the direct genome-wide association approach. The basic principle of this approach is the association of a genetic polymorphism or mutation with the clinical phenotype. Although this approach has been and will continue to be useful, it is important to consider that the immediate significance of any positive association may be limited because the finding(s) necessarily may not lead to a complete understanding of the relationship between the genetic variant and CAD/MI.[9] But nevertheless this approach does provide a beginning point in that genes from various physiologic pathways which can influence either protein structure/function or vascular wall function, can be selected for DNA analysis. In a case–control study, any identified variant could quickly be analyzed to determine whether or not it was associated with the clinical phenotype. Microarrays, another potentially highly informative molecular approach will be discussed later.

Most of the genetic studies to date have focused on candidate genes that appear to be involved in the pathophysiology of ischemic heart disease.[5–7,10–19] These genes can be loosely grouped in physiologic categories and include: (i) inflammatory, (ii) coagulation, (iii) fibrinolytic, (iv) vascular tone, (v) vascular wall, (vi) lipid metabolism and (vii) platelet receptors (Box 4.2). In most cases, these genes have been analyzed as single genes in the context of a clinically documented CAD/MI irrespective of plaque morphology or stability. Although there is little doubt that many of these genes listed in these categories may have a role in plaque stability and/or instability as well as in the vulnerable plaque, there is paucity of information regarding which genes are directly involved in the pathophysiologic process that leads to development of the vulnerable plaque as well as to plaque rupture and its aftermath. Just as important, there is limited information concerning what effects environmental influences as well as gene–gene and gene–environment interactions have on the vulnerable plaque. The importance of environmental influences is perhaps best illustrated by plaque erosion in premenopausal women as compared to plaque rupture in similar aged males and postmenopausal females.[1,20] Plaque erosion was associated with smoking in premenopausal females, while hypercholesterolemia was linked to rupture in postmenopausal females.[20] This relationship between age and plaque evasion/rupture was not seen in males.[20] For the sake of both simplicity and argument, it will be assumed by the author that genes involved in the development of the vulnerable plaque will also be involved in the development of the unstable plaque and subsequent rupture.

Vulnerable plaque: genetic implications

Although there are many issues surrounding the vulnerable plaque,[21] there are at least four questions which merit attention with respect to the development of a genetic profile for its detection:

1 What controls the evolution of a stable plaque to a vulnerable then to the unstable plaque

---

Box 4.2 Categories and examples of candidate genes

Inflammatory
IL-6
    -174G→C
    -572G→C
MCP-1
    -2518A→G
TNF-α
    -308G→A

TGF-β
    G74→C
    T29→C

Coagulation
Factor VII
    $Arg^{353}Gln$
Tissue factor
    -1208 D→I (deletion→insertion)
Tissue factor pathway inhibitor
    874G→A
Fibrinogen
    -455G→A

Fibrinolytic
PAI-1
    4G/5G
    -844A→G

Vascular wall
ACE
    I/D

AT_1R
    A1166C
Vascular tone

ecNOS
    a/b (27-bp repeat)
    -786T→C

Platelet receptors
GP IIIa PLA^1/PLA^2
GP Ia C807T

Lipid metabolism
Per

IL, interleukin; AT_1R, angiotensin receptor type 1; MCP, monocyte chemoattractant protein; TNF, tumor necrosis factor; TGF, transforming growth factor; PAI, plasminogen activator inhibitor; ACE, angiotensin converting enzyme; eNOS, endothelial nitric oxide synthase gene; GP, glycoprotein.

2   What causes one plaque to become vulnerable/unstable and rupture as compared to other plaques within the coronary bed?

3   Which gene–gene, gene–environment interaction(s) influence inter-individual differences with respect to development and rupture of the vulnerable plaque?

4   What regulates the magnitude of thrombus formation at the site of plaque rupture?

In pathophysiologic terms, these issues are interrelated, but for the sake of identifying molecular targets that can be used for both risk assessment and intervention, it may be useful to consider these questions as separate areas of investigation. As previously indicated, the most commonly used molecular approach has revolved around the identification of candidate genes involved in the pathobiology of CAD/MI. Because these genes are identified in a physiologic context of the disease, it is crucial to have at least some understanding of the disease process. In terms of the vulnerable plaque, this knowledge would not only include the atherosclerotic process throughout the disease continuum, but would also include the molecular immunobiology of the vulnerable and unstable plaque and forces involved in coagulation, fibrinolysis, inflammation and endothelial function/vascular tone.

It is not the purpose here to fully discuss the pathobiology of the vulnerable plaque or the atherosclerotic process that leads to the vulnerable plaque, but rather to focus on relevant areas of current knowledge that have known or potential genetic information. Since the pivotal event of the ACS is thrombus formation at the site of a ruptured plaque, Virchow's triad provides a conceptual basis for the appreciation of the multiple biological interactions that must occur during clot initiation and propagation.[22] Genetic variations in genes that encode for proteins that are indirectly or directly involved in the dynamics of thrombus formation could significantly influence the biokinetics of the vulnerable plaque.

Dynamics of the vulnerable plaque

Over a century ago, Virchow defined the critical parameters of thrombus formation as endothelial damage, stasis and hypercoagulability.[23] In an attempt to reflect the pathophysiology of the vulnerable plaque, these parameters have recently been modified and referred to as vessel wall substrates, rheology and systemic metabolic factors by Rauch and colleagues (Box 4.3).[22] In their adaption, endothelial damage could be a consequence of clinical interventional vessel wall injury, local inflammation and most importantly, the components of the atherosclerotic plaque. The core of the vulnerable plaque contains many elements that could act as substrates for arterial thrombosis and include lipid-derived particles, cellular debris and tissue factor.[9,24–26] Although the basic pathologic process that leads to plaque formation and progression appears to be essentially the same for both the stable and vulnerable plaque, the plaque endpoint or composition differs significantly between the two plaque types. While the stable plaque is characterized by smooth muscle proliferation and collagen synthesis, the vulnerable and unstable plaque is defined by a thin fibrous cap, a large lipid core, inflammatory cells, loss of smooth muscle cells and proteolytic activity within the lesion.[2] Risk factors for plaque rupture are thought to include

---

Box 4.3 Adaptation of Vichow's triad to the acute coronary syndrome

Vessel wall substrates (endothelial damage)
Plaque components and type of plaque disruption (i.e erosion, rupture)
Vascular wall inflammation
Exogenous vascular wall injury (PCI)

Rheology (stasis)
High shear stress (i.e vasconstriction, endothelial dysfunction)
Local stasis
Oscillatory shear stress (artery bifurcation)

Systemic factors (hypercoagulability):
Metabolic/hormonal (i.e lipids, renin–angiotensin system)
Coagulation/fibrinolysis
Cellular components

(Reproduced with permission from U Rauch et al. *Ann Intern Med* 2001; **134**:224–38.[22])

---

the size of the lipid core, patterns and degree of inflammation and proteinase expression.[2,27,28]

Vessel wall substrates

The macrophage, which is found in abundance in the vulnerable and unstable plaque, releases a variety of bioactive proteins that can affect plaque architecture and these include the matrix metalloproteinases (MMPs) and inflammatory cytokines.[29] There are at least 20 members of the MMPs grouped into four subfamilies all of which function to degrade components of the vascular wall.[30,31] For example, MMP-1, MMP-8 and MMP-13 function to degrade collagen, while MMP-3, MMP-10 and MMP-13 can degrade a variety of other vascular wall constituents such as lamin, elastins and proteoglycans.[30,31] Degradation or loss of the extracellular matrix, which is most commonly seen at the shoulder region, has been associated with plaque rupture and, in addition, histopathologic analysis has demonstrated an increase in MMPs in the vulnerable plaque.[31,32]

One working hypothesis has been that any genetic alterations in the MMPs could influence vascular remodeling and, as a consequence, the rate of lesion progression may be changed and the plaque could be destabilized thus rendering it vulnerable to rupture.[30,31] An insertion-deletion polymorphism, 5A/6A, has been identified in the promoter region of the MMP-3 (stromelysin-1) gene. In vitro studies have indicated that homozygosity for 5A allele was associated with increased transcriptional activity thereby suggesting that this allele may be linked to an increase in proteolytic activity.[30,33,34] When this variant was investigated in the STARS and REGRESS clinical trials, no association with MI was found, but quantitative coronary angiography in the REGRESS trial did show that homozygosity for the 6A allele was associated with an increased risk for the development of new atherosclerotic lesions.[30,33] These findings led to a model that proposed that 6A homozygosity would cause a decrease in transcription which would lead to an increase in matrix production in early plaque development, while homozygosity for 5A would lead to in an increase in proteolytic activity within the lesion that could contribute to plaque instability.[30] But in contrast to the STARS and REGRESS trials, which were conducted among US whites, a recent Japanese case–control study found that the 6A allele was associated with MI in Japanese women but not men.[14] But in an earlier Japanese study, investigators had found an association between acute MI and the 5A allele.[35] However, this latter study had only 330 subjects (59 women), whereas the former study enrolled 909 subjects (458 women). These different 5A/6A results suggest the importance of sex, ethnicity and sample size. The importance of defining vessel characteristics along with disease is highlighted by a French study that found an association between the 5A allele and coronary aneurysms.[36]

Another matrix metalloproteinase, MMP-9, which has been shown to cause plaque destabilization in animal models,[37] has not only been reported to be associated with unstable angina but has also been found in macrophage-derived foam cells that can accumulate at the site of plaque rupture.[31,32] One polymorphism found in MMP-9 (gelatinase B), the C-1562/T variant, has been shown to correlate with disease severity in which 26% of the T allele carriers had stenosis greater than 50% in three coronary arteries as compared to 15% in patients with the C allele.[38] These observations suggested that the C-1562/T variant may have a role in minor rupture as opposed to deep plaque rupture.[38] This finding indicated that there may be an age–genotype interaction with respect to the coronary artery stenosis score.[38] In addition the CC genotype was also correlated with increased plasma levels of MMP-9. In another clinical study, MMP-9 plasma levels but not the C-1562/T variant, were linked to CAD mortality.[39] The same study did however find an association between another MMP-9 variant, R2279Q and future events in patients with stable angina.[39]

The synthesis and MMP-induced degradation of the extracellular matrix is a continuous, dynamic process which is tightly regulated by proinflammatory cytokines.[40] Collagen, the major component controlling the strength of the fibrous cap is regulated by γ-interferon, while other proinflammatory cytokines such as interleukin (IL)-1, IL-6 and tumor necrosis factor-α (TNF-α) induce transcription of the MMPs.[40,41] The activity of the MMPs is controlled by tissue inhibitors of metalloproteinases (TIMPs) whose regulation appears to be less dependent on inflammatory cytokines.[40] Interestingly enough, the anti-inflammatory cytokine, IL-10, has been reported to be a regulator of TIMP-1, and transforming growth factor (TGF)-β, a pleiotrophic growth factor and reported inhibitor of smooth muscle proliferation has been shown to regulate TIMP-3.[40] Consequently, any DNA polymorphism that could cause an increase in proinflammatory cytokine production and/or cause a decrease in TIMP production or one that would upset the MMP/TIMP balance could be considered a possible genetic determinant or risk factor not only for the development and progression of atherosclerosis, but also for the vulnerable plaque. Conversely, a variant that would lead to a decrease in proinflammatory cytokine production may be protective or could contribute to plaque stabilization.

Increased or altered proinflammatory cytokine production as a consequence of inflammation, is thought to have a pivotal role via multiple mechanisms in atherosclerosis as well as in the pathobiology of the vulnerable plaque.[40-46] Pathologic cytokine production may not only be due to a prolonged or chronic stimulus, but may also be due to genetic polymorphisms or a combination. There have been reports of genetic alterations that have been linked to an increase in cytokine production as well as to CAD/MI.[47] The monocyte chemoattractant protein-1 (MCP-1) chemokine functions to attract monocytes to the site of injury.[50,51] Because of the fundamental role that monocytes/macrophages have in inflammation and atherosclerotic plaque development, it is believed that MCP-1 may be one of the more significant chemokines. Studies have found that increased MCP-1 plasma levels were higher in patients with ACS as compared to those with stable coronary disease and were an independent predicator of outcome.[52] There has been at least one MCP-1 genetic polymorphism, -2518 A/G, that has been reported not only to cause an increase in MCP-1 plasma levels but was also associated with CAD, and conversely that a polymorphism in the receptor for MCP-1, CCR2-64I, appeared to be linked to a reduced risk for CAD.[53]

Two genetic variants located in the IL-6 promoter region, -174G→C and -572G→C, have been correlated with increased IL-6 plasma levels, which in turn have been linked to unstable angina, CAD and increased risk for MI.[54-56] These findings, however, have led to different interpretations. In the ECTIM study, it was found that the -174C allele was more common in MI survivors with two or fewer stenosed vessels.[57] Based in part on an Apo E/IL-6 double knockout mice study in which these mice has less fibrotic plaques and decreased collagen staining, the ECTIM investigators proposed low IL-6 levels could lead to plaque destabilization.[57] However, in another study, the -174C allele was associated with an IL-6 increase following coronary artery bypass surgery.[54] It was noted however, that IL-6 levels associated with the -174C allele peaked earlier than levels linked to the G allele thus providing some possible insights into the published discrepancies.[54] These findings, concomitantly with other findings of increased IL-6 levels in unstable angina, are not only indicative of the complexity of cytokine effects in atherosclerosis but also support the concept of multiple polymorphisms in the IL-6 promoter region regulating IL-6 production.[58]

TNF-α, which as previously noted, plays a role in the upregulation of MMP expression has been found to be increased after an acute MI.[59] One TNF polymorphism, -308G/A has been reported to be associated with an increase in TNF-α production, but its association with CAD/MI is not clear.[60]

Inflammation of the vascular wall

In addition to inflammatory cytokines and other growth factors which may control the expression of MMPs, TIMPs, collagen expression and other extracellular matrix proteins, inflammation of the vascular wall has also been included by Rauch and colleagues as a contributor to endothelial damage or as a substrate for thrombosis. Consequently, in addition to the genetic variants previously mentioned, other DNA variants in genes that encode for cytokines or growth factors may also have a role in the development and rupture of the vulnerable plaque. As indicated earlier, TGF-β has been reported to be an inhibitor of smooth muscle proliferation but its role in CAD/MI as well as in vascular restenosis is controversial.[61] But, nevertheless, because of its reported role in the inhibition of smooth muscle proliferation and extracellular matrix production, it may be important in the pathobiology of the vulnerable plaque. At least two TGF-β genetic variants, G74→C and T29→C, have been implicated in CAD/MI.[49,62,63] Both variants which were analyzed in the ECTIM study, found that although the G74→C variant was associated with MI, this association appeared to be regional. No such association was found with the TGF-β T29→C variant.[62] In contrast, a similar study in Japan found the opposite, in which there was an association of MI with T29→C but not with G74→C variant.[63] Of special interest was that the MI association of the TGF-β T29→C variant was seen only in Japanese males.[63] Another study conducted in the United Kingdom found no link with MI.[49] Although these studies were relatively small, they do nevertheless again point out what impact that sex and differences in allele frequencies may have on genetic associations with disease. Members of the cytokine and growth factor family may also act as modifiers in that they can enhance or attenuate the effect(s) of other cytokines.

Genetics of thrombogenicity

The type and degree of plaque disruption are pivotal determinants that influence the magnitude of local thrombogenicity.[22] Plaque erosion, which has been reported to be more common in young women, induces thrombus formation as consequence of exposure to collagen and tissue factor (TF).[20] The more common type of disruption is a tear or crack in the fibrous cap. Once ruptured and exposed to blood flow, the contents of the plaque can act as substrates for the formation of the thrombus. The lipid core of the plaque contains apoptotic cells, free cholesterol crystals, cellular debris and TF.[22] Other than possibly young age and the female sex, no predicative genetic determinants have been identified for either plaque erosion or rupture.[20] However, there are genetic variants in genes that encode for proteins involved in the coagulation cascade that may have an effect of the magnitude of thrombus formation.

Tissue factor and tissue factor pathway inhibitor

TF is perhaps one of the most pivotal proteins in coagulation because of its role in thrombin generation following vessel injury. At the site of injury, TF binds to activated factor VIIa and as a consequence, factor Xa becomes activated to initiate the rapid conversion of prothrombin into thrombin. Function of both the TF-factor-VIIa complex and Xa is inhibited by a serine proteinase inhibitor known as tissue factor pathway inhibitor (TFPI), functions as a negative regulator by inhibiting the activity of both factor Xa and TF–factor VIIa.[65,66] As compared to individuals with a wild type or referent genotype, variations in genes that encode for any of these proteins could perhaps not only lead to an increase in amplification and prolongation of thrombin generation but could also significantly diminish thrombin generation as well. Genetic polymorphisms have been described for TF, TFPI as well as factor VII.[64–69] Although polymorphisms in both TF and TFPI have been linked to their respective plasma levels, no consistent relationship has yet been established with MI or with the vulnerable plaque. It has been noted, however, that one cannot exclude the possible association of these polymorphisms with subtypes of the ACS and in addition, other undetected TF and TFPI genetic variants may yet be linked to MI or the vulnerable plaque.[66]

While increased levels of the coagulant factor VII were reported to be associated with fatal CAD in the Northwick Park Heart Study, other studies have either failed to clearly define this relationship or were unable to document it at all.[16,70–72] Despite the inconsistent findings with respect to increased factor VII coagulant activity and disease, several factor VII polymorphisms such as the Arg^{353}Gln have been associated with both factor VII clotting activities and plasma antigen levels.[16,68] In one study, it was reported that the Gln^{353} allele was not only associated with a decrease in factor VII plasma levels, but also decreased the risk of familial MI.[16,67] While this factor VII genotype relationship with the coagulant phenotype has been found in other studies, the correlation with risk of MI has yet to be confirmed. The complexity of factor VII as it relates to the genetics of cardiovascular disease is further underscored by the fact that the effect of environmental factors (i.e. age, body mass index, menopausal status) on factor VII plasma levels may also be genetically determined and there may be geographic differences with respect to allele frequencies of the different factor VII genetic polymorphisms.[16,70,71] Based on the genetic complexity of this coagulation protein, it could be argued that the magnitude and dynamic of thrombus as the site of plaque rupture can in part depend on the factor VII genotype as well at its interaction with other genetic variants such as those found in TF and TFPI. This interaction could be modified by environmental factors such as age and sex.

Fibrinogen and platelets

Components of the intracoronary thrombus include fibrin and platelets. The association between increased fibrinogen levels and CAD/MI has been the most reproducible finding among all of the coagulant proteins.[16,73,74] Several genetic variants have been identified in the fibrinogen β-chain which have corresponded to increased plasma levels. One such polymorphism, the -455G/A variant which is located in the promoter region, has been associated with fibrinogen levels in several studies including REGRESS, but its relationship with CAD/MI is not clear and is controversial.[75] Despite the lack of a clear-cut association with the disease phenotype, this polymorphism has been of special interest because it is in linkage disequilibrium with another variant, -148C/T, found near the IL-6 consensus sequence.[48,76] The finding does suggest a mechanism in which IL-6 upregulation of fibrinogen could significantly amplify the functional effect of the -455G/A and the -148C/T variant.[48] In addition it could also be argued that the IL-6 variant such as -174G/C or -572G/C that causes an increase in IL-6 production could further augment fibrinogen levels.[48] Both mutations if occurring in tandem, would perhaps contribute to the magnitude of thrombus formed at the disrupted plaque. Fibrinogen will be further discussed in the section on Systemic factors.

Platelet adhesion and aggregation, both of which are fundamental to normal and pathologic clot formation, may be influenced not only by IL-6, but also by genetic variations in platelet receptors. Perhaps the best known and controversial platelet receptor polymorphism, PL^{A1}/PL^{A2}, is found in the gene that encodes for GP IIIa in the GP IIb/IIIa complex.[12,77] In the initial report involving 71 patients and 68 controls, the PL^{A2} variant was found to be associated with unstable angina and MI.[77] Although this finding was not confirmed by investigators in several subsequent larger studies, other studies which focused on the combination of PL^{A2} with other risk factors did however find an association.[18,78] At least two studies found an association with young age (47 years or younger) in MI survivors, while other studies found that in PL^{A2} carriers, the co-inheritance of the endothelial nitric oxide synthase (eNOS) 393 allele[79] or high cholesterol increased the risk of MI.[78] Yet another study that found a mild, independent association for both PL^{A2} and the PAI-1 4G/5G polymorphism with MI, also found that the MI risk was significantly increased for individuals who had both variants.[80] This additive risk was most prominent in males. In an autopsy study, it was ascertained that despite the lack of association between MI and the PL^{A2} variant, homozygosity for PL^{A1} was associated with more stenotic, stable plaques, while the PL^{A2} allele was linked to coronary thrombosis and the vulnerable plaque.[81]

While the PL[A2] variant has been reported to cause an increase in platelet aggregation through the binding of fibrinogen,[12] another platelet receptor polymorphism found in the GP Ia gene, C807T, has been linked to an increase in collagen receptor density.[82] Similar to PL[A2], the association between C807T and CAD/MI is controversial, but in at least one study, this variant was linked to young MI survivors who smoke.[12,83,84] In addition, polymorphisms in the platelet receptor complex GP Ib-V-IX, which binds von Willebrand factor, has also been linked to MI in some but not all studies and these include the Thr/Met 145 variant, a variable number of tandem repeat (VNTR) and the Kozak (-5 C/T) polymorphism.[12,85,86] Given the fundamental importance of platelets in clot formation, the identification of any gene that can either directly or indirectly affect activation and aggregation may be useful in predicting the dynamics and magnitude of clot formation in the acute coronary syndrome. Consequently, any genetic polymorphism that would help define the 'acuity' of platelet-mediated thrombosis could have therapeutic implications.[87]

The endpoint of the coagulation cascade, the fibrin clot, is stabilized through the cross-linking of fibrin monomers which is mediated by factor XIII. Several studies have begun to link changes in circulating factor XIII levels to CAD/MI.[88,89] While it has been long recognized that mutations in factor XIII can lead to bleeding disorders, recent genetic investigations with respect to MI have identified one polymorphism, factor XIII Val[34]Leu, which in some[90,91] but not all reports has appeared to decrease the risk of MI.[92] Because this polymorphism occurred near the activation cleavage site it was thought that a decrease in factor XIII enzymatic activity could reduce clot stability and make it more susceptible to fibrinolysis.[93,94] However, more recent studies while finding no functional correlations between the polymorphism and decreased enzyme activity or with clot structure,[95] did find a relationship between the [34]Leu and thrombin activation.[96] Findings from a recent genetic analysis in a genetically isolated Newfoundland population, further supported the importance of sex, geography and interactions in CAD/MI genetics.[97] These investigators found that although there was no significant relationship between factor XIII Val[34]Leu and MI risk in the overall population, there was however, higher prevalence of the [34]Leu allele in male MI patients as compared to female patients and male controls.[97] In the same study, it was found that while the prothrombin G20210A variant alone conferred a 3.2-fold risk with no observed sex differences, it synergized with [34]Leu to increase the MI risk by almost 12-fold.[97] The penetrance of these two alleles was calculated to be 92.3% thereby suggesting that these combinations of alleles represent a strong predisposing factor for MI.[97] Since both prothrombin and factor XIII are physiologically interrelated and intimately involved in the formation and stabilization of the fibrin clot, these two genetic variants or other yet unidentified variants within the same genes could play a major role in determining the magnitude of thrombus formation at the site of plaque rupture.

Further underscoring the complexity of clot structure with respect to gene—environment interactions was a recent in vitro study that found that the effect of the factor XIII Val[34]Leu polymorphisms was dependent on fibrinogen concentrations.[98] It was found that as compared to the [34]Val allele, the [34]Leu allele was associated with increased clot permeability and looser clot structures with thicker fibers, thus providing a protective effect.[98] This effect was seen at the fibrinogen concentration of 10–11.2 μmol/l and higher.

Rheology

There are many genetic and non-genetic factors that could alter or impede blood flow within the lumen of the coronary artery. These include size of thrombus, vascular tone and lesion location.[20] The magnitude of thrombus formation by the previously discussed determinants, can influence the clot size which in turn can change the shear force of the circulating blood. In addition to vessel occlusion by the plaque/thrombus, thrombin and other platelet-derived proteins can contribute to ischemic events by inducing vasoconstriction. A hallmark of· endothelial dysfunction, impaired vasodilation, is found in both coronary and peripheral atherosclerosis.[4,20] Through the production and release of a variety of locally acting bio-active proteins, the vascular endothelium is pivotal in the control of vascular tone. Nitric oxide (NO), which was initially known as a 'endothelial relaxation factor', functions among other things as a vasodilator as well as an inhibitor of both platelet aggregration and leukocyte adhesion.[99,100] In ACS, endothelial dysfunction not only would lead to increased platelet aggregation but also to vasoconstriction.[4] There are several different mechanisms that could cause endothelial dysfunction and many of these revolve around NO. Nitric oxide is produced from Nitric Oxide Synthese (NOS) of which there are at least three different isoforms: endothelial NOS, inducible NOS and neuronal NOS.[101] Endothelial NOS or better known as eNOS is found within the endothelium and produces constitutive levels of NO. Since NO is involved in both platelet aggregation and vascular tone, and inhibits smooth muscle proliferation, it can be argued that eNOS or the other NOS genes may be intimately involved in the pathogenesis of ACS.[101–103]

Genetic polymorphisms which have been identified in eNOS have been linked to CAD/MI in several studies. One interesting polymorphism in the eNOS gene is a 27-base-pair (bp) repeat in intron 4 near the end of the 5′ region.[104] The most common or referent allele has five 27-bp repeats which correspond to 420 bp, while the rare allele or disease-associated allele has four 27-bp repeats corresponding to 393 bp.[104] These alleles have been referred to as 'a' and 'b' corresponding to the four 27-bp and five 27-bp repeats respectively in some reports, while other reports have used fragment size for allele designation with the 393-bp fragment corresponding to the four 27-bp repeat or 'a' allele.[105] Wang and colleagues found that homozygosity for the 'a' or 393-bp allele was associated with CAD/MI in an Australian white population.[104] This link was only seen in smokers. A more recent Japanese study reported a similar association but it was seen in smokers as well as non-smokers.[106] This same study also found that the relationship with the 393 (a) allele was the strongest in patients without other cardiovascular disease risk factors.[106] However, in the prospective Edinburgh Artery Study, an association of the 393 (a) allele was found with CAD which was confined to non-smokers.[107] In a study focused on African-Americans, this same allele was reported to be linked with MI.[105] It was also noted that the 393 (a) allele was significantly associated with MI occurrence in individuals 45 years of age or younger. This particular allele frequency was more common in African-Americans (26%) as compared to whites (14%) and Japanese (10%).[105] The study further reported a possible interaction between the eNOS 393 (a) allele and the platelet receptor GP IIIa PL^{A2} allele in African-Americans.[105] It was observed, however, that the PL^{A2} allele alone was not linked to MI. If these findings could be validated, not only would the PL^{A2}-393 (a) interaction may be predicative of the vulnerable plaque, especially in the young, but would also be suggestive that a variant with no apparent relation to disease may become significant in tandem with other genetic variants. This latter point should not be surprising since CAD/MI is a polygenic disease.

Although there is currently no explanation as to why the 393 (a) allele was only associated with MI in whites, but not in Japanese, smokers, it can, however, be suggested that certain gene–environment interactions may differ among populations. This issue will only be resolved through large prospective studies, but nevertheless it does appear that the 393 (a) allele does play a role in CAD/MI. At least two other eNOS variants have been linked to CAD/MI. The eNOS Glu^{298}Asp polymorphism located in exon 7 has similarly been linked to CAD/MI in some[102,108,109] but not all studies.[110,111] As was the case for the eNOS 393 (a) allele, there do appear to be ethnic/racial differences in allele frequencies in which the ^{298}Asp allele was much lower in Japanese as compared to whites. Another variant, eNOS -786T/C found in the promoter region has been linked to coronary artery spasm in the Japanese,[112] CAD in whites[113] and MI in African-Americans (Hooper et al, unpublished data). As has been suggested for the IL-6 promoter variants, it could be argued that two or more eNOS variants may have a greater impact on NO production.

The renin–angiotensin system plays a pivotal role in maintaining and controlling cardiovascular hemostasis both directly and indirectly. Given its central role, it could be argued that dysregulation of this pathway may be a key determinant for the formation and rupture of the vulnerable plaque. There are two distinct but functionally similar systems, one is endocrine-related while the other is within the vascular wall.[114] Three key proteins in this pathway, angiotensinogen, angiotensin converting enzyme (ACE) and angiotensin receptor type-1 (AT$_1$R) have been shown to have cardiovascular disease-associated

63

polymorphisms.[114–116] ACE is responsible for converting angiotensin I into the effector protein, angiotensin II, and it also functions to inactivate bradykinin. Increased ACE levels would lead to increased angiotensin II levels and increased bradykinin degradation. Consequently, any genetic variant that would lead to increased ACE levels would be important to identify. The biological effects of increased angiotensin II levels and bradykinin degradation would include vascoconstriction, decreased NO production and changes in smooth muscle proliferation.[114] Based on the observations that (i) angiotensin II may increase stress on the shoulder region of the plaque, (ii) localization of angiotensin II in macrophages at the site of plaque rupture and (iii) angiotensin II can lead to increased production of reactive oxygen species,[117,118] investigators have proposed that angiotensin II is intimately involved in the pathobiology of the vulnerable plaque. In a recent immunohistochemical study that has looked at the renin–angiotensin system in atherosclerotic plaques, Schieffer and colleagues found that expression of ACE, angiotensin II and AT_1R was enhanced in the unstable plaque.[117] In addition, angiotensin II was co-localized with IL-6 near the site of plaque rupture. Although these same proteins were found in stable plaques, it is important to remember that increased macrophage accumulation is a characteristic of the vulnerable plaque and consequently it would be expected that expression levels of ACE, angiotensin II and AT_1R would also be significantly increased. Based on the data, the investigators suggested that macrophage-associated ACE is the major producer of angiotensin II within the atherosclerotic plaque.[117] Consequently, it could easily be envisioned that this pathophysiological occurrence through increased inflammation, vasoconstriction, impaired fibrinolysis and decreased NO production, could either contribute to the development and/or rupture of the vulnerable plaque. It could also be surmised that functional genetic variants within the renin–angiotensin system that could lead to increased angiotensin II levels or activity would significantly accelerate this process.

The intronic insertion/deletion (I/D) polymorphism of the ACE gene which has been linked to increased ACE levels, has perhaps been the most analyzed genetic polymorphism in cardiovascular disease.[114] It has been suggested that since this polymorphism probably has no functional effects as a consequence of its location in an intron, it may be in strong linkage disequilibrium with another genetic variant that influences ACE levels.[119] The first study which investigated the relationship between the ACE I/D polymorphism and cardiovascular disease found that the prevalence of the DD genotype was significantly higher in MI survivors and the association was strongest in the absence of other risk factors.[119] This finding led to the suggestion that increased ACE levels might be a contributing cause of CAD/MI and investigators in the ECTIM study did indeed find a relationship between ACE levels and MI in patients 55 years old and younger.[120] There was no association in older individuals. Despite similar findings in other studies, including an MI autopsy study,[121] there have been negative findings with respect to the DD genotype as well as to ACE plasma levels.[122] For example, the large prospective US Physicians' Health Study found no association between CAD/MI and the DD genotype.[122,123] Some of the more obvious reported reasons that may have contributed to the differences, include case selection and definition, length of time between study enrollment and MI occurrence, and geographic-related allele or genetic differences that were seen among the various studies.[114] The latter reason which is often overlooked, is important in comparing results from a relatively homogeneous population to a more heterogeneous population. This point was recently underscored by Carluccio et al who noted that a purported linkage disequilibrium between the ACE I/D polymorphism and a causative gene may vary among populations,[114] and that the US population is probably more heterogeneous than those in Europe. Although females were underrepresented in the majority of studies, some reports were suggestive of a possible sex-based difference.[124]

The gene that encodes angiotensinogen, the precursor to angiotensin II, has been reported to have at least two polymorphisms, T174M and M235T, which have been linked to CAD/MI in some but not all studies.[115,125,126] One of the more interesting studies correlated homozygosity for the rare allele from both angiotensinogen polymorphisms to disease severity as defined by the Gensini score in individuals younger than 62 years.[115] However, no relationship was found with the number of disease vessels or with an increased risk for MI.[115] Although the reasons underlying the association with atherosclerotic burden but not with MI are not clear, it nevertheless can be suggested that genes involved in atherosclerotic progression necessarily may not be involved in formation and rupture of the vulnerable plaque.

Several polymorphisms have been found in the receptor for angiotensin II, AT_1R. The most frequently studied AT_1R polymorphism, A1166C, has been linked to CAD/MI as well as to increased coronary artery vasoconstriction in some but not all studies.[114] Similar to ACE, geography and ethnicity may have a role in the differing AT1R results. For example, the prevalence of the CC genotype is significantly higher in whites as compared to African-Americans. Also similar to ACE, are possible sex-based differences with respect to what impact this receptor may have on disease.[127]

As discussed earlier, gene–gene interactions are a major component of cardiovascular disease and these interactions do happen within and outside the renin–angiotensin system. In addition to interactions within the same gene as noted with angiotensinogen, several reports have found that interactions between the ACE DD and the AT_1R 1166CC genotypes significantly increased the risk of MI.[128,129] This interaction was not seen in all studies.[130] One report found this interaction to increase risk of recurrent ischemic events in the absence of increased coronary atherosclerosis.[129] The interaction between these two polymorphisms could not only lead to increased vasoconstriction and increased oxidative stress, but also to the increased production of both inflammatory cytokines and adhesion molecules that would lead to plaque destabilization. Possible renin–angiotensin interactions with genes outside the system include eNOS polymorphisms.

One report found that an interaction between the ACE DD and eNOS - 786CC genotype was associated with early onset of CAD,[112] while a Japanese study found that the combination of the ACE I/D and eNOS 393/420 (a/b) genotypes did not increase risk.[131] The Cholesterol and Recurrent Events study found that GP IIIa PlA1,A2 genotype increased the risk for recurrent events and the ACE DD genotype conferred an additive effect and it was further observed that this genotype combination had the greatest benefit from pravastatin therapy.[132] Although this observation does require confirmation, it can nevertheless be suggested that plaque which has the greatest risk for rupture might also be the most amenable to pharmacological intervention.

Systemic factors

Factors which contribute to a systemic hypercoagulable state include alterations in fibrinolysis and hemostasis as well as lipid and hormonal changes.[20] Many of the genetic variants that encode for these systemic factors have already been previously discussed and in addition, many factors which have not been discussed will interact and overlap with those previously discussed in the earlier sections on vessel wall substrates and rheology. Although many of these factors have long been considered risk factors for CAD/MI, it has only been recently appreciated that patients with these systemic hypercoagulable risk factors eventually developed coronary thrombosis on plaque erosions.

Although genetic variations may not be the cause of increased plasma levels for many of these factors, they nevertheless may interact with other proteins encoded by a genetic variant. Perhaps the best example of this was the interaction between elevated fibrinogen levels and the factor XIII Val[34]Leu polymorphisms previously discussed.[98] Fibrinogen levels can not only be increased by genetic variation, but also by environmental influences such as smoking and oral contraceptives. As described by Humphries, elements that influence fibrinogen levels can be divided in extrinsic (i.e. smoking, oral contraceptives) and intrinsic (i.e diabetes, hypertension) factors.[133] The influence of these factors does vary significantly among individuals and it is thought that genetic variation may be the major contributor to this inter-individual variability.[133] Studies in the past have suggested that genetics may contribute to the plasma variation anywhere from 0.5 to 0.30, but defining to what extent plasma fibrinogen levels are regulated by genes cannot be clearly discerned because these levels can be affected by changes in rates of both synthesis and degradation.[134,135]

Several genetic polymorphisms found in the β-chain of the fibrinogen protein have been shown to be associated with an increase in plasma levels.[133–136] One such polymorphism in the promoter region in which a guanine to adenine substitution occurred at -455 has been associated with increased plasma fibrinogen levels.[137] Several studies have reported that the relation between the -455 polymorphism and fibrinogen plasma levels was greater in smokers compared to non-smokers.[138–139] Studies which investigated a possible link between the G-455-A polymorphism and cardiovascular disease have been controversial.[16,136,139] Nevertheless it is clear that carriers of A allele of the G-455-A polymorphism have higher plasma fibrinogen levels.[136,138,140] As previously discussed, the G-455-A variant is in complete allelic association with the C 148T polymorphism which is located by the consensus sequence of the IL-6 element.[48,134,140] These observations led to the hypothesis that smoking indirectly increased fibrinogen transcription through the induction of IL-6 from pulmonary monocytes and macrophages.[141] In further support of the relationship between cytokines and fibrinogen was the observation that the A allele of the G-455-A polymorphism was statistically linked to higher fibrinogen levels in healthy males following an acute phase response induced by exercise.[140]

Increased plasma levels of fibrinogen, factor VII, von Willebrand factor and plasminogen activator inhibitor type 1 (PAI-1) have been associated with MI. PAI-1 which is produced by the liver, and endothelium function to inhibit plasminogen activation. Several studies have linked high plasma levels of PAI-1 to CAD/MI and at least two of these studies have documented this relationship in young males.[142–144] Immunohistochemical analysis has documented increased PAI-1 expression in severely atherosclerotic coronary vessels as compared to normal vessels thus leading to the suggestion that local PAI-1 production could facilitate thrombus formation after plaque rupture.[144,145] This association appears to be strongest in individuals with type 2 diabetes.[144] Although several polymorphisms have been identified in the PAI-1 gene, the 4G/5G variant found in the promoter region has been the most studied. It has been shown that individuals homozygous for the 4G allele have approximately a 25% increase in PAI-1 levels as compared to those homozygous for the 5G allele[146] and in vitro analysis has shown that the 4G allele is associated with increased transcription.[146,147] There have been some findings showing that the 4G allele can be regulated by triglycerides, thus providing a link between the PAI-1 genotype and CAD/MI.[144,148] Despite numerous studies, the relationship between the PAI-1 4G/5G polymorphism is somewhat controversial and a meta-analysis found only a small effect on MI.[149] It could be argued as with the other genes discussed within this chapter that the effect of 4G/5G polymorphism is the most profound as an interactive gene, not as a single gene. One report found that carriers of both the 4G allele and the GP IIIa Pl[A2] allele have a significantly greater increase in MI risk as compared to carriers of only one variant.[80] It was further noted that this finding was strongest in males.[80] Another report found that the protective effect of the factor XIII Val[34]Leu polymorphism was abolished in the presence of high

PAI-1 levels, which in turn was linked to the 4G/4G genotype.[90] These latter observations did suggest a role for the PAI-1 4G/5G variant in thrombus formation at the site of plaque rupture, erosion or fissure.

Future directions

Future directions not only include the candidate gene approach, but also the incorporation of macroarray technology. The array technology can not only be expressed in multiple formats, but both RNA and DNA can be utilized. Although the application of this approach is constantly being expanded, its current uses include the detection of gene mutations/polymorphisms, differential gene RNA expression and determining the binding sites for transcriptional factors.[150] The essence of this technology revolves around the spotting or placement of hundreds to thousands of either oligonucleotides or cDNAs on a filter with subsequent hybridization to the target probe. The hybridization signal is subsequently analyzed by a fluorescent detector.[150] Although it is outside the scope of this chapter to discuss this methodology, some examples on how this technology can be used for analysis of the vulnerable plaque will be briefly highlighted.

One recent study used directional coronary atherectomy and cDNA arrays to investigate differences in gene expression between stable and unstable plaques. In essence, cDNA which was generated from RNA extracted from patient samples, was hybridized to a panel of 482 genes that represented subsets of inflammation, adhesion and hemostasis.[151] As compared to the stable plaque, the expression of tissue factor was increased while that of the anticoagulant, protein S, was decreased. This finding was suggestive of a 'local' hypercoagulable state.[151] In the stable plaque, increased expression of cyclooxygenase (COX)-1, MCP-1, MCP-2, IL-7 as compared to the unstable plaque was observed.[151]

A similar study used subtractive hybridization to investigate expression differences between the stable and ruptured plaque.[152] The exclusive expression of perilipin in the ruptured plaque was perhaps the most significant finding. The phosphorylation of perilipin, a phosphoprotein found on the surface layer of intracellular lipid droplets, is thought to facilitate the lipolysis. It has been suggested that the non-phosphorylation form of perilipin may act to suppress enzymes involved in lipolysis and this could lead to plaque instability because of an increase in lipid retention.[152] Furthermore, an increase in lipid within the plaque core could lead to a more robust thrombus formation. Although an A→T substitution in the 5′ region of the perilipin gene has been identified, there is no information available on its relationship to CAD/MI.[153] Although both of these studies used expression arrays, these findings still could be invaluable in determining the genetics of the vulnerable plaque because the results do suggest candidate genes.

References

1. Farb A, Burke AP, Tang AL et al. Coronary plaque erosion without rupture into a lipid core. *Circulation* 1996; **93**:1354–63.

2. Davies MJ. Stability and instability: two faces of coronary atherosclerosis. *Circulation* 1996; **94**:2013–20.

3. Rioufol G, Finet G, Ginon I et al. Multiple atherosclerotic plaque rupture in acute coronary syndrome. *Circulation* 2002; **106**:804–8.

4. Fuster V, Fernandez-Ortiz A. Pathophysiology of ischemic syndromes. In: Loscalzo J, Creager MA, Dzau VJ, eds, *Vascular Medicine*, 2nd edn. Boston: Little, Brown, 1996.

5. Krause WE. Genetic approaches for the investigation of genes associated with coronary heart disease. *Am Heart J* 2000; **140**:S27–S35.

6. Daley GQ, Cargill M. The heart SNPs a beat: polymorphisms in candidate genes for cardiovascular disease. *Trends Cardiovasc Med* 2001; **11**:60–6.

7. Day INM, Wilson DI. Genetics and cardiovascular risk. *BMJ* 2001; **323**:1409–12.

8. Jukema JW, Kastelein JJP. Tailored therapy to fit individual profiles: genetic and coronary artery disease. *Ann NY Acad Sci* 2000; **902**:17–24.

9. Hauser ER, Pericak-Vance MA. Genetic analysis for complex disease. *Am Heart J* 2000; **140**:S36–S44.

10. Manzoli A, Andreotti F, Leone AM et al. Vascular and hemostatic gene polymorphisms associated with non-fatal myocardial infarction: a critical review. *Ital Heart J* 2000; **1**:184–93.

11. Winkelmann BR, Hager J. Genetic variation in coronary heart disease and myocardial infarction: methodological overview and clinical evidence. *Pharmacogenomics* 2000; **1**:73–94.

12. Williams MS, Bray PF. Genetics of arterial prothrombotic risk states. *Exp Biol Med* 2001; **226**:409–19.

13. Franco RF, Reistma PH. Gene polymorphisms of the haemostatic system and the risk of arterial thrombotic disease. *Br J Haematol* 2001; **115**:491–506.

14. Yamada Y, Izawa H, Ichihara S, Takatsu F et al. Prediction of the risk of myocardial infarction from polymorphisms in candidate genes. *N Engl J Med* 2003; **347**:1916–23.

15. Sykes TCF, Fegan C, Mosquera D. Thrombophilia, polymorphisms, and vascular disease. *J Clin Pathol Mol Pathol* 2000; **53**:300–6.

16. Lane DA, Grant PJ. Role of hemostatic gene polymorphisms in venous and arterial thrombotic disease. *Blood* 2000; **95**:1517–32.

17. Boekholdt SM, Bijsterveld NR, Moons AHM et al. Genetic variation in coagulation and fibrinolytic proteins and their relation with acute myocardial infarction. *Circulation* 2001; **104**:3036–68.

18. Ardissino D, Mannucci PM, Merlini PA et al. Prothrombotic genetic risk factors in young survivors of myocardial infarction. *Blood* 1999; **94**:46–51.

19. Winkelmann BK, Hager J, Kraus WE et al. Genetics of coronary heart disease: current knowledge and research principles. *Am Heart J* 2000; **140**:S11–S26.

20. Burke AP, Farb A, Malcom GT et al. Effect of risk factors on the mechanism of acute thrombosis and sudden coronary death in women. *Circulation* 1998; **97**:2110–6.

21. Maseri A, Fuster V. Is there a vulnerable plaque. *Circulation* 2003; **107**:2068–71.

22. Rauch U, Osende JI, Fuster V et al. Thrombus formation on atherosclerotic plaques: pathogenesis and clinical consequences. *Ann Intern Med* 2001; **134**:224–38.

23. Virchow R. *Gesammelte Abhandlungen zur wissenschaftlichen Medicin*. Frankfurt: AM von Meidinger Sohn, 1856:520–5.

24. Fernandez-Ortiz A, Badimon JJ, Falk E et al. Characterization of the relative thrombogenicity of atherosclerotic plaque components: implications for plaque rupture. *J Am Coll Cardiol* 1994; **23**:1562–9.

25. Toschi V, Gallo R, Lettino M et al. Tissue factor modulates the thrombogenicity of human atherosclerotic plaques. *Circulation* 1997; **95**:594–9.

26. Mallet Z, Hugel B, Ohan J et al. Shed membrane microparticles with procoagulant potential in human atherosclerotic plaques: a role for apoptosis in plaque thrombogenicity. *Circulation* 1999; **26**:348–53.

27. Falk E, Shah PK, Fuster V. Coronary plaque disruption. *Circulation* 1995; **92**:657–71.

28. Corti R, Farkouh ME, Badimon JJ. The vulnerable plaque and acute coronary syndromes. *Am J Med* 2002; **113**:668–80.

29. Moreno PR, Falk E, Palacios IF et al. Coronary heart disease/myocardial infarction/peripheral vascular disease: macrophage infiltration in acute coronary syndromes: implications for plaque rupture. *Circulation* 1994; **90**:775–8.

30. Henney AM, Ye S, Zhang B et al. Genetic diversity in the matrix metalloproteinase family. *Ann NY Acad Sci* 2000; **902**;27–37.

31. Ikeda U, Shimada K. Matrix metalloproteinases and coronary artery diseases. *Clin Cardiol* 2003; **26**:55–9.

32. Henny AM, Wakeley PR, Davies MJ et al. Localization of stromelysin gene expression in atherosclerotic plaques by in situ hybridization. *Proc Natl Acad Sci USA* 1991; **88**:8154–54.

33. Ye S, Watts GF, Mandalia S, Humphries SE, Henney AM. Preliminary report: genetic variation in the human stromelysin promoter is associated with progression of coronary atherosclerosis. *Br Heart J* 1995; **73**:209–15.

34. Ye S, Eriksson P, Hamsten A et al. Progression of coronary atherosclerosis is associated with a common genetic variant of the human stromelysin-1 promoter which results in reduced gene expression. *J Biol Chem* 1996; **271**:13055–60.

35. Masahiro T, Hozuka A, Kenji K et al. Stromelysin promoter 5A/6A polymorphism is associated with acute myocardial infarction. *Circulation* 1999; **99**:2717–19.

36. Lamblin N, Bauters C, Herman X et al. Polymorphisms in the promoter regions of MMP-2, MMP-3, MMP-9 and MMP-12 genes as determinants of aneurysmal coronary artery disease. *J Am Coll Cardiol* 2002; **40**:43–8.

37. Galis ZS, Asanuma K, Godin D, Meng X. N-acetyl-cysteine decreases the matrix-degrading capacity of macrophage-derived foam cells: new target for antioxidant therapy. *Circulation* 1998; **97**:2445–53.

38. Zhang B, Ye S, Herrmann S-M et al. Functional polymorphism in the regulatory region of gelatinase B gene in relation to severity of coronary atherosclerosis. *Circulation* 1999; **99**:1788–94.

39. Blankenberg S, Rupprecht HJ, Poirer O, Bicket C. Plasma concentrations and genetic variation of matrix metalloproteinase 9 and prognosis of patients with cardiovascular disease. *Circulation* 2003; **107**:1579–85.

40. Loftus IM, Naylor AR, Bell PRF, Thompson MM. Matrix metalloproteinases and atherosclerotic plaque instability. *Br J Surg* 2002; **89**:680–94.

41. Libby P. Current concepts of the pathogenesis of the acute coronary syndromes. *Circulation* 2001; **104**:365–72.

42. Meuwissen M, van der Wal AC, Koch KT, van der Loos CM, Chamuleau AJ. Association between complex coronary artery stenosis and unstable angina and the extent of plaque inflammation. *Am J Med* 2003; **114**:521–7.

43. Willerson JT. Systemic and local inflammation in patients with unstable atherosclerotic plaques. *Prog Cardiovasc Diseases* 2002; **44**:469–78.

44. Buffon A, Biasucci LM, Liuzzo G et al. Widespread coronary inflammation in unstable angina. *N Engl J Med* 2002; **347**:5–12.

45. Young JL, Libby P, Schonbeck U. Cytokines in the pathogenesis of atherosclerosis. *Throm Haemost* 2002; **88**:554–67.

46. Liuzzo G, Buffon A, Biasucci LM et al. Enhanced inflammatory response to coronary angioplasty in patients with severe unstable angina. *Circulation* 1998; **98**:2370–6.

47. Ross R. Atherosclerosis – an inflammatory disease. *N Engl J Med* 1999; **340**:115–26.

48. Woods A, Brull DJ, Humphries SE, Montgomery HE. Genetics of inflammation and risk of coronary artery disease: the central role of interleukin-6. *Eur Heart J* 2001; **21**:1574–83.

49. Andreotti F, Porto I, Crea F, Maseri A. Inflammatory gene polymorphisms and ischaemic heart disease: review of population association studies. *Heart* 2002; **87**:107–12.

50. Reape TJ, Groot PHE. Chemokines and atherosclerosis. *Atherosclerosis* 1999; **147**:213–25.

51. Baggiolini M. Chemokines in pathology and medicine. *J Intern Med* 2001; **250**:91–104.

52. de Lemos JA, Morrow DA, Sabatine MS et al. Association between plasma levels of monocyte chemoattractant protein-1 and long-term clinical outcomes in patients with acute coronary syndromes. *Circulation* 2003; **107**:690–5.

53. Szalai C, Duba J, Prohaszka Z et al. Involvement of polymorphisms in the chemokine system in the susceptibility for coronary artery disease (CAD). Coincidence of elevated Lp(a) and MCP-1-2518 G/G genotype in CAD patients. *Atherosclerosis* 2001; **158**:233–9.

54. Brull DJ, Montgomery HE, Sanders J et al. Interleukin-6 gene -174G→C and -572G→C promoter polymorphisms are strong predicators of plasma interleukin-6 levels after coronary artery bypass surgery. *Arterioscler Thromb Vasc Biol* 2001; **21**:1458–63.

55. Biasucci LM, Giovanna L, Fantuzzi G et al. Increasing levels of interleukin (IL)-1Ra and IL-6 during the first 2 days of hospitalization in unstable angina are associated with increased risk of in-hospital coronary events. *Circulation* 1999; **99**:2079–84.

56. Liuzzo G, Buffon A, Biasucci LM et al. Enhanced inflammatory response to coronary angioplasty in patients with severe unstable angina. *Circulation* 1998; **98**:2370–6.

57. Georges J-L, Loukaci V, Poirer O et al. Interleukin-6 gene polymorphisms and susceptibility to myocardial infarction: the ECTIM study. *J Mol Med* 2001; **79**:300–5.

58. Terry CF, Loukaci V, Green FR. Cooperative influence of genetic polymorphisms on interleukin-6 transcriptional regulation. *J Biol Chem* 2000; **257**:18138–44.

59. Ridker PM, Rifai N, Pfeffer M et al. Elevation of tumor necrosis factor-α and increased risk of recurrent coronary events after myocardial infarction. *Circulation* 2000; **101**:2149–53.

60. Wilson AG, Symons JA, McDowell TL et al. Effects of a polymorphism in the human tumor necrosis factor-α promoter on transcriptional activation. *Proc Natl Acad Sci USA* 1997; **94**:3195–9.

61. McCaffrey TA. TGF-βs and TGF-β receptors in atherosclerosis. *Cytokine Growth Factor Rev* 2000; **11**:103–14.

62. Cambien F, Ricard S, Troesch A et al. Polymorphisms of the transforming growth factor-beta 1 gene in relation to myocardial infarction and blood pressure. The etude cas-temoin de l'infarctus du myocarde (ECTIM) study. *Hypertension* 1996; **28**:881–7.

63. Yokota M, Ichihara S, Lin T-L, Nakashima N, Yoshiji Y. Association of a T29→C polymorphism of the transforming growth factor-β1 gene with genetic susceptibility to myocardial infarction in Japanese. *Circulation* 2000; **101**:2783–7.

64. Arnaud E, Barbalat V, Nicaud V et al. Polymorphisms in the 5′ regulatory region of the tissue factor gene and the risk of myocardial infarction and venous thrombosis: the ECTIM and PATHROS studies. *Arterioscler Thromb Vasc Biol* 2000; **20**:892–8.

65. Moatti D, Seknadi P, Galand C et al. Polymorphisms of the tissue factor pathway inhibitor (TFPI) gene in patients with acute coronary syndromes and in healthy subjects: impact of the V264M substitution on plasma levels of TFPI. *Arterioscler Thromb Vasc Biol* 1999; **19**:862–9.

66. Moatti D, Haidar B, Fumeron F et al. A new T-287C polymorphism in the 5′ regulatory region of the tissue factor pathway inhibitor gene. Association study of the T-287C and C-399T polymorphisms with coronary artery disease and plasma TFPI levels. *Thromb Haemost* 2000; **84**:244–9.

67. Iacoviello L, Di Casteinuovo A, de Knijff P et al. Polymorphisms in the coagulation factor VII gene and the risk of myocardial infarction. *N Engl J Med* 1998; **338**:79–84.

68. van't Hooft FM, Silveira A, Tornvall P et al. Two common functional polymorphisms in the promoter region of the coagulation factor VII gene determining plasma factor VII activity and mass concentration. *Blood* 1999; **93**:3432–6.

69. Lane A, Cruikshank JK, Mitchell J et al. Genetic and environmental determinants of factor VII coagulant activity in ethnic groups at different risk of coronary heart disease. *Atherosclerosis* 1992; **94**:43–8.

70. Meade TW, Mellow S, Brozovic M et al. Haemostatic function and ischaemic heart disease: principal results of the Northwick Park Heart Study. *Lancet* 1986; **2**:533–5.

71. Heywood DM, Ossei-Gerning N, Grant PJ. Association of factor VII: C levels with environmental and genetic factors in patients with ischaemic heart disease and coronary atheroma characterised by angiography. *Thromb Haemost* 1996; **76**:161–5.

72. Junker R, Heinrich J, Schite H, van der Loo J, Assman G. Coagulation factor VII and the risk of coronary heart disease in healthy men. *Arterioscol Thromb Vasc Biol* 1997; **17**:1539–42.

73. Heinrich J, Balleisen L, Schulte H, Assmann G, van de Loo J. Fibrinogen and factor VII in the prediction of coronary risk factor. *Arterioscler Thromb* 1994; **14**:54–9.

74. Behague I, Poirer O, Nicaud V et al. β-fibrinogen gene polymorphisms are associated with plasma fibrinogen and coronary artery disease in patients with myocardial infarction. *Circulation* 1996; **93**:440–6.

75. de Maat MPM, Kastelein JJP, Jukema JW et al. -455G/A polymorphism of the β-fibrinogen gene is associated with the progression of coronary atherosclerosis in symptomatic men: proposed role for an acute phase reaction pattern of fibrinogen. *Arterioscler Thromb Vasc Biol* 1998; **18**:265–72.

76. Baumann RE, Henschen AH. Linkage disequilibrium relationships among four polymorphisms within the human gene cluster. *Hum Genet* 1994; **94**:165–70.

77. Weiss EJ, Bray PF, Tayback M et al. A polymorphism of a platelet receptor as an inherited risk factor for coronary thrombosis. *N Engl J Med* 1996; **334**:1090–4.

78. Carter AM, Gerning-Ossei N, Wilson IJ et al. Association of the platelet Pl[A] polymorphism of glycoprotein IIb/IIIa the fibrinogen-β 488 polymorphism with myocardial infarction and extent of coronary artery disease. *Circulation* 1997; **96**:1424–31.

79. Hooper WC, Lally C, Austin H et al. The relationship between polymorphisms in the endothelial cell nitric oxide synthase gene and the platelet GP IIIa gene with myocardial infarction and venous thromboembolism in African-Americans. *Chest* 1999; **116**:880–6.

80. Pastinen T, Perola M, Ninni P et al. Array-based multiplex analysis of candidate genes reveals two independent and additive genetic risk factors for myocardial infarction in the Finnish population. *Hum Mol Genet* 1998; **7**:1453–62.

81. Mikkelsson J, Perola M, Laippala P et al. Glycoprotein IIIa Pl[A] polymorphism associates with progression of coronary disease and with myocardial infarction in an autopsy series of middle-aged men who died suddenly. *Arterioscler Thromb Vasc Biol* 1999; **19**:2573–8.

82. Kritzik M, Savage B, Nugent DJ et al. Nucleotide polymorphism in the α2 gene define multiple alleles that are associated with differences in platelet α2β1 density. *Blood* 1998; **92**:2382–8.

83. Santoso S, Kunicki TJ, Kroll H, Haberbosch W, Gardemann A. Association of the platelet glycoprotein Ia C807T gene polymorphism with nonfatal myocardial in younger patients. *Blood* 1999; **93**:2449–53.

84. Croft SA, Hampton KK, Sorrell JA et al. The GPIa C807T dimorphism associated with platelet receptor density is not a risk factor for myocardial infarction. *Br J Haematol* 1999; **106**:771–6.

85. Gonzalez-Conejero R, Lozano ML, Riveria J et al. Polymorphisms of platelet membrane glycoprotein Ibα associated with arterial thrombotic disease. Blood 1998; **92**:2771–6.

86. Murata M, Matsubara Y, Kawano T et al. Coronary artery disease polymorphisms in a receptor mediating shear stress-dependent platelet activation. *Circulation* 1997; **96**:3281–6.

87. Quinn MJ, Plow EF, Topol EJ. Platelet glycoprotein IIb/IIIa inhibitors. *Circulation* 2002; **106**:379–85.

88. Kohler HP, Ariens RAS, Mansfield MW, Whitaker P, Grant PJ. Factor XIII activity and antigen levels in patients' coronary artery disease. *Thromb Haemost* 2001; **85**:569–70.

89. Kohler HP, Ariens RAS, Catto AJ et al. Factor XIII-subunit concentration predicts outcome in stroke subjects and vascular outcome in healthy, middle-aged men. *Br J Haematol* 2002; **118**:825–32.

90. Kohler HP, Strickland MH, Ossei-Gerning N et al. Association of a common polymorphism in the factor XIII gene with myocardial infarction. *Thromb Haemost* 1998; **79**:8–13.

91. Wartiovaara U, Perola M, Mikkola H et al. Association of FXIII Val34Leu with decreased risk of myocardial infarction in Finnish males. *Atherosclerosis* 1999; **142**:295–300.

92. Aleksic N, Ahn C, Wang Y-W et al. Factor XIIIA Val34Leu polymorphism does not predict risk of coronary heart disease. *Arterioscler Thromb Vasc Biol* 2002; **22**:348–54.

93. Ariens RAS, Phillipou H, Nagaswami C et al. The factor XIII V34L polymorphism accelerates thrombin activation of factor XIII and affects cross-linked fibrin structure. *Blood* 2000; **96**:988–95.

94. Trumbo TA, Maurer MC. Examining thrombin hydrolysis of the factor XIII activation peptide segment leads to a proposal for explaining the cardioprotective effects observed with the factor V34L mutation. *J Biol Chem* 2000; **275**:20627–31.

95. Mills JD, Ariens RAS, Mansfield MW, Grant PJ. Altered fibrin clot structure in the healthy relatives of patients with premature coronary artery disease. *Circulation* 2002; **106**:1938–42.

96. Undas A, Sydor WJ, Brummel K et al. Aspirin alters the cardioprotective effects of the factor XIII Val34Leu polymorphism. *Circulation* 2003; **107**:17–20.

97. Butt C, Zheng H, Randell E et al. Combined carrier status of prothrombin 20210A and factor XIII-A Leu34 alleles as a strong risk factor for myocardial infarction: evidence of a gene–gene interaction. *Blood* 2003; **101**:3037–41.

98. Lim BCB, Ariens RAS, Carter AM, Weisel JW, Grant PJ. Genetic regulation of fibrin structure and function: complex gene–environment interactions may modulate vascular risk. *Lancet* 2003; **361**:1424–31.

99. Hingorani AD, Vallance P. Endothelial nitric oxide. In: Vallance PJT, Web DJ, eds, *Vascular Endothelium in Human Physiology and Pathophysiology*. New York: Harwood, 2000:3–28.

100. Cooke JP, Dzau VJ. Nitric oxide synthesis: role in the genesis of vascular disease. *Annu Rev Med* 1997; **48**:489–509.

101. Moncada S, Higgs A. The L-arginine-nitric oxide pathway. *N Engl J Med* 1993; **329**:2002–12.

102. Hingorani AD. Polymorphisms in endothelial nitric oxide synthase and atherogenesis. *Atherosclerosis* 2000; **154**:521–7.

103. Maxwell AJ. Mechanisms of dysfunction of the nitric oxide pathway in vascular diseases. *Nitric Oxide* 2002; **6**;101–24.

104. Wang XL, Sim AS, Badenhop et al. A smoking-dependent risk of coronary artery disease associated with a polymorphism of the endothelial nitric oxide synthase gene. *Nat Med* 1996; **2**:41–5.

105. Hooper WC, Lally C, Austin H et al. The relationship between polymorphisms in the endothelial cell nitric oxide synthase gene and the platelet GPIIIa gene with myocardial infarction and venous thromboembolism in African-Americans. *Chest* 1999; **116**:880–6.

106. Ichihara S, Yamada Y, Fujimura T et al. Association of a polymorphism of the endothelial constitutive nitric oxide synthase with myocardial infarction in the Japanese population. *Am J Cardiol* 1998; **81**:83–6.

107. Fowkes FGR, Lee AJ, Hau CM et al. Methylene tetrahydrofolate reductase (MTHFR and nitric oxide synthase (ecNOS) genes and risks of peripheral arterial disease and coronary heart disease: Edinburgh artery study. *Atherosclerosis* 2000; **150**:179–85.

108. Hibi K, Ishigami T, Tamura K et al. Endothelial nitric oxide synthase gene polymorphism and acute myocardial infarction. *Hypertension* 1998; **32**:521–6.

109. Hingorani AD, Liang CF, Fatibene J et al. A common variant for the endothelial nitric synthase (Glu298→Asp) is a major risk factor for coronary artery disease in the UK. *Circulation* 1999; **100**:1515–20.

110. Poirer O, Mao C, Mallet C et al. Polymorphisms of the endothelial nitric oxide synthase gene – no consistent association with myocardial infarction in the ECTIM study. *Eur J Clin Invest* 1999; **29**:284–90.

111. Nassar B, Bevin LD, Johnstone DE et al. Relationship of the Glu298Asp polymorphism of the endothelial nitric oxide synthase gene and early-onset coronary artery disease. *Am Heart J* 2001; **142**:586–9.

112. Nakayama M, Yasue H, Yoshimura M et al. T-786→C mutation in the 5'-flanking region of the endothelial nitric oxide synthase gene is associated with coronary spasm. *Circulation* 1999; **99**:2864–70.

113. Alvarez R, Gonzalez P, Batalla A et al. Association between the NOS3 (-786 T/C) and the ACE (I/D) genotypes and early coronary artery disease. *Nitric Oxide* 2001; **5**:343–8.

114. Carluccio M, Soccio M, De Caterina R. Aspects of gene polymorphisms in cardiovascular diseases: the renin–angiotensin system. *Eur J Clin Invest* 2001; **31**:476–88.

115. Gardemann A, Stricker J, Humme J et al. Angiotensinogen T174M and M235T gene polymorphisms are associated with the extent of coronary atherosclerosis. *Atherosclerosis* 1999; **145**:309–14.

116. Bonnardeaux A, Davis E, Jeunemaitre X et al. Angiotensin II type 1 receptor gene polymorphism in human essential hypertension. *Hypertension* 1994; **24**:63–9.

117. Schieffer B, Schieffer E, Kleiner-Hilfiker D et al. Expression of angiotensin II and interleukin 6 in human coronary atherosclerotic plaques. *Circulation* 2000; **101**:1372–8.

118. Brasier AR, Recinos A, Eledrisi et al. Vascular inflammation and the renin–angiotensin system. *Arterioscler Thromb Vasc Biol* 2002; **22**:1257–66.

119. Cambein F, Poirier O, Lecerf L et al. Deletion polymorphism in the gene for angiotensin-converting enzyme is a potent risk factor for myocardial infarction. *Nature* 1992; **359**:641–4.

120. Cambein F, Costerousse O, Tiret L et al. Plasma level and gene polymorphism of angiotensin-converting enzyme in relation to myocardial infarction. *Circulation* 1994; **90**:669–76.

121. Evans AE, Poirer O, Kee F et al. Polymorphisms of the angiotensin-converting enzyme gene in subjects who die from coronary heart disease. *QJM* 1994; **87**:211–4.

122. Bohn M, Berge L, Bakken A, Erikssen J, Berg K. Insertion/deletion polymorphism at the locus of ACE and myocardial infarction. *Clin Genet* 1993; **44**:292–7.

123. Lindpaintner K, Pfeffer MA, Kreutz R et al. A prospective evaluation of an angiotensin-converting-enzyme gene polymorphism and the risk of ischemic heart disease. *N Eng J Med* 1995; **332**:706–11.

124. Schuster H, Weinker TF, Stremmler et al. An angiotensin-converting enzyme gene variant is associated with acute myocardial infarction in women but not men. *Am J Cardiol* 1995; **76**:601–3.

125. Katsuuya T, Koike G, Yee TW et al. Association of angiotensinogen gene T235 variant with increased risk of coronary artery disease. *Lancet* 1995; **345**:1600–3.

126. Yamakawa-Kobayashi K, Arinami T, Hamaguchi H. Absence of association of angiosinogen gene T235 allele with increased risk of coronary heart disease in Japanese. *Lancet* 1995; **346**:515.

127. Reich H, Duncan JA, Weinstein J et al. Interactions between gender and the angiotensin type receptor gene polymorphism. *Kidney Int* 2003; **63**:1443–9.

128. Tiret L, Bonnardeaux A, Poirer O et al. Synergistic effects of angiotensin-converting enzyme and angiotensin-II type 1 receptor gene polymorphism on risk of myocardial infarction. *Lancet* 1994; **334**:910–3.

129. van Geel PP, Pinto YM, Zwinderman AH et al. Increased risk for ischaemic events is related to combined RAS polymorphism. *Heart* 2001; **85**:458–62.

130. Steeds RP, Wardle A, Smith PD et al. Analysis of the postulated interaction between the angiotensin II sub-type receptor gene A1166C polymorphism and the insertion/deletion polymorphism of the angiotensin converting enzyme gene on risk of myocardial infarction. *Atherosclerosis* 2001; **154**:123–8.

131. Nakagami H, Ikeda U, Maeda Y et al. Coronary artery disease and endothelial nitric oxide synthase and angiotensin-converting enzyme gene polymorphisms. *J Thromb Thrombolysis* 1999; **8**:191–5.

132. Bray PF, Cannon CP, Goldschmidt-Clermont P et al. The platelet Pl^{A2} and angiotensin-converting enzyme (ACE) D allele polymorphisms and the risk of recurrent events after acute myocardial infarction. *Am J Cardiol* 2002; **88**:347–52.

133. Humphries SE. Genetic regulation of fibrinogen. *Eur Heart J* 1995; **16**:16–20.

134. Humphries SE, Luong L-A, Montgomery HE et al. Gene–environment interaction in the determination of levels of plasma fibrinogen. *Thromb Haemost* 1999; **82**:818–25.

135. Thomas AE, Green FR, Kelleher CH et al. Variation in the promoter region of the β-fibrinogen gene is associated with plasma fibrinogen levels in smokers and non-smokers. *Thromb Haemost* 1991; **65**:487–90.

136. Tybjaerg-Hansen A, Angerholm-Larsen B, Humphries SE et al. A common mutation (G-455→A) in the β-fibrinogen promoter is an independent predicator of plasma fibrinogen, but not of ischemic heart disease. *J Clin Invest* 1997; **99**:3034–9.

137. Thomas AE, Green FR, Kelleher CH et al. Variation in the promotor region of the β fibrinogen gene is associated with plasma fibrinogen levels in smokers and non-smokers. *Thromb Haemost* 1991; **65**:487–90.

138. Green FR, Hamsten A, Blomback M et al. The role of β-fibrinogen genotype in determining plasma fibrinogen levels in young survivors of myocardial infarction and healthy controls from Sweden. *Thromb Haemost* 1993; **70**:915–20.

139. Behague I, Porier O, Nicaud V et al. β-fibrinogen gene polymorphisms are associated with plasma fibrinogen and coronary artery disease in patients with myocardial infarction (The ECTIM Study). *Circulation* 1996; **93**:440–9.

140. Humphries SE, Panahloo AP, Montgomery HE, Green F, Yudkin J. Gene–environment interaction in the determination of levels of hemostatic variables involved in thrombosis and fibrinolysis. *Thromb Haemost* 1997; **78**:457–61.

141. Churg A, Dai J, Tai H, Xie C, Wright JL. Tumor necrosis factor-α is central to acute cigarette smoke-induced inflammation and connective tissue breakdown. *Am J Respir Crit Care Med* 2002; **202**:849–54.

142. Hamsten A, de Faire U, Walldius G et al. Plasminogen activator inhibitor in plasma: risk factor for recurrent myocardial infarction. *Lancet* 1987; **2**:3–9.

143. Hamsten A, Wiman B, de Faire U, Blomback M. Increased plasma levels of a rapid inhibitor of tissue plasminogen activator in young survivors of myocardial infarction. *N Engl J Med* 1985; **313**:1557–63.

144. Kohler HP, Grant PJ. Plasminogen-activator inhibitor type I and coronary artery disease. *N Engl J Med* 2000; **342**:1792–1801.

145. Scheiderman J, Sawdy MS, Keeton MR et al. Increased type 1 plasminogen activator inhibitor gene expression in atherosclerotic human arteries. *Proc Natl Acad Sci USA* 1992; **89**:6998–7002.

146. Eriksson P, Kallin B, van't Hooft FM, Bavenholm P, Hamsten A. Allele-specific increase in basal transcription of the plasminogen-activator inhibitor 1 gene is associated with myocardial infarction. *Proc Natl Acad Sci USA* 1995; **92**:1851–5.

147. Dawson SJ, Winman B, Hamsten A et al. The two allele sequences of a common polymorphism in the promoter of the plasminogen activator-1 (PAI-1) gene respond differently to interleukin-1 in HepG2 cells. *J Biol Chem* 1993; **268**:10739–45.

148. Eriksson P, Nilsson L, Karpe F, Hamsten A. Very-low density lipoprotein response element in the promoter region of the human plasminogen activator inhibitor-1 gene implicated in the impaired fibrinolysis of hypertriglyceridemia. *Arterioscler Thromb Vasc Biol* 1998;**18**:20–6.

149. Iacoviello L, Burzotta F, Di Castelnuovo A et al. The 4G/5G polymorphism of the PAI-1 gene and risk of myocardial infarction: a meta-analysis. *Thromb Haemost* 1998; **80**:1029–30.

150. Napoli C, Lerman LO, Sica V et al. Macroarray analysis: a novel research tool of cardiovascular scientists and physicians. *Heart* 2003; **89**:597–604.

151. Randi AM, Biguzzi B, Falciani F et al. Identification of differentially expressed genes in coronary atherosclerotic plaques from patients with stable or unstable angina by cDNA array analysis. *J Thromb Haemost* 2003; **1**:829–35.

152. Faber BCG, Cleutjens KBJM, Niessen RLJ et al. Identification of genes potentially involved in rupture of human atherosclerotic plaques. *Circ Res* 2001; **89**:547–54.

153. NCBI SNP Cluster ID: rs 1052700.

5. DIAGNOSING THE VULNERABLE PLAQUE IN THE CARDIAC CATHETERIZATION LABORATORY

Johannes A Schaar, Evelyn Regar, Francesco Saia, Chourmouzios A Arampatzis, Angela Hoye, Frits Mastik, Rob Krams, Cornelis J Slager, Frank J Gijsen, Jolanda J Wentzel, Pim J de Feyter, Anton FW van der Steen and Patrick W Serruys

Rupture of vulnerable plaques is the main cause of acute coronary syndrome (ACS) and myocardial infarction (MI). Identification of vulnerable plaque is therefore essential to enable the development of treatment modalities to stabilize such plaque, and because MI and its consequences are so important, options to identify those areas that will be responsible for future events must be investigated. This chapter discusses the current statement of development of imaging techniques that have the potential to detect vulnerable plaques.

A wide range exists in the stability of coronary atherosclerotic plaques. A plaque may be stable for years, however abrupt disruption of its structure is the main cause of ACS.[1] The vulnerable plaque has certain features that could be diagnosed by various specialized methods. The ideal technique would provide morphologic, mechanical and chemical information, however at present, no diagnostic modality providing such an all-embracing assessment is available. The characteristics of vulnerable plaque have been described by numerous reviewers[2,3] and are as follows:

- size of the lipid core (40% of the entire plaque)
- thickness of the fibrous cap
- presence of inflammatory cells
- amount of remodeling and extent of plaque free vessel wall
- three-dimensional morphology.

Angiography

Coronary angiography has been the gold standard to assess the severity of obstructive luminal narrowing. Furthermore, it serves as a decision tool to direct therapy such as PTCA (percutaneous coronary angiography) or CABG (coronary artery bypass graft).

With coronary angiography we can assess the lumen boundaries, but cannot assess the plaque burden, and its delineation and components. The predictive power of occurrence of MI is rather low since 70% of acute coronary occlusions are in areas that were previously angiographically normal, and only a minority occur where there was severe stenosis.[4] Other studies have affirmed that the culprit lesion prior to an MI has, in 48–78% of all cases, a stenosis smaller than 50%.[5–7] Coronary angiograms also often fail to identify the culprit lesion of non-transmural MI.[8] The majority of ulcerated plaques are not big enough to be detected by angiography, but can be well assessed pathologically.[9]

Furthermore, we have to take into account that the predictive power of angiography is strongly dependent on the time interval between the angiogram and the MI, because both time and interim therapy can influence atherosclerosis. In one study, the angiograms were performed between 1 and 77 months before the event[4] and showed that atherosclerosis can be a rapidly progressive process. A recent study evaluated angiograms done 1 week before acute MI and showed that signs of thrombosis and rupture were present in a majority of patients.[10] During the year after the MI, the presence of multiple complex plaques is associated with an increased incidence of recurrent ACS.[11]

Thus, patients with silent non-obstructive coronary atherosclerosis harbor vulnerable plaques that cannot be detected by angiograms, but which are associated with adverse clinical outcomes. If a disrupted ulcerated plaque is seen on angiography, the existence of additional rupture-prone plaques is to be expected. Angiography therefore, has a low discriminatory power to identify the vulnerable plaque, but does provide information about the entire coronary system and serves as guide for invasive imaging techniques and therapy.

In the future, our current view of angiography may totally change when non-invasive coronary imaging with MRI (magnetic resonance imaging) or CT (computed tomography) becomes available for routine use.[12]

Angioscopy

Intracoronary angioscopy offers direct visualization of the plaque surface and intraluminal structures like tears and thrombi. It allows assessment of the color of the plaque and thrombus[13] with higher sensitivity compared to angiography.[14] Angioscopic plaque rupture and thrombus have been shown to be associated with adverse clinical outcomes in patients with complex lesions.[15] Furthermore, yellow plaques seem to have an increased instability, in comparison between IVUS (intravascular ultrasound) and angioscopy.[16] In patients with MI all three coronary arteries are widely diseased and have multiple yellow plaques.[17] In a 12-month follow-up study of 157 patients with stable angina, ACS occurred more frequently in patients with yellow plaques than in those with white plaques. These results indicate that ACS occur more frequently in patients with yellow plaques, which can be imaged with angioscopy, but not with angiography.[18] However, angioscopy is difficult to perform, is invasive and only a limited part of the vessel tree can be investigated. Most importantly, to enable clear visualization of the vessel wall, the vessel has to be occluded and the remaining blood flushed away with saline, thereby potentially inducing ischemia. Information regarding the degree of plaque extension into the vessel wall is not provided by angioscopy.

Intravascular ultrasound

IVUS provides real-time high-resolution images of the vessel wall and lumen.[19] The size of IVUS catheters is between 2.9 and 3.5 Fr (French). Depending on the distance from the catheter the axial resolution is about 150 μm and the lateral 300 μm. The images appear real-time at a frequency of up to 30 frames/s. Features of the vessel can be detected based on the echogenicity and the thickness of the material. Small structures can be visualized, however only those over 160 μm can be estimated accurately. The normal thickness of the media is about 125–350 μm.

IVUS provides some insight into the composition of coronary plaques. In IVUS images, calcification is characterized by a bright echo signal with distal shadows which hide plaque components and deeper vessel structures. In comparative studies of histology and IVUS, plaque calcification can be detected with a sensitivity of between 86 and 97%.[20,21] The sensitivity of detection of microcalcification is around 60%.[22]

In IVUS images lipid depositions are described as echolucent zones and can be detected with a sensitivity of between 78 and 95% and specificity of 30%.[23,24] This sensitivity is dependent on the amount of lipid and can drop down further if the echolucent area is smaller than a quarter of the plaque. Echolucent zones can also be caused by loose tissue and shadowing from calcium, which makes the interpretation of echolucent areas difficult. The sensitivity to differentiate between fibrous and fatty tissue is between 39 and 52%.[25]

The detection of vulnerable plaques by IVUS is mainly based on a series of case reports.[26,27] The main focus of these reports is the detection of already ruptured plaques. To evaluate the role of IVUS in detecting plaque rupture, a study was conducted on 144 patients with angina. Ruptured plaques were characterized by a cavity (echolucent area within the plaque) and a tear of the thin fibrous cap. These were identified in 31 patients of whom 23 (74%) presented with unstable angina. Plaque rupture was confirmed by injecting contrast medium and seeing filling of the plaque cavity on IVUS. Of the patients without plaque rupture (n = 108), only 19 (18%) had unstable angina. The echolucent area (cavity) to total plaque area ratio was larger in the unstable group than in the stable group. The thickness of the fibrous cap in the unstable group was found to be smaller than in the stable group.[28]

The problem with such studies is that they are not prospective with adequate follow-up. Only Yamagishi et al have performed a prospective study with a follow-up period of about 2 years.[29] Large eccentric plaques containing an echolucent zone on IVUS were found to be at increased risk of instability even though the lumen area was preserved at the time of the initial study.[29]

It has been demonstrated that unstable plaques are associated with positive remodeling. IVUS assessment of vascular remodeling may help to classify plaques with the highest probability of spontaneous rupture.[30]

A number of investigators have studied the potential of ultrasound radiofrequency signal analysis for tissue characterization.[31–37] Many of the studies revealed the potential to identify calcified plaques, but although promising, no one has yet produced a technique with sufficient spatial and parametric resolution to identify a lipid pool covered by a thin fibrous cap.

Intravascular elastography/palpography

In 1991, a new technique was introduced to measure the mechanical properties of tissue using ultrasound: elastography.[38] The underlying concept is that upon uniform loading, the local relative amount of deformation (strain) of a tissue is related to the local mechanical properties of that tissue. If we apply this concept to determine the local properties of arterial tissue, blood pressure acts as a stressor. At a given pressure difference, soft plaque components will deform more than hard components. Measurement of local plaque deformation in the radial direction can be obtained with ultrasound. For intravascular purposes, a derivative of elastography called palpography may be a suitable tool.[39] In this approach, one strain value per angle is determined and plotted as a color-coded contour at the lumen vessel boundary. Since radial strain is obtained, the technique may have the potential to detect regions with elevated stress: increased circumferential stress results in increased radial deformation of the plaque components. In vitro studies with histologic confirmation have shown that there are differences of strain normalized to pressure between fibrous, fibro-fatty and fatty components of the plaque of coronary as well as femoral arteries.[40] This difference was mainly evident between the fibrous and fatty tissue. The plaque types could not be differentiated by echo-intensity on the IVUS echogram.

It is possible to apply intravascular palpography during interventional catheterization procedures. In a recent study, data were acquired in patients ($n =$ 12) during PTCA procedures with echo apparatus equipped with radiofrequency output. The systemic pressure was used to strain the tissue, and the strain was determined using cross-correlation analysis of sequential frames acquired at different pressures. A likelihood function was determined to obtain the frames with minimal motion of the catheter in the lumen since motion of the catheter impairs accuracy of strain estimation. Minimal motion was observed near the end of the passive filling phase. Reproducible strain estimates were obtained within one and over several pressure cycles. Validation of the results was limited to the information provided by the echogram. Significantly higher strain values were found for non-calcified plaques than for calcified plaques.[41] Another in vivo validation study in atherosclerotic Yucatan pigs showed that fatty plaques have an increased mean strain value. High-strain spots were also associated with the presence of macrophages, another feature of vulnerable plaques.[42]

Palpography reveals information not seen on IVUS. To differentiate between hard and soft tissue may be important for the detection of an deformable plaque that is prone to rupture. Since palpography is based on clinically available IVUS catheters, the technique can be easily introduced into the catheterization laboratory. Elastography has a high sensitivity and specificity to detect vulnerable plaques in vitro.[42a] By acquiring data at the end of the filling phase, when catheter motion is minimal, the quality and reliability of the palpogram is increased. The clinical value of this technique is currently under investigation.

Thermography

Inflammation produces a rise in temperature in the affected tissue. Since atherosclerosis is accompanied by inflammation a hypothesis was set up that a temperature rise could be measured at the surface of a plaque. As vulnerable plaque is a very active metabolic area, the hypothesis was extended that vulnerable plaques may have an even higher rise in temperature.

Casscells et al reported that carotid plaques taken at endarterectomy from 48 patients showed temperature heterogeneity.[43] The temperature difference between different areas was up to 2.2 °C, and correlated with cell density ($R^2 = -0.47$, $P = 0.0001$). There was a negative correlation between temperature difference and cap thickness ($R2 = -0.34$, $P=0.0001$). The same group reported approximately the same findings in vitro in atherosclerotic rabbits.[44] A correlation between temperature rise and macrophage infiltration has also been suggested in an in vivo rabbit trial.[45] Stefanadis et al performed studies in humans.[46] Patients with stable angina, unstable angina, and acute MI were studied. The thermistor of the thermography catheter has a temperature accuracy of 0.05 °C, a time constant of 300 ms, and a spatial resolution of 0.5 mm. The thermistor of the catheter was driven against the vessel wall by the force of blood flow, without the help of a mechanical device like a balloon. Temperature was constant within the arteries of the control subjects, whereas most atherosclerotic plaques showed higher temperatures compared with healthy vessel walls. Temperature differences between atherosclerotic plaque and healthy vessel walls increased progressively from patients with stable angina to patients with acute MI with a maximum difference of 1.5±0.7 °C.[46] Furthermore, patients with a high temperature gradient have a significantly worse outcome than patients with a low gradient.[47] However, these data have yet to be confirmed prospectively in other centers, and the influence of parameters such as coronary blood flow or catheter design has to be studied further.

Optical coherence tomography

Optical coherence tomography (OCT) can provide images with ultrahigh resolution. The technique measures the intensity of back-reflected light in a similar way as IVUS measures acoustic waves.[48] It is an invasive technique with a catheter advanced over a 0.014" wire. With a Michelson interferometer light is split into two signals. One is sent into the tissue and the other to a reference arm with a mirror. Both signals are reflected and cross-correlated by interfering with the light beams. To achieve cross-correlation at incremental penetration depths in the tissue, the mirror is dynamically translated. The intensity of the interfering signals at a certain mirror position represents backscattering at a corresponding depth. High-resolution images with a resolution ranging from 4 μm to 20 μm can be achieved[49] with a penetration depth up to 2 mm. Images can be acquired real-time at 15 frames/s.

Early attempts were made to validate OCT using histology. A lipid pool generates decreased signal areas, and a fibrous plaque produces a homogeneous signal-rich lesion.[50] In vitro comparison of OCT with IVUS demonstrated superior delineation by OCT of structural details like thin caps or tissue proliferation.[51]

Limitations of OCT include the low penetration depth, which hinders studying large vessels, and the light absorbance by blood that currently needs to be overcome by saline infusion or balloon occlusion with associated potential for ischemia. Special techniques like index matching may improve imaging through blood.[52]

Raman spectroscopy

Raman spectroscopy is a technique that characterizes the chemical composition of biological tissue by utilizing the Raman effect.[53] This effect occurs when incident light (wavelength 750–850 nm) excites molecules in a tissue sample, which back-scatter the light while changing wavelength. This change in wavelength is the Raman effect.[54] The wavelength shift and the signal intensity are dependent on the chemical components of the tissue sample. Due to this unique feature, Raman spectroscopy can provide quantitative information about the molecular composition of the sample.[55] The spectra obtained from tissue require post-processing to differentiate between plaque components.

Even in the presence of blood, Raman spectra have been obtained in vivo from the aortic arch of sheep.[56] In a study using mice that received a high-fat/high-cholesterol (HFC) diet for 0, 2, 4, or 6 months, Raman spectroscopy showed good correlation between cholesterol accumulation and total serum cholesterol exposure (R approximately 0.87, $P<0.001$). In female mice ($n = 10$) that were assigned to an HFC diet, with or without 0.01% atorvastatin, a strong reduction in cholesterol accumulation (57%) and calcium salts (97%) ($P<0.01$) was demonstrated in the atorvastatin-treated group. Raman spectroscopy can therefore be used to quantitatively study the size and distribution of cholesterol deposition and calcification.[57]

Limitations of the technique are the limited penetration depth (1–1.5 mm), the long acquisition time and the absorbance of the light by blood. Raman spectroscopy gives no geometrical information.

Near-infrared spectroscopy

Near-infrared (NIR) spectroscopy also provides information of the chemical components of the coronary vessel wall. Molecular vibrational transitions measured in the NIR region (750–2500 nm) give qualitative and quantitative results on plaque composition. NIR spectroscopy sensitivity and specificity for the histologic features of plaque vulnerability were 90% and 93% for lipid pool, 77% and 93% for thin cap, and 84% and 89% for inflammatory cells, respectively.[58] A differentiation between vulnerable and non-vulnerable carotid plaques could be achieved ex vivo.[59] Future studies will address the question whether NIR spectroscopy is feasible in vivo. Problems like acquisition time, blood scattering, influence of pH and temperature must be addressed.

Magnetic resonance imaging

High-resolution MRI is a non-invasive modality to characterize atherosclerotic plaques. Combining information from T1- and T2-weighted imaging permits in vitro identification of the atheromatous core, collagenous cap, calcification, media, adventitia and perivascular fat.[60] In a small number of patients ($n = 6$) a matching between the in vivo and in vitro measurements of carotid arteries was seen.[61] Yuan et al determined the accuracy of in vivo MRI for measuring the cross-sectional maximum wall area of atherosclerotic carotid arteries in a group of 14 patients undergoing carotid endarterectomy. The authors showed that paired in vivo and ex vivo measurements strongly agreed using a Bland and Altman's analysis.[62] Although not perfect, it may be possible to identify carotid plaques at high risk for stroke using MRI.[63] Images of carotid arteries can be further improved using a coil placed close to the carotid artery at the surface of the neck.[64] An in-plane resolution of 0.4×0.4 mm and a slice thickness of 3 mm may allow an assessment of fibrous cap thickness and integrity.[65]

Imaging of coronary arteries with MRI is more difficult than imaging carotid plaques since cardiac and respiratory motion, the small plaque size, and the location of the coronary arteries can cause acquisition problems. Nevertheless, high-resolution MRI of the human coronary wall of angiographically normal and abnormal vessels has been shown to be feasible. In a study by Botnar et al the coronary wall thickness and wall area were significantly enlarged in patients with coronary artery disease demonstrated by angiography.[66] Small plaque structures like fibrous caps cannot be assessed using current MRI techniques. Thinner slices and higher in-plane resolution are needed to better delineate coronary plaques.

Shear stress imaging

High-resolution reconstruction of three-dimensional coronary lumen and wall morphology is obtained by combining angiography and IVUS (ANGUS).[67] Briefly, a biplane angiogram of a sheath-based IVUS catheter taken at end-diastole allows reconstruction of the three-dimensional pullback trajectory of the catheter. Combining this path with lumen and wall information derived from IVUS images that are successively acquired during catheter pullback at end-diastole gives accurate three-dimensional lumen and wall reconstruction with resolution determined by IVUS. Filling the three-dimensional lumen space with a high-resolution three-dimensional mesh allows calculation of the detailed blood velocity profile in the lumen.[68]

For this purpose absolute flow and blood viscosity need to be provided as boundary conditions. From the blood velocity profile local wall shear stress on the endothelium can be accurately derived. Wall shear stress is the frictional force, normalized to surface area that is induced by the blood passing the wall. Although from a mechanical point of view shear stress is of a very small magnitude compared to blood pressure-induced tensile stress it has a profound influence on vascular biology[69] and explains the localization of atherosclerotic plaque in the presence of systemic risk factors.[70] Many of these biological processes also influence the stability of the vulnerable plaque including inflammation, thrombogenicity, vessel remodeling, intimal thickening or regression and smooth muscle cell proliferation. Therefore, the study of this parameter as derived by image-based modeling is of utmost importance.

Conclusions

Assessment of atherosclerosis by imaging techniques is essential for in vivo identification of vulnerable plaques. Several invasive and non-invasive imaging techniques are currently under development.

OCT has the advantage of high resolution, thermography measures metabolism and NIR spectroscopy provides information on chemical

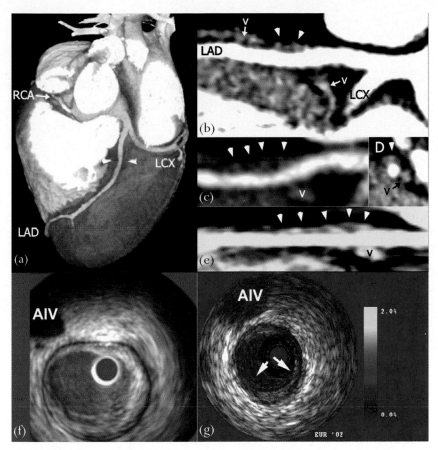

Figure 5.1 *Non-invasive coronary imaging, using a 16-slice spiral computed tomography scanner (MSCT) (Sensation 16, Siemens AG, Forchheim, Germany) suggested a non-obstructive lesion in the mid left anterior descending (LAD) artery (b), (c), (d) (arrowheads), which was confirmed with coronary angiography. The attenuation value of the plaque was measured as 80 HU (Hounsfield units), suggesting a mixed plaque composition without calcification (c, d, arrowheads). The entire segment can be shown in a single plane by means of vessel tracking (e, arrowhead). The great cardiac vein can be differentiated from the plaque by the higher and homogeneous attenuation of the venous lumen (v). Palpography (g) delivers strain information of this plaque's surface. At the right a scale ranging from 0 (blue) to 2% (yellow) characterizes the strain pattern. The strain images are colour-coded, blue indicates stiff (low strain) material and red indicates softer (higher strain) material. In this cross-section, which is in exactly the same position as the IVUS image (f), an eccentric soft plaque is visible with shoulders of high strain (arrows) on either side of the otherwise stable cap. Between 22.00 and 24.00 hrs the palpogram appears to show an area of high strain, however, this is caused by the nearby cardiac vein (AIV). RCA, right coronary artery; LCX, left circumflex.*

components. IVUS and IVUS-palpography are easy to perform and assess morphology and mechanical instability. Shear stress is an important mechanical parameter deeply influencing vascular biology. MRI and CT have the advantage of non-invasive imaging.

Nevertheless all techniques are still under development and at present, none of them can identify a vulnerable plaque alone or predict its further development. This is related to fundamental methodological insufficiencies that may be resolved in the future. From a clinical point of view, most techniques currently assess only one feature of the vulnerable plaque. Thus the combination of several modalities (Figure 5.1)[71] will be of importance in the future to ensure high sensitivity and specificity in detecting vulnerable plaque.

References

1. Libby P. Molecular bases of the acute coronary syndromes. *Circulation* 1995; **91**:2844–50.

2. Falk E. Stable versus unstable atherosclerosis: clinical aspects. *Am Heart J* 1999; **138**:S421–S425

3. Virmani R, Burke AP, Farb A et al. Pathology of the unstable plaque. *Prog Cardiovasc Dis* 2002; **44**:349–56.

4. Little WC, Constantinescu M, Applegate RJ et al. Can coronary angiography predict the site of a subsequent myocardial infarction in patients with mild-to-moderate coronary artery disease? *Circulation* 1988; **78**:1157–66.

5. Nobuyoshi M, Tanaka M, Nosaka H et al. Progression of coronary atherosclerosis: is coronary spasm related to progression? *J Am Coll Cardiol* 1991; **18**:904–10.

6. Ambrose JA, Tannenbaum MA, Alexopoulos D et al. Angiographic progression of coronary artery disease and the development of myocardial infarction. *J Am Coll Cardiol* 1988; **12**:56–62.

7. Giroud D, Li JM, Urban P et al. Relation of the site of acute myocardial infarction to the most severe coronary arterial stenosis at prior angiography. *Am J Cardiol* 1992; **69**:729–32.

8. Kerensky RA, Wade M, Deedwania P et al. Revisiting the culprit lesion in non-Q-wave myocardial infarction. Results from the VANQWISH trial angiographic core laboratory. *J Am Coll Cardiol* 2002; **39**:1456–63.

9. Frink RJ. Chronic ulcerated plaques: new insights into the pathogenesis of acute coronary disease. *J Invasive Cardiol* 1994; **6**:173–85.

10. Ojio S, Takatsu H, Tanaka T et al. Considerable time from the onset of plaque rupture and/or thrombi until the onset of acute myocardial infarction in humans: coronary angiographic findings within 1 week before the onset of infarction. *Circulation* 2000; **102**:2063–9.

11. Goldstein JA, Demetriou D, Grines CL et al. Multiple complex coronary plaques in patients with acute myocardial infarction. *N Engl J Med* 2000; **343**:915–22.

12. Kim WY, Danias PG, Stuber M. Coronary magnetic resonance angiography for the detection of coronary stenoses. *N Engl J Med* 2001; **345**:1863–9.

13. Mizuno K, Satomura K, Miyamoto A et al. Angioscopic evaluation of coronary-artery thrombi in acute coronary syndromes. *N Engl J Med* 1992; **326**:287–91.

14. Sherman CT, Litvack F, Grundfest W et al. Coronary angioscopy in patients with unstable angina pectoris. *N Engl J Med* 1986; **315**:913–19.

15. Feld S, Ganim M, Carell ES et al. Comparison of angioscopy, intravascular ultrasound imaging and quantitative coronary angiography in predicting clinical outcome after coronary intervention in high risk patients. *J Am Coll Cardiol* 1996; **28**:97–105.

16. Takano M, Mizuno K, Okamatsu K et al. Mechanical and structural characteristics of vulnerable plaques: analysis by coronary angioscopy and intravascular ultrasound. *J Am Coll Cardiol* 2001; **38**:99–104.

17. Asakura M, Ueda Y, Yamaguchi O et al. Extensive development of vulnerable plaques as a pan-coronary process in patients with myocardial infarction: an angioscopic study. *J Am Coll Cardiol* 2001; **37**:1284–8.

18. Uchida Y, Nakamura F, Tomaru T et al. Prediction of acute coronary syndromes by percutaneous coronary angioscopy in patients with stable angina. *Am Heart J* 1995; **130**:195–203.

19. Bom N, Li W, van der Steen AF et al. Intravascular imaging. *Ultrasonics* 1998; **36**:625–8.

20. Di Mario C, The SH, Madretsma S et al. Detection and characterization of vascular lesions by intravascular ultrasound: an in vitro study correlated with histology. *J Am Soc Echocardiogr* 1992; **5**:135–46.

21. Sechtem U, Arnold G, Keweloh T et al. In vitro diagnosis of coronary plaque morphology with intravascular ultrasound: comparison with histopathologic findings. *Z Kardiol* 1993; **82**:618–27.

22. Friedrich GJ, Moes NY, Muhlberger VA et al. Detection of intralesional calcium by intracoronary ultrasound depends on the histologic pattern. *Am Heart J* 1994; **128**:435–41.

23. Potkin BN, Bartorelli AL, Gessert JM et al. Coronary artery imaging with intravascular high-frequency ultrasound. *Circulation* 1990; **81**:1575–85.

24. Rasheed Q, Dhawale PJ, Anderson J et al. Intracoronary ultrasound-defined plaque composition: computer-aided plaque characterization and correlation with histologic samples obtained during directional coronary atherectomy. *Am Heart J* 1995; **129**:631–7.

25. Hiro T, Leung CY, Russo RJ et al. Variability of a three-layered appearance in intravascular ultrasound coronary images: a comparison of morphometric measurements with four intravascular ultrasound systems. *Am J Card Imaging* 1996; **10**:219–27.

26. Ge J, Haude M, Gorge G et al. Silent healing of spontaneous plaque disruption demonstrated by intracoronary ultrasound. *Eur Heart J* 1995; **16**:1149–51.

27. Jeremias A, Ge J, Erbel R. New insight into plaque healing after plaque rupture with subsequent thrombus formation detected by intravascular ultrasound. *Heart* 1997; **77**:293.

28. Ge J, Chirillo F, Schwedtmann J et al. Screening of ruptured plaques in patients with coronary artery disease by intravascular ultrasound. *Heart* 1999; **81**:621–7.

29. Yamagishi M, Terashima M, Awano K et al. Morphology of vulnerable coronary plaque: insights from follow-up of patients examined by intravascular ultrasound before an acute coronary syndrome. *J Am Coll Cardiol* 2000; **35**:106–11.

30. von Birgelen C, Klinkhart W, Mintz GS et al. Plaque distribution and vascular remodeling of ruptured and nonruptured coronary plaques in the same vessel: an intravascular ultrasound study in vivo. *J Am Coll Cardiol* 2001; **37**:1864–70.

31. Nair A, Kuban BD, Obuchowski N et al. Assessing spectral algorithms to predict atherosclerotic plaque composition with normalized and raw intravascular ultrasound data. *Ultrasound Med Biol* 2001; **10**:1319–31.

32. Landini L, Sarnelli R, Picano E et al. Evaluation of frequency dependence of backscatter coefficient in normal and atherosclerotic aortic walls. *Ultrasound Med Biol* 1986; **5**:397–401.

33. Wilson LS, Neale ML, Talhami HE et al. Preliminary results from attenuation-slope mapping of plaque using intravascular ultrasound. *Ultrasound Med Biol* 1994; **20**:529–42.

34. Jeremias A, Kolz ML, Ikonen TS et al. Feasibility of in vivo intravascular ultrasound tissue characterization in the detection of early vascular transplant rejection. *Circulation* 1999; **100**:2127–30.

35. Wickline SA, Miller JG, Recchia D et al. Beyond intravascular imaging: quantitative ultrasonic tissue characterization of vascular pathology. IEEE Ultrasonics Symposium, Cannes, 1994; **3**:1589–97.

36. Bridal SL, Beyssen B, Fornes P, Julia P, Berger G. Multiparametric attenuation and backscatter images for characterization of carotid plaque. *Ultrason Imaging* 2000; **22**:20–34.

37. Spencer T, Ramo MP, Salter DM et al. Characterisation of atherosclerotic plaque by spectral analysis of intravascular ultrasound: an in vitro methodology. *Ultrasound Med Biol* 1997; **23**:191–203.

38. Ophir J, Cespedes I, Ponnekanti H et al. Elastography: a quantitative method for imaging the elasticity of biological tissues. *Ultrason Imaging* 1991; **13**:111–34.

39. Doyley MM, Mastik F, de Korte CL et al. Advancing intravascular ultrasonic palpation toward clinical applications. *Ultrasound Med Biol* 2001; **27**:1471–80.

40. de Korte CL, Pasterkamp G, van der Steen AF et al. Characterization of plaque components with intravascular ultrasound elastography in human femoral and coronary arteries in vitro. *Circulation* 2000; **102**:617–23.

41. de Korte CL, Carlier SG, Mastik F et al. Morphological and mechanical information of coronary arteries obtained with intravascular elastography; feasibility study in vivo. *Eur Heart J* 2002; **23**:405–13.

42. de Korte CL, Sierevogel MJ, Mastik F et al. Identification of atherosclerotic plaque components with intravascular ultrasound elastography in vivo: a Yucatan pig study. *Circulation* 2002; **105**:1627–30.

42a. Schaar JA, de Korte CL, Mastik F et al. Characterizing vulnerable plaque features with intravascular elastography. *Circulation* 2003; **108**:2636–41.

43. Casscells W, Hathorn B, David M et al. Thermal detection of cellular infiltrates in living atherosclerotic plaques: possible implications for plaque rupture and thrombosis. *Lancet* 1996; **347**:1447–51.

44. Casscells W, David M, Bearman G et al. Thermography. In: Fuster V, ed. *The Vulnerable Atherosclerotic Plaque*. New York: Futura Publishing Company, 1999:231–42.

45. Verheye S, De Meyer GR, Van Langenhove G et al. In vivo temperature heterogeneity of atherosclerotic plaques is determined by plaque composition. *Circulation* 2002; **105**:1596–601.

46. Stefanadis C, Diamantopoulos L, Vlachopoulos C et al. Thermal heterogeneity within human atherosclerotic coronary arteries detected in vivo: a new method of detection by application of a special thermography catheter. *Circulation* 1999; **99**:1965–71.

47. Stefanadis C, Toutouzas K, Tsiamis E et al. Increased local temperature in human coronary atherosclerotic plaques: an independent predictor of clinical outcome in patients undergoing a percutaneous coronary intervention. *J Am Coll Cardiol* 2001; **37**:1277–83.

48. Huang D, Swanson EA, Lin CP et al. Optical coherence tomography. *Science* 1991; **254**:1178.

49. Boppart SA, Bouma BE, Pitris C et al. In vivo cellular optical coherence tomography imaging. *Nat Med* 1998; **4**:861–5.

50. Jang IK, Bouma BE, Kang DH et al. Visualization of coronary atherosclerotic plaques in patients using optical coherence tomography: comparison with intravascular ultrasound. *J Am Coll Cardiol* 2002; **39**:604–9.

51. Brezinski ME, Tearney GJ, Weissman NJ et al. Assessing atherosclerotic plaque morphology: comparison of optical coherence tomography and high frequency intravascular ultrasound. *Heart* 1997; **77**:397–403.

52. Brezinski M, Saunders K, Jesser C et al. Index matching to improve optical coherence tomography imaging through blood. *Circulation* 2001; **103**:1999–2003.

53. Baraga JJ, Feld MS, Rava RP. In situ optical histochemistry of human artery using near-infrared Fourier transform Raman spectroscopy. *Proc Natl Acad Sci USA* 1992; **89**:3473–7.

54. Van de Poll SWE, Motz JT, Kramer JR. Prospects of laser spectroscopy to detect vulnerable plaque. In: Brown DL, ed. *Cardiovascular Plaque Rupture*. New York: Dekker, 2002.

55. Hanlon EB, Manoharan R, Koo TW et al. Prospects for in vivo Raman spectroscopy. *Phys Med Biol* 2000; **45**:R1–59.

56. Buschman HP, Marple ET, Wach ML et al. In vivo determination of the molecular composition of artery wall by intravascular Raman spectroscopy. *Anal Chem* 2000; **72**:3771–5.

57. van De Poll SW, Romer TJ, Volger OL et al. Raman spectroscopic evaluation of the effects of diet and lipid-lowering therapy on atherosclerotic plaque development in mice. *Arterioscler Thromb Vasc Biol* 2001; **21**:1630–5.

58. Moreno PR, Lodder RA, Purushothaman KR et al. Detection of lipid pool, thin fibrous cap, and inflammatory cells in human aortic atherosclerotic plaques by near-infrared spectroscopy. *Circulation* 2002; **105**:923–7.

59. Wang J, Geng YJ, Guo B et al. Near-infrared spectroscopic characterization of human advanced atherosclerotic plaques. *J Am Coll Cardiol* 2002; **39**:1305–13.

60. Toussaint JF, Southern JF, Fuster V et al. T2-weighted contrast for NMR characterization of human atherosclerosis. *Arterioscler Thromb Vasc Biol* 1995; **15**:1533–42.

61. Toussaint JF, LaMuraglia GM, Southern JF *et al*. Magnetic resonance images lipid, fibrous, calcified, hemorrhagic, and thrombotic components of human atherosclerosis in vivo. *Circulation* 1996; **94**:932–8.

62. Yuan C, Beach KW, Smith LH Jr et al. Measurement of atherosclerotic carotid plaque size in vivo using high resolution magnetic resonance imaging. *Circulation* 1998; **98**:2666–71.

63. Yuan C, Mitsumori LM, Beach KW et al. Carotid atherosclerotic plaque: noninvasive MR characterization and identification of vulnerable lesions. *Radiology* 2001; **221**:285–99.

64. Hayes CE, Mathis CM, Yuan C. Surface coil phased arrays for high-resolution imaging of the carotid arteries. *J Magn Reson Imaging* 1996; **6**:109–12.

65. Hatsukami TS, Ross R, Polissar NL et al. Visualization of fibrous cap thickness and rupture in human atherosclerotic carotid plaque in vivo with high-resolution magnetic resonance imaging. *Circulation* 2000; **102**:959–64.

66. Botnar RM, Stuber M, Kissinger KV et al. Noninvasive coronary vessel wall and plaque imaging with magnetic resonance imaging. *Circulation* 2000; **102**:2582–7.

67. Slager CJ, Wentzel JJ, Schuurbiers JCH et al. True 3-dimensional reconstruction of coronary arteries in patients by fusion of angiography and IVUS (ANGUS) and its quantitative validation. *Circulation* 2000; **102**:511–16.

68. Thury A, Wentzel JJ, Schuurbiers JC et al. Prominent role of tensile stress in propagation of a dissection after coronary stenting: computational fluid dynamic analysis on true 3d-reconstructed segment. *Circulation* 2001; **104**:E53–4.

69. Malek AM, Alper SL, Izumo S. Hemodynamic shear stress and its role in atherosclerosis. *JAMA* 1999; **282**:2035–42.

70. Asakura T, Karino T. Flow patterns and spatial distribution of atherosclerotic lesions in human coronary arteries. *Circ Res* 1990; **66**:1045 66.

71. Arampatzis CA, Ligthart JMR, Schaar JA et al. Images in Cardiovascular Medicine. Detection of a vulnerable coronary plaque: a treatment dilemma. *Circulation* 2003 **108**:34–5.

6. MRI AND OTHER NON-INVASIVE IMAGING MODALITIES FOR ATHEROTHROMBOTIC PLAQUE

Konstantin Nikolaou, Robin P Choudhury,
Christoph R Becker, Valentin Fuster and Zahi A Fayad

Non-invasive imaging of atherosclerosis

Atherosclerosis is a systemic disease of the vessel wall that occurs in the aorta and in the carotid, coronary and peripheral arteries. It has been shown that plaque composition plays an important role in the risk of plaque rupture and acute clinical complications of atherosclerotic vessel disease.[1–3] Assessment of atherothrombotic vessel wall changes through non-invasive imaging techniques may enhance the understanding of the natural history and of the pathophysiologic mechanisms of atherosclerosis. This would allow for a better risk stratification of the disease, for identification and follow-up of patients at risk and for selecting appropriate therapeutic strategies.[4] Therefore, imaging tools that can detect various stages of atherothrombotic disease in different vessels and characterize the composition of plaques are clinically desirable.[5] Currently, a number of invasive and non-invasive imaging modalities are used to study atherosclerosis. Most of the techniques available can specify the luminal diameter and can detect stenoses, and some are able to assess vessel wall thickness and plaque volume. In this context, the ultimate goal is the non-invasive identification of the high-risk or 'vulnerable' plaque.[6]

Among others, the two most promising non-invasive imaging modalities that have been introduced to the study of atherosclerosis are magnetic resonance imaging (MRI) and computed tomography (CT).[5,6] Both techniques have been shown to be capable of imaging vessel wall structures and differentiating various stages of atherosclerotic wall changes. MRI has been applied in various in vivo human studies to image atherosclerotic plaques in coronary,[7] carotid[8] and aortic[9] arterial disease. The latest generation of multidetector-row computed tomography (MDCT) systems allows for the non-invasive characterization of different plaque components in various vascular structures including the carotid arteries,[10] coronary arteries[11] and the aorta[12] at high speed and with high spatial resolution, including quantitative measurements of calcified[13] and non-calcified atherosclerotic burden.[14] Using either technique, the repeatable, non-invasive study of atherosclerotic disease during its natural history and after therapeutic intervention will enhance our understanding of disease progression and regression and aid in selecting appropriate treatments.

Plaque imaging: methods

MR plaque imaging

High-resolution MRI has emerged as the potential leading non-invasive in vivo imaging modality for atherosclerotic plaque characterization. MRI differentiates plaque components on the basis of biophysical and biochemical parameters such as chemical composition and concentration, water content, physical state, molecular motion or diffusion.[15] MRI provides imaging without ionizing radiation and can be repeated over time. In vivo MR plaque imaging and characterization have been performed utilizing a multi-contrast approach with high-resolution black blood spin echo and fast spin echo (FSE)-based MR sequences. The signal from the blood flow is rendered black through preparatory pulses (e.g. radiofrequency spatial saturation or inversion recovery pulses) to better image the adjacent vessel wall.[9] However, bright blood imaging (i.e. three-dimensional fast time of flight) can be employed in assessing fibrous cap thickness and morphologic integrity of the carotid artery plaques.[16] This sequence enhances the signal from flowing blood, and a mixture of T1 and proton density contrast-weighting highlights (as a 'dark band') the fibrous cap. Atherosclerotic plaque characterization by MRI is generally based on the signal intensities and morphologic appearance of the plaque on T1-weighted proton density-weighted and T2-weighted images.[6,17] Table 6.1 gives an overview of characteristic signal intensities for different plaque components as assessed by a multi-contrast MRI approach.

CT plaque imaging

Both MDCT and electron-beam CT (EBCT) allow image acquisition at a faster rate than conventional spiral CT.[19] Primary requisites for sufficient delineation and depiction of atherosclerotic calcified and non-calcified plaques are simultaneous high-spatial and high-temporal resolution. MRI, x-ray angiography and ultrasound can identify calcified deposits in blood vessels; however, EBCT and spiral CT (single or multidetector) can measure the amount or volume of calcium.[20,21] Comparison of coronary calcium assessment by EBCT and non-EBCT systems demonstrated good correlation.[22] With the advent of faster and higher-resolution imaging and soft-tissue delineation using these new multidetector CT systems, the detection of non-calcified plaques is now being explored. In 2002, newly developed 16 detector-row CT (16DCT) systems were introduced to clinical practice allowing for even faster data acquisition with improved spatial resolution.[22] Using 16DCT, isotropic sub-millimeter voxels can now be acquired. Based on the improved spatial resolution, beam-hardening artifacts of calcium deposits in the vessel wall are reduced due to reduced partial

Table 6.1 Plaque characterization with MRI and CT. Imaging parameters for MRI and CT and typical appearance of different plaque types according to the composition of the plaque.

| | Modality | | | | |
| | CT (HU) | MR (SI)* | | | |
	C/E	T1-w	PD-w	T2-w	ToF
Thrombus[†]	~20	Variable	Variable	Variable	Variable
Lipids	~50	+	+	−	±
Fibrous	~100	± to +	± to +	± to +	− to ±
Calcium	>300	−	−	−	−

(Modified from ZA Fayad et al. *Circulation* 2002; **106**:2026–34[5] and CR Becker et al. *Eur Radiol.* 2003; **13**:1094–8[18])

*SI relative to adjacent muscle.
[†]SI of thrombus depends on thrombus age.
HU, Hounsfield units; CT, computed tomography; MR, magnetic resonance; SI, signal intensity; C/E, contrast-enhanced; T1w, T2w PDw, ToF, multi-contrast MRI sequences; −, hypointense; ±, isointense; +, hyperintense.

volume effects. This allows for improved depiction and delineation of calcified and non-calcified plaques. Optimization of vessel contrast-to-noise (CNR) is mandatory for sufficient visualization of non-calcified plaques. Because non-enhanced blood on CT has similar attenuation (50–70 HU (Hounsfield units)) to non-calcified plaques, this type of lesion can only be detected after administration of a contrast medium. Therefore, vessel enhancement significantly above the CT values of non-calcified lesions must be achieved to allow for reliable detection of non-calcified plaques. A target attenuation of 200 HU seems best suited to fulfill this requirement. With this vessel enhancement, calcified coronary lesions remain detectable because their attenuation is significantly higher.[24]

Other non-invasive imaging methods

Surface and transesophageal ultrasound

Measurements of carotid and aortic wall thickness as well as qualitative and quantitative analysis of plaque can be determined by surface ultrasound (US), or from the esophagus (transesophageal echo, TEE). Echogenicity of the plaque reflects its characteristics. Hypoechoic heterogeneous plaque is associated with both intraplaque hemorrhage and lipids, whereas hyperechoic homogeneous plaque is mostly fibrous.[25] High-resolution, real-time B-mode US with Doppler flow imaging has emerged as the modality of choice for examining the carotid arteries.[26] Because of the physical principles of a diagnostic US, the measurement is reliable only at the far arterial wall and does not indicate whether the thickening is due to intima or media infiltration and/or hypertrophy.[27] As with other US methods, this technique is operator-dependent and has rather low reproducibility. Examinations of the aorta by B-mode US and TEE have been used as predictors of coronary artery disease (CAD) and cardiovascular risk.[12,28] Ultrasonic contrast agents have been introduced to improve image resolution and specificity.[29] For example, acoustic liposomes conjugated with monoclonal antibodies can be used for plaque component targeted imaging.[30]

Plaque imaging: applications

Plaque imaging of the coronary arteries

Coronary artery vulnerable plaques

Rupture-prone plaques in the coronary arteries, the so-called 'vulnerable plaques,' tend to have a thin fibrous cap (cap thickness 65–150 µm) and a large lipid core. Acute coronary syndromes (ACS) often result from rupture of a modestly stenotic vulnerable plaque, not visible on x-ray angiography.[31,32] According to the criteria of the American Heart Association (AHA) Committee on Vascular Lesions, lesion types depend in part on the phase of progression.[33,34] Coronary 'vulnerable' type IV and type Va lesions and the 'complicated' type VI lesions are the most relevant to ACS. Type IV and Va lesions, although not necessarily stenotic at angiography, are prone to disruption.[35] Type IV lesions consist of extracellular lipid intermixed with fibrous tissue covered by a fibrous cap, whereas type Va lesions possess a predominant extracellular lipid core covered by a thin fibrous cap. Disruption of a type IV or Va lesion leads to the formation of a thrombus or 'complicated' type VI lesion, as the lipid core is highly thrombogenic. Relatively small type IV and Va coronary lesions may account for as many as two-thirds of cases of unstable angina or other ACS.[36] In contrast, the most severely stenotic plaques at angiography, which have a high content of smooth muscle cells and collagen, and little lipid, are less susceptible to rupture.[37]

MR plaque imaging of the coronary arteries

With a combination of multi-contrast MRI sequences, differentiation of fibrocellular, lipid-rich and calcified regions of the atherosclerotic coronary plaque is feasible, as shown in an ex vivo study on human coronary arteries with correlation to histopathology (Figure 6.1).[38] Calcifications are well defined by signal loss in all sequences (T1w, T2w, PDw), due to the low mobile proton density within the calcified area. Fibrocellular regions are typically characterized by intermediate to high signal intensities in all weightings, being well distinguishable from fatty lesions, as these are identified as areas of low signal intensity in T2w and hyperintense signal in T1w sequences (see Table 6.1).

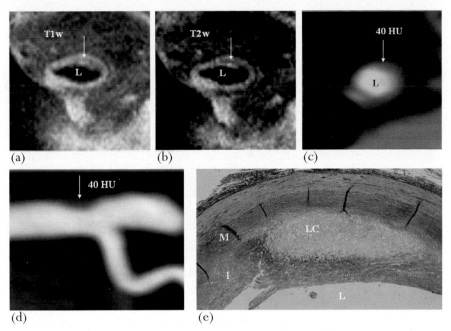

Figure 6.1 *Ex vivo MR and MDCT coronary plaque. Type IV atherosclerotic lesion. MRI in T1w (a) and T2w (b) shows vessel wall thickening with a signal-intense fibrous cap and a signal-loss in T2w in the area of the lipid core (arrow). Lumen (L) is dark in MR images due to contrast medium. The corresponding MDCT images (cross-sectional (c) and MIP (d) reconstruction) with bright lumen (L) show a soft tissue lesion with a mean density of 40 HU (arrow). Histopathology (e) proves presence of extensive lipid accumulation (LC, lipid core) within the atherosclerotic widened intima (I) and media (M) cell layer (L, lumen). (MDCT, multidetector-row computed tomography). (Reproduced with permission from K Nikolaou et al[44] and CR Becker et al,[18] Ludwig-Maximilians-University, Munich, Germany.)*

In vivo studies of coronary artery plaques are obviously more challenging. Preliminary studies in a pig model showed that the difficulties of coronary wall imaging are the result of a combination of cardiac and respiratory motion artifacts, non-linear course, small size, and location.[39] Fayad et al extended the black blood MRI methods used in the human carotid artery and aorta to the imaging of the coronary arterial lumen and wall (Figure 6.2).[7] The method was validated in swine coronary lesions induced by balloon angioplasty.[39] High-resolution black blood MRI of both normal and atherosclerotic human coronary arteries was performed for direct assessment of coronary wall thickness and the visualization of focal atherosclerotic plaque in the wall. The difference in maximum wall thickness between the normal subjects and patients (>40% stenosis) was statistically significant. At the same time, no significant change in the lumen diameter was found when comparing healthy subjects and patients with

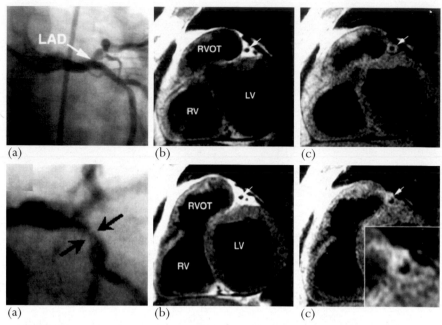

Figure 6.2 *In vivo MR coronary plaque. Upper row: x-ray angiogram of a 78-year-old female patient with mild disease on x-ray angiography in proximal LAD (a, arrow). BB-MR cross-sectional lumen image reveals circular lumen (b); wall shows uniformly thickened LAD wall (b) with concentric plaque (c). Lower row: x-ray angiogram of a 76-year-old male patient shows high-grade stenosis in proximal LAD (a, arrows). In vivo cross sectional BB-MR images of LAD lumen (b) shows obstructed lumen (elliptical lumen shape); wall image (c) shows large eccentric plaque with heterogeneous signal intensity. (BB, black blood; LAD, left anterior descending artery; RV, right ventricle; LV, left ventricle; RVOT, right ventricular outflow tract.) (Reproduced with permission from ZA Fayad et al,[5] Radiology/Cardiology Imaging Science Laboratories, Mount Sinai School of Medicine, New York, USA.)*

non-significant CAD, due to positive coronary remodeling effects, as confirmed for the first time by an in vivo MRI study. The coronary MR plaque imaging study by Fayad et al[7] was performed during breath holding to minimize respiratory motion with a resolution of $0.46 \times 0.46 \times 2.0$ mm^3. To alleviate the need for the patient to hold his or her breath, Botnar et al[40] have combined the black blood FSE method and a real-time navigator for respiratory gating and real-time slice position correction. A near isotropic spatial resolution ($0.7 \times 0.7 \times 0.8$ mm^3) was achieved with the use of a 2D local inversion and black blood preparatory pulses.[40] This method provided a quick way to image a long segment of the coronary artery wall and may be useful for rapid coronary plaque burden measurements. Future studies need to address these possibilities.

CT plaque imaging of the coronary arteries

CT possesses a high sensitivity for the detection of calcified plaques, due to its inherent high sensitivity for calcifications caused by the high CT attenuation values of these lesions (type Vb lesions). Therefore, CT has become an established method for the non-invasive detection of coronary artery calcifications.[41] According to Virmani et al[3] calcified plaques are likely the result of repetitive plaque rupture and healing, causing shrinkage of the vessel lumen with consecutive stenosis. Earlier stages of atherosclerosis without calcifications might be more prone to acute rupture, resulting in acute cardiovascular events,[42] though this is contentious.[43]

In an ex vivo study on human coronary arteries, it was shown that various imaging features of non-calcified and calcified plaques depicted with CT correlate well with histopathologic stages of atherosclerosis defined by the AHA.[18] Lipid-rich, fibrous and calcified plaques could be differentiated reliably. However, sensitivity has been reported to be lower for earlier stages of atherosclerosis (type III and IVa plaques), mainly due to lack of in-plane spatial resolution and partial volume effects. Heavy coronary calcifications may prevent adequate assessment of complex plaques with calcified and soft plaque components in direct vicinity of each other. The reasons for this are considerable beam hardening artifacts and partial volume effects of calcium on CT. Table 6.1 gives an overview on typical morphological appearance and CT attenuation (in HU) for various plaque components as described in this chapter.

Recently, it was shown that CT has the potential to identify non-calcified plaques in the coronary arteries in vivo (Figure 6.3).[45,46] For plaques with and without signs of calcification detected on intravascular ultrasound (IVUS), EBCT without contrast enhancement yielded a sensitivity of 97% and 47% and a specificity of 80% and 75%, respectively.[47] In an in vivo study using contrast-enhanced MDCT Schroeder et al reported a good correlation in differentiation between soft, intermediate and calcified plaques, as compared to IVUS.[24] Acute intravascular thrombi can also be detected in vivo, with a typical appearance of the irregular thrombus with typically low attenuation numbers in the range of 20–30 HU. Additionally, new image analysis software may enable in vivo quantification of non-calcified atherosclerotic lesions.[14] However, further validation studies will be necessary before broad usage.

Ultrasound imaging of the coronary arteries

The proximal coronary arteries, specifically the left main coronary artery and its proximal branches, have been identified with two-dimensional transthoracic echocardiography (2DTTE) using short-axis views.[48] Successful application of this technique to the detection of left main and left anterior descending coronary (LAD) artery atherosclerosis has been described.[49] Recent advances in imaging technique and technology have increased the potential for successful visualization

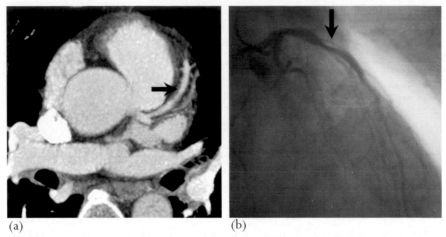

(a)   (b)

Figure 6.3 *In vivo MDCT coronary plaque. Contrast-enhanced coronary CT angiography. The use of maximum-intensity-projection plane allows the visualization of the proximal course of the left anterior descending coronary artery (a). In the middle segment distal to the first diagonal branch a non-calcified lesion can be detected (arrow), corresponding to a significant stenosis in the conventional angiogram (b, arrow). (MDCT, multidetector-row CT). (Reproduced with permission from CR Becker et al,[11] Ludwig-Maximilians-University, Munich, Germany.)*

of the coronary arteries. It could be shown, that using a transthoracic technique in the parasternal long-axis view, relatively long segments of the LAD can be seen.[50] Image quality also has improved due to new broadband, high-resolution transducers, making measurements more reliable. Gradus-Pizlo et al demonstrated, that with the use of such high-resolution broadband transducers and HR-2DTTE, the penetration and resolution was sufficient to evaluate the vessel wall of the proximal LAD.[51] Increased wall thickness and external diameter of the LAD are indicative of subclinical coronary atherosclerosis.[52] Gradus-Pizlo et al compared HR-2DTEE with high-frequency epicardial echocardiography (HFEE), which was performed during open-heart surgery. They found greater wall thickness in patients with coronary atherosclerosis than in those with normal coronary arteries by both HR-2DTTE and HFEE.[53] HR-2DTTE and HFEE measurements of the wall thickness correlated well. It could be proved, that on HR-2DTTE, the wall thickness measured consisted of intima, media and a third layer, which represents the adventitia. The average thickness of adventitia was greater in patients with coronary atherosclerosis than in those with normal coronary arteries.

Adventitia and different imaging modalities
The inclusion of adventitia is responsible for the discrepancy between coronary artery wall thickness reported by studies using IVUS[54] or histologic

morphometry,[55] in which measurements are obtained within the area of external elastic lamina and include only intima and media. The vessel diameter and wall thickness measured with this transthoracic US technique correlated and agreed well with those obtained by MRI studies.[7]

Plaque imaging of the carotid arteries

Carotid arteries high-risk plaques

Carotid artery plaques that are more prone to disruption, fracture, or fissuring may be associated with a higher risk of embolization, occlusion, and consequent ischemic neurologic events.[56] Various findings emphasize the importance of accurate delineation of the morphology of the carotid bifurcation, as well as the degree of stenosis. The inability of conventional x-ray angiography to depict plaque ulceration is well documented, because it is an imaging technique for depicting the vessel lumen only and it also suffers from the limited number of two-dimensional projections that are typically obtained.[57]

In contrast to coronary artery vulnerable plaques characterized by high lipid content and a thin fibrous cap, high-risk plaques in carotid arteries typically are severely stenotic. The term 'high-risk' is used rather than the classic term 'vulnerable', which only implies the presence of a lipid-rich core. High-risk carotid plaques are heterogeneous, very fibrous, and not necessarily lipid-rich. Rupture often represents an intramural hematoma or dissection, probably related to the impact of blood during systole against the resistance of such a stenotic lesion.[58] Because they are superficial, with predictable course and not subject to cardiac and respiratory motion, carotid arteries are more amenable to imaging and plaque characterization than are coronary arteries.[15]

MR plaque imaging of the carotid arteries

Magnetic resonance imaging has been shown to reliably identify plaque composition in the carotid artery vessel wall, using multi-contrast high-resolution spin echo based MR sequences.[8,15,59,60] For black-blood sequences, the signal from the blood flow is rendered black by the use of preparatory pulses to better visualize the adjacent vessel wall. Hatsukami et al introduced the use of bright blood time-of-flight imaging for the visualization of the fibrous cap thickness and morphological integrity.[61] This sequence provides enhancement of the signal from flowing blood and a mixture of T1 and proton density contrast-weighting that highlights the fibrous cap. MR angiography (MRA) and high-resolution black-blood imaging of the vessel wall can be combined. Improvements in spatial resolution have been possible with the design of new phased-array coils tailored for carotid imaging[62] and new imaging sequences such as long echo train FSE with 'velocity-selective' flow suppression.[9] Some of the MRI studies of carotid arterial plaques include the imaging and characterization of atherosclerotic plaques,[15,63] the quantification of plaque size,[8] and the detection of fibrous cap 'integrity'.[16]

Typically, the images are acquired with a resolution of $0.25 \times 0.25 \times 2.0$–$0.4 \times 0.4 \times 3.0$ mm^3 by use of a carotid phased-array coil to improve signal-to-noise ratio and image resolution (Figure 6.4).

CT plaque imaging of the carotid arteries

Several precedent studies in animals and humans in vascular territories other than the coronary arteries have demonstrated the ability of CT to differentiate calcified, fibrous and lipid-rich plaque components based on CT attenuation (HU). CT is an accurate, non-invasive means for studying detailed plaque morphology and composition in the carotid arteries. CT has been shown to differentiate different tissue types in the carotid artery wall[10,64] and to reliably assess vessel wall thickness.[65] Contrast-enhanced MDCT was able to differentiate between calcified, fibrous and lipid plaque components with moderate to high sensitivity and specificity.[10] Yet, it does not reach the potential of tissue characterization that is inherent to MRI, and in-plane spatial resolution will still have to be improved for more reliable assessment of plaque components and for identification of plaques at risk. According to Estes et al, CT accurately defined

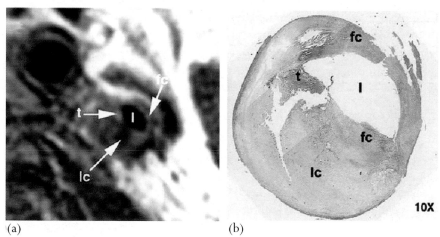

(a)   (b)

Figure 6.4 *In vivo MR carotid plaque. In vivo transverse T2-weighted FSE MRI of a left internal carotid artery. Plaque characterization was based on information obtained from T1, intermediate, and T2-weighted MR images. (a) T2-weighted MR image (repetition time, two R-R intervals; echo time, 55 ms; 3-mm section thickness; 450-mm in-plane resolution) shows low signal intensity lipid core (lc), high signal intensity fibrous cap (fc), and very high signal intensity thrombus (t). (l, arterial lumen.) (b) Corresponding histopathologic section. (fc, fibrous cap, l, arterial lumen, lc, lipid core, t, thrombus). (Reproduced with permission from ZA Fayad et al,[44] Radiology/ Cardiology Imaging Science Laboratories, Mount Sinai School of Medicine, New York, USA.)*

106

plaque features containing calcium, fibrous stroma, and lipids in carotid arteries.[64] Using tissue attenuation values, CT distinguished between lipid and fibrous stroma (means 39 ± 12 HU and 90 ± 24 HU, respectively, $P<0.001$). Oliver et al tried to assess, whether features seen at CT angiography might be used to predict carotid plaque stability by comparing CT angiograms with histopathologic examinations of the carotid artery bifurcation.[10] They concluded that CT angiography is a promising method for assessing the lumen and wall of the carotid artery and that the apparent correlation between histologic appearance and plaque density on CT angiograms could have important implications for the prediction of plaque stability (Figure 6.5).

Plaque imaging of the aorta

Aortic plaques

Thoracic aortic atherosclerosis has been proven to be an important cause of severe morbidity and mortality. Autopsy studies have shown that the amount of atherosclerotic plaque in the thoracic aorta directly correlates with the degree of atherosclerotic disease in the coronary arteries. Furthermore, thoracic aortic atherosclerosis is a stronger predictor of coronary artery disease than conventional risk factors and is also a marker of increased mortality, stroke and visceral thromboembolic events.[66–68] Parameters such as aortic wall thickness, luminal irregularities and plaque composition are strong predictors of future vascular events.[24,69]

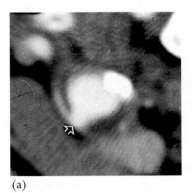
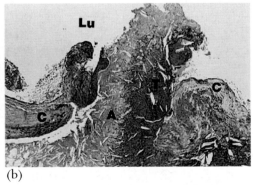

(a)   (b)

Figure 6.5 In vivo MDCT carotid plaque ulceration. (a) CT angiogram of the common carotid artery 1 cm below the bifurcation shows circumferential arterial wall thickening, with a focal contrast containing defect interpreted as an ulcer (arrow). (b), Corresponding histologic section shows a ruptured fibrous cap (C) with a mixture of necrotic debris (A) and thrombus (T) projecting into the lumen (Lu). (MDCT, multidetector-row CT). (Reproduced with permission from TB Oliver et al,[10] Department of Neuroradiology, Western General Hospital, Edinburgh, Scotland.)

MRI plaque imaging of the aorta

The principal challenges associated with MRI of the thoracic aorta are obtaining sufficient sensitivity for sub-millimeter imaging and exclusion of artifacts caused by respiratory motion and blood flow. In vivo black blood MRI atherosclerotic plaque characterization of the human aorta has been reported recently.[70] It could be shown, that MRI findings compare well with those obtained from TEE imaging. Thoracic aortic plaque composition and size was assessed using T1w, T2w, and PDw images. The acquired images had an in-plane resolution of $0.8 \times 0.8\,mm^2$ using a torso phased-array coil. Rapid high-resolution imaging was performed with an FSE sequence in conjunction with velocity-selective flow suppression preparatory pulses. Matched cross-sectional aortic imaging with MR and TEE showed a strong correlation for plaque composition and mean maximum plaque thickness. Figure 6.6 shows MR imaging from a patient with a complex plaque in the descending thoracic aorta. A recent study using MRI in asymptomatic subjects from the Framingham Heart Study demonstrated that aortic plaque burden increased significantly with age, and was higher in the abdominal aorta compared with the thoracic aorta. Results ascertained that long-term measures of risk factors and Framingham Heart Study coronary risk score are strongly associated with asymptomatic aortic atherosclerosis as detected by MRI.[71] Other approaches

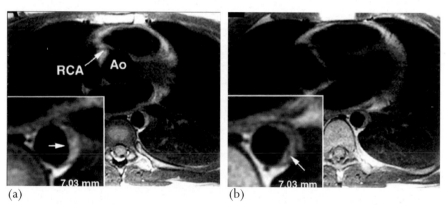

(a)   (b)

Figure 6.6 In vivo MR aortic plaque. A female patient with history of peripheral embolic disease and severe atherosclerosis of the descending thoracic aorta. Representative plaques are different in appearance and can be characterized on the basis of T1, proton density, and T2-weighted MR images. Inserts represent magnified views of the descending thoracic aorta. Axial T2-weighted MR image shows 7-mm fibrocellular stable plaque (a, arrows). Note origin of right coronary artery (RCA) from the aortic root (Ao). Axial T2-weighted MR image at different level than (a) shows 7-mm fibrocellular unstable lipid-rich plaque (b). Hypointense area in plaque (arrow) corresponds to the lipid-rich core. (Reproduced with permission from ZA Fayad et al,[70] Radiology/Cardiology Imaging Science Laboratories, Mount Sinai School of Medicine, New York, USA.)

for the non-invasive detection of plaque in aorta are gadolinium-enhanced three-dimensional MRA,[72] or new semi-invasive procedures like transesophageal MRI.[73] In conclusion, MRI may be a powerful non-invasive imaging tool for direct non-invasive assessment of aortic atherosclerotic plaque thickness, extent and composition, and may thereby allow the serial evaluation of progression and therapy-induced regression of atherosclerotic plaques.

CT plaque imaging of the aorta

The development of EBCT to quantify coronary artery calcification and coronary atherosclerotic plaque burden has paralleled similar developments using conventional CT to quantify calcifications of the aortic wall.[74] Unlike coronary artery imaging, the larger-sized aorta lends itself to easier quantification of non-calcified plaque, particularly with contrast-enhanced CT. This approach has been proposed as a valuable non-invasive method for following the progression and regression of atherosclerotic disease.[75] Tenenbaum et al. used unenhanced dual-helical CT to assess calcium deposits and areas of hypoattenuation adjacent to the aortic wall in 32 patients with recent stroke or embolic events.[76] The authors found that defining a threshold of 4-mm thickness for protruding atheromatous plaques resulted in the best sensitivity (87%) and specificity (82%) for CT when compared with TEE. This corresponds well to the threshold of 4 mm that was found in the French Aortic Plaque in Stroke study to predict a significantly increased risk of stroke.[69] Tenenbaum et al also found that although unenhanced CT is suitable for screening studies, unenhanced dual-helical CT with positive results should be followed with contrast-enhanced CT or TEE (Figure 6.7). Compared to TEE, CT (as well as MRI) provides complete imaging of the thoracic aorta. New MDCT scanners with short image acquisition times and higher spatial resolution are promising, as the acquisition of true isotropic voxel sizes allows for high-quality three-dimensional reconstructions of the aorta in any desirable plane. Additionally, ECG-gated, synchronous imaging with the cardiac cycle will reduce artifacts associated with cardiac motion in the ascending aorta and the aortic root.

Transesophageal ultrasound imaging of the aorta

TEE has been the procedure of choice for identifying thoracic aortic atheromas.[68] Using TEE, the French Aortic Plaque in Stroke investigators determined increased risk of all vascular events (stroke, MI, peripheral embolism and cardiovascular death) for patients who had non-calcified aortic plaques >4 mm thick.[69] TEE-detected aortic plaque has been correlated with a higher prevalence of CAD and the presence of significant angiographic coronary artery stenosis.[68] In addition, the lack of aortic plaque on TEE has been shown to be predictive of the absence of CAD.[77] A new non-invasive method has been developed to image aortic arch plaque employing transcutaneous real-time B-mode ultrasonography with color flow duplex Doppler. B-mode imaging has an 86% accuracy for

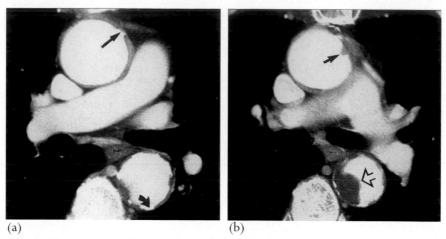

(a)   (b)

Figure 6.7 *In vivo MDCT aortic plaque. An 82-year-old male patient with severe atherosclerotic disease. (a) Contrast-enhanced helical CT scan at level of right main pulmonary artery reveals ulcerated plaque in ascending aorta (straight arrow) and descending thoracic aorta (curved arrow). (b) Contrast-enhanced helical CT scan at level of bifurcation of main pulmonary artery shows protruding atheromas of the ascending (solid arrow) and descending (open arrow) thoracic aorta. (Reproduced with permission from PA Tunick et al,*[12] *Department of Medicine, New York University School of Medicine, New York, USA.)*

identifying complex aortic arch plaques as compared with TEE. Non-invasive imaging of the aortic arch can be employed in diagnosing the etiology of cerebrovascular disease in patients with stroke or transient ischemic attack in conjunction with duplex B-mode sonography of the extracranial carotid arteries. It also provides a non-invasive method for studying atherosclerotic plaque in the aortic arch which is applicable for investigational studies of the mechanisms of atherosclerosis and evaluation of pharmacological agents designed to treat atherosclerotic disease.[78]

Today, TEE is an easy, reliable and widely available imaging modality for imaging of aortic atherosclerosis. However, TEE is a semi-invasive procedure. Actual technical advances in MR and CT seem to allow for a less invasive and more complete evaluation of aortic atherosclerosis, particularly using the potential of MR plaque characterization and the use of plaque specific contrast agents, in the near future. Furthermore, both CT and MRI are better suited to evaluate penetrating atherosclerotic ulcers and their complications such as intramural hematoma, pseudoaneurysm formation and aortic rupture.

Future perspectives

Future improvements in non-invasive imaging modalities

Future potentials – MR plaque imaging

Thinner slices, such as those obtained with three-dimensional MR acquisition techniques, could further improve artery wall imaging.[40] Details on the impact of spatial resolution on plaque characterization in the coronary arteries using MRI have recently been reported.[79] It was shown that low spatial resolution is clearly associated with an overestimation of the wall area and underestimation of the lumen area. Additional MR techniques, such as water diffusion weighting,[80] magnetization transfer weighting,[17] steady-state free precession sequences,[81] contrast enhancement,[82] and molecular imaging[83,84] may provide complementary structural information and allow more detailed plaque characterization. New and improved blood suppression methods[40] are necessary for accurate plaque imaging, especially in the carotid artery bifurcation region. Contrast-enhanced MRA with the use of gadolinium-based contrast agents may provide additional information for plaque characterization by identifying neovascularization in the atherosclerotic plaque and potentially improve the differentiation between necrotic core and fibrous tissue.[82] Furthermore, other non-specific and specific contrast agents may facilitate accurate plaque constituent characterization and the identification of specific molecular and biological activity.[83,84] An example of promising specific contrast agents are fibrin-specific contrast agents, allowing for reliable detection of thrombotic material and for longitudinal study of thrombus progression or regression (Figure 6.8).[85]

Monitoring of atherosclerotic disease with MRI

As shown in animal studies,[86,87] MRI is also a powerful tool to serially and non-invasively investigate the progression and regression of atherosclerotic lesions in vivo. In asymptomatic, untreated, hypercholesterolemic patients with carotid and aortic atherosclerosis, Corti et al have shown that MRI can be used to measure the efficacy of lipid-lowering therapy (statins).[88] Atherosclerotic plaques were assessed with MRI at different times after lipid-lowering therapy. Significant regression of atherosclerotic lesions was observed. As with previous experimental studies, there was a decrease in the vessel wall area and no alteration in the lumen area after 12 months.[86,87] A case–control study demonstrated substantially reduced carotid plaque lipid content (but no change in overall lesion area) in patients treated for 10 years with an aggressive lipid-lowering regimen compared with untreated controls.[89] As yet, there are no reports of longitudinal human in vivo studies on the alteration of coronary atherosclerotic plaques over time.

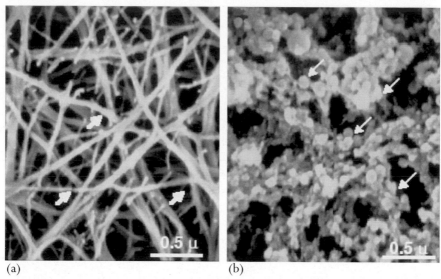

(a)   (b)

Figure 6.8 *Molecular imaging. Scanning electron micrographs (×330 000) of control fibrin clot (a) and fibrin targeted paramagnetic nanoparticles bound to clot surface (b). Arrows indicate (a) fibrin fibril and (b) fibrin-specific nanoparticle-bound fibrin epitopes. (Reproduced with permission from S Flacke et al,[84] Radiologische Klinik, University of Bonn, Germany.)*

Future potentials – CT plaque imaging

The next generation of MDCT scanners will most probably allow for even faster gantry rotation and simultaneous acquisition of more than 16 slices. The breath hold time may decrease to <10 s thus reducing the necessary volume of the contrast medium (e.g. 60 ml) needed for sufficient enhancement of the coronary arteries. The temporal and spatial resolution may most likely further decrease to ideally 100 ms and 0.6-mm slice thickness for true isotropic voxel sizes. These enhancements may help in the detection, differentiation and reliable quantification of calcified and non-calcified coronary artery plaques. Reduction of spatial resolution and new image reconstruction algorithms should further reduce beam hardening artifacts and partial volume effects caused by calcifications and improve the assessment of complex mixed plaques. Further optimization of multisegmental reconstruction algorithms[90,91] may allow the investigation of patients with higher heart rates without any loss in image quality.

Molecular imaging of atherosclerosis

Images obtained from CT, US and MRI reflect the inherent physicochemical properties of plaques. An alternative approach is to image plaque through the introduction of contrast agents that are targeted to specific cells, molecules or processes that can be precisely localized and quantified.[92] Examples might include macrophage imaging, targeting molecules mediating vascular inflammation and functional assays of proteolytic enzyme activity. Our expanding understanding of cellular and molecular events within atherosclerotic plaque has been accompanied by imaginative application of imaging tools leading to a new field of 'molecular imaging'.[93-96]

Nuclear scintigraphic techniques

Radioisotopes offer potential for imaging atherosclerotic lesions and have been evaluated in animal models and in humans.[97] For example, ^{99m}Tc (technetium 99-m)-labeled oxidized low density lipoprotein particles[98] localize to human carotid atherosclerotic plaque and can be identified with non-invasive tomographic scintigraphy. Autoradiography of endarterectomized carotid artery showed radiolabeled oxidized LDL localized to macrophages.[99] Alternative approaches have used radiolabeled peptide fragments[100] and monoclonal antibodies[101] directed at plaque components. In vivo, nuclear techniques can be impaired where labeled particles are cleared slowly from circulating blood, contributing to a low target to background scintigraphic ratio. A further disadvantage of in vivo scintigraphy is relatively poor spatial resolution and paucity of anatomical information about the plaque, although anatomical information can be enhanced by co-registration of scintigraphic images with CT or MRI (both discussed above).[102]

Positron emission tomography (PET) and single photon emission computed tomography (SPECT) benefit from imaging agents that can be detected in extremely low concentration (picomolar range) and provide excellent sensitivity for application to molecular imaging, but with lower spatial resolution than other technologies.[103] After intravenous injection of [^{18}F]-fluorodeoxyglucose (^{18}FDG), a glucose analog that signals active glycolysis, Rudd et al demonstrated its accumulation in the plaques of patients with symptomatic carotid atherosclerosis and confirmed their non-invasive ^{18}FDG-PET findings by autoradiography following carotid endarterectomy.[102] Others have shown correlation between plaque macrophage content and signal from ^{18}FDG-PET.[104]

Targeted contrast-enhanced MRI

In contrast to PET, MRI provides excellent spatial resolution but is inherently limited by the available signal-to-noise ratio. To address this limitation, much work has been directed to the development of contrast-enhancing molecular probes for use in high-resolution MRI.[93,105] Contrast agents that specifically identify components of atherothrombotic plaque could help to predict pathophysiological behavior of individual plaques. For instance, macrophage-rich areas are found in unstable plaque.[106] Small superparamagnetic particles of iron oxide (SPIO) and ultrasmall SPIO (USPIO) are taken up avidly by macrophages. Injection of USPIO into hyperlipidemic rabbits was associated with accumulation in macrophages and, after 2 hours[107] to 5 days,[83] the appearance of signal voids studded on the luminal surface of the aorta. Similar appearances have been observed incidentally in humans in the aorta and intrapelvic arteries of patients who have received USPIO for oncological imaging[108] and in carotid arteries, where subsequent histologic examination of endarterectomized material showed particle accumulation predominantly in ruptured and rupture-prone plaque.[109] This type of specific cellular targeting is potentially powerful; indeed magnetic particle labeling has enabled the identification of *individual* cells in vitro[110] and in vivo.[111]

MRI and molecular imaging

Louie et al have developed an MR contrast agent (EgadMe) capable of reporting activity of a β-galactosidase.[112] In the resting state, interaction of gadolinium with water is prevented by the attachment of galactopyranose, a 'blocking group' that is susceptible to enzymatic cleavage by β-galactosidase. The subsequent association of water with the gadolinium core results in an increase of T1 signal by ~60%. Using this approach it was possible to localize the lineage of a cell injected with β-galactosidase mRNA in early embryonic development. The ability to image areas in which β-galactosidase is active may be useful in mapping sites of expression in therapeutic gene therapy. Furthermore, this technique may represent a paradigm of intelligent contrast agents that are activated in response to specific biological events. Successors of EgadMe may contain cleavage–activation sites that are substrates for other enzymes. In the context of atherosclerosis, matrix metalloproteinases (MMPs) digest collagen, elastin and other matrix components. MMPs have the additional advantage of extracellular activity, thus avoiding the problem of intracellular access by contrast agents.

Some endothelial cell surface proteins, such as vascular cell adhesion molecule-1 (VCAM-1) or intercellular adhesion molecule-1 (ICAM-1), are upregulated in atherosclerotic plaque[113,114] and in areas of arteries prone to lesion formation.[115] Direct contact with circulating blood renders such molecules potential targets for monoclonal antibody-conjugated intravascular MR contrast agents. Antibodies conjugated to paramagnetic liposomes have been used to image ICAM expression in a murine model of multiple sclerosis, ex vivo,[116] and $\alpha_v\beta_3$ integrin expression as a marker of angiogenesis.[117] Where cells are accessible to blood, perhaps as a consequence of abnormal vascular permeability in plaques, imaging specific receptor expression using contrast-ligand constructs may also be feasible.[118]

Enzyme activity

Chen et al have developed fluorescent imaging probes that can be injected intravenously in an inactive or 'quenched' form. Following site-specific cleavage by proteolytic enzymes, the probe becomes brightly fluorescent and can be imaged by near-infrared spectroscopy. This technique imaged cathepsin B activity in the atherosclerotic plaques of apolipoprotein E deficient mice, but is amenable to modification for broader application.[119] indeed the same principle has been applied to image the activity of thrombin, a serine protease that plays a key role in thrombosis.[120] With suitable adaptation, such techniques may be transferable to intravascular imaging in humans.

New imaging strategies discussed in this section should build on our expanding understanding of vascular pathobiology and add an important functional dimension to imaging atherothrombotic plaque.

Conclusions

Assessment of atherosclerotic plaques by imaging techniques is essential for in vivo identification of atherothrombotic plaques. Several invasive and non-invasive imaging techniques are available. Most techniques identify luminal diameter or stenosis, some of them assess wall thickness and/or plaque volume, but the ultimate goal is the identification of the high-risk plaques that are vulnerable to rupture and thrombosis.

MR and CT imaging are emerging as the most promising imaging modalities for atherosclerotic disease detection. They identify flow-limiting stenoses in various vessel areas with high accuracy, are able to directly image the atherosclerotic lesions, measure atherosclerotic burden, characterize the plaque components and may be used to assess progression and regression of atherosclerosis. Application of MRI opens new areas for diagnosis, prevention and treatment of atherosclerosis in many arterial locations. However, there are still disadvantages of MRI concerning in vivo plaque imaging in the coronary arteries, as the technique suffers from patient movement and breathing artifacts due to relatively long acquisition times and limited spatial resolution. This is the main reason why, in an in vivo setting, a detailed analysis of coronary artery plaques is not routinely feasible yet, and only limited regions of the coronary artery tree can be depicted.[7]

Modern MDCT scanners allow for in vivo investigation of various vascular systems within short acquisition times, achieving a nearly isotropic sub-millimeter voxel size, with typically better out-of-plane resolution compared to MRI. This makes MDCT easier to perform especially in the in vivo assessment of coronary artery plaques. However, MDCT is not able to provide such detailed information on plaque composition as multi-contrast MRI can, and it applies a considerable amount of ionizing radiation to the patient combined with the useage of iodine-containing contrast agents.

In future, imaging atherothrombotic plaque may be enhanced by the application of new techniques that combine developing imaging technology and innovative targeted contrast agents with an expanding understanding of plaque pathology at the molecular and cellular level.

Further clinical investigation is needed to define the technical requirements for optimal imaging, develop accurate image analysis methods, outline criteria for interpretation, delineate the clinical indications for which MR and/or CT imaging should be used as an adjunct to conventional imaging and address the issue of cost-effectiveness. Finally, imaging may address the high-risk plaque, but it does not take into account the blood hypercoagulable state or markers of inflammation. Therefore, the goal for the clinicians should be the identification of the high-risk patient through a combination of strategies such as assessment of conventional risk factors, blood markers and imaging.

References

1. Fuster V, Badimon L, Badimon JJ, Chesebro JH. The pathogenesis of coronary artery disease and the acute coronary syndromes (1). *N Engl J Med* 1992; **326**:242–50.

2. Fuster V, Badimon L, Badimon JJ, Chesebro JH. The pathogenesis of coronary artery disease and the acute coronary syndromes (2). *N Engl J Med* 1992; **326**:310–8.

3. Virmani R, Kolodgie FD, Burke AP, Farb A, Schwartz SM. Lessons from sudden coronary death: a comprehensive morphological classification scheme for atherosclerotic lesions. *Arterioscler Thromb Vasc Biol* 2000; **20**:1262–75.

4. Pasterkamp G, Falk E, Woutman H, Borst C. Techniques characterizing the coronary atherosclerotic plaque: influence on clinical decision making? *J Am Coll Cardiol* 2000; **36**:13–21.

5. Fayad ZA, Fuster V, Nikolaou K, Becker C. Computed tomography and magnetic resonance imaging for noninvasive coronary angiography and plaque imaging: current and potential future concepts. *Circulation* 2002; **106**:2026–34.

6. Fayad ZA, Fuster V. Clinical imaging of the high-risk or vulnerable atherosclerotic plaque. *Circ Res* 2001; **89**:305–16.

7. Fayad ZA, Fuster V, Fallon JT et al. Noninvasive in vivo human coronary artery lumen and wall imaging using black-blood magnetic resonance imaging. *Circulation* 2000; **102**:506–10.

8. Yuan C, Beach KW, Smith LH, Jr., Hatsukami TS. Measurement of atherosclerotic carotid plaque size in vivo using high resolution magnetic resonance imaging. *Circulation* 1998; **98**:2666–71.

9. Fayad ZA, Nahar T, Fallon JT et al. In vivo MR evaluation of atherosclerotic plaques in the human thoracic aorta: a comparison with TEE. *Circulation* 2000; **101**:2503–9.

10. Oliver TB, Lammie GA, Wright AR et al. Atherosclerotic plaque at the carotid bifurcation: CT angiographic appearance with histopathologic correlation. *AJNR Am J Neuroradiol* 1999; **20**:897–901.

11. Becker CR. Assessment of coronary arteries with CT. *Radiol Clin North Am* 2002; **40**:773–82.

12. Tunick PA, Krinsky GA, Lee VS, Kronzon I. Diagnostic imaging of thoracic aortic atherosclerosis. *AJR Am J Roentgenol* 2000; **174**:1119–25.

13. Becker CR, Schoepf UJ, Reiser MF. Coronary artery calcium scoring: medicine and politics. *Eur Radiol* 2003; **13**:445–7.

14. Nikolaou K, Becker CR, Wintersperger BJ, Sagmeister S, Reiser MF. Multidetector-row computed tomography of the coronary arteries: predictive value and quantitative assessment of non-calcified vessel-wall changes. *Eur Radiol;* **13**:2505–12.

15. Toussaint JF, LaMuraglia GM, Southern JF, Fuster V, Kantor HL. Magnetic resonance images lipid, fibrous, calcified, hemorrhagic, and thrombotic components of human atherosclerosis in vivo. *Circulation* 1996; **94**:932–8.

16. Hatsukami TS, Ross R, Polissar NL, Yuan C. Visualization of fibrous cap thickness and rupture in human atherosclerotic carotid plaque. In vivo with high-resolution magnetic resonance imaging. *Circulation* 2000; **102**:959–64.

17. Yuan C, Mitsumori LM, Beach KW, Maravilla KR. Carotid atherosclerotic plaque: noninvasive MR characterization and identification of vulnerable lesions. *Radiology* 2001; **221**:285–99.

18. Becker CR, Nikolaou K, Muders M et al. Ex vivo coronary atherosclerotic plaque characterization with multi-detector-row CT. *Eur Radiol* 2003; **13**:1094–8.

19. Klingenbeck-Regn K, Flohr T, Ohnesorge B, Regn J, Schaller S. Strategies for cardiac CT imaging. *Int J Cardiovasc Imaging* 2002; **18**:143–51.

20. Budoff MJ, Raggi P. Coronary artery disease progression assessed by electron-beam computed tomography. *Am J Cardiol* 2001; 19; **88**:46E–50E.

21. Becker CR, Knez A, Ohnesorge B et al. Visualization and quantification of coronary calcifications with electron beam and spiral computed tomography. *Eur Radiol* 2000; **10**:629–35.

22. Becker CR, Jakobs TF, Aydemir S et al. Helical and single-slice conventional CT versus electron beam CT for the quantification of coronary artery calcification. *AJR Am J Roentgenol* 2000; **174**:543–7.

23. Wintersperger BJ, Herzog P, Jakobs TF, Reiser MF, Becker CR. Initial experience with the clinical use of a 16 detector row CT system. *Crit Rev Comput Tomogr* 2002; **43**:283–316.

24. Schroeder S, Kopp AF, Baumbach A et al. Noninvasive detection and evaluation of atherosclerotic coronary plaques with multislice computed tomography. *J Am Coll Cardiol* 2001; **37**:1430–5.

25. Cohen A, Tzourio C, Bertrand B et al. Aortic plaque morphology and vascular events: a follow-up study in patients with ischemic stroke. FAPS Investigators. French Study of Aortic Plaques in Stroke. *Circulation* 1997; **96**:3838–41.

26. Weinberger J, Tegeler CH, McKinney WM, Wechsler LR, Toole J. Ultrasonography for diagnosis and management of carotid artery atherosclerosis. A position paper of the American Society of Neuroimaging. *J Neuroimaging* 1995; **5**:237–43.

27. Pignoli P, Tremoli E, Poli A, Oreste P, Paoletti R. Intimal plus medial thickness of the arterial wall: a direct measurement with ultrasound imaging. *Circulation* 1986; **74**:1399–406.

28. Weinberger J, Azhar S, Danisi F, Hayes R, Goldman M. A new noninvasive technique for imaging atherosclerotic plaque in the aortic arch of stroke patients by transcutaneous real-time B-mode ultrasonography: an initial report. *Stroke* 1998; **29**:673–6.

29. Lindner JR, Dayton PA, Coggins MP et al. Noninvasive imaging of inflammation by ultrasound detection of phagocytosed microbubbles. *Circulation* 2000; **102**:531–8.

30. Tiukinhoy SD, Mahowald ME, Shively VP et al. Development of echogenic, plasmid-incorporated, tissue-targeted cationic liposomes that can be used for directed gene delivery. *Invest Radiol* 2000; **35**:732–8.

31. Falk E, Shah PK, Fuster V. Coronary plaque disruption. *Circulation* 1995; **92**:657–71.

32. Fuster V. Mechanisms leading to myocardial infarction: insights from studies of vascular biology. *Circulation* 1994; **90**:2126–46.

33. Stary HC, Chandler AB, Dinsmore RE et al. A definition of advanced types of atherosclerotic lesions and a histological classification of atherosclerosis. A report from the Committee on Vascular Lesions of the Council on Arteriosclerosis, American Heart Association. *Arterioscler Thromb Vasc Biol* 1995; **15**:1512–31.

34. Stary HC. Natural history and histological classification of atherosclerotic lesions: an update. *Arterioscler Thromb Vasc Biol* 2000; **20**:1177–8.

35. Libby P. Molecular bases of the acute coronary syndromes. *Circulation* 1995; **91**:2844–50.

36. Falk E, Fernandez-Ortiz A. Role of thrombosis in atherosclerosis and its complications. *Am J Cardiol* 1995; **75**:3B–11B.

37. Fuster V, Fayad ZA, Badimon JJ. Acute coronary syndromes: biology. *Lancet* 1999; **353** (Suppl 2):5–9.

38. Nikolaou K, Becker CR, Muders M. High-resolution magnetic resonance and multi-slice CT imaging of coronary artery plaques in human ex vivo coronary arteries. *Radiology* 2001; **221**:503.

39. Worthley SG, Helft G, Fuster V et al. Noninvasive in vivo magnetic resonance imaging of experimental coronary artery lesions in a porcine model. *Circulation* 2000; **101**:2956–61.

40. Botnar RM, Kim WY, Bornert P et al. 3D coronary vessel wall imaging utilizing a local inversion technique with spiral image acquisition. *Magn Reson Med* 2001; **46**:848–54.

41. Becker CR, Knez A, Jakobs TF et al. Detection and quantification of coronary artery calcification with electron-beam and conventional CT. *Eur Radiol* 1999; **9**:620–4.

42. Virmani R, Burke AP, Farb A. Sudden cardiac death. *Cardiovasc Pathol* 2001; **10**:211–18.

43. Burke AP, Taylor A, Farb A, Malcom GT, Virmani R. Coronary calcification: insights from sudden coronary death victims. *Z Kardiol* 2000; **89**(Suppl 2):49–53.

44. Nikolaou K, Becker CR, Muders M, Loehrs U, Reiser M. High resolution magnetic resonance and multi slice CT imaging of coronary artery plaques in human ex vivo coronary arteries. *Radiology* 2001; **221**(P):503.

45. Becker CR, Knez A, Leber A et al. [Angiography with multi-slice spiral CT. Detecting plaque, before it causes symptoms]. *MMW Fortschr Med* 2001; **143**:30–2.

46. Becker CR, Knez A, Ohnesorge B, Schoepf UJ, Reiser MF. Imaging of noncalcified coronary plaques using helical CT with retrospective ECG gating. *AJR Am J Roentgenol* 2000; **175**:423–4.

47. Baumgart D, Schmermund A, Goerge G et al. Comparison of electron beam computed tomography with intracoronary ultrasound and coronary angiography for detection of coronary atherosclerosis. *J Am Coll Cardiol* 1997; **30**:57–64.

48. Weyman AE, Feigenbaum H, Dillon JC, Johnston KW, Eggleton RC. Noninvasive visualization of the left main coronary artery by cross-sectional echocardiography. *Circulation* 1976; **54**:169–74.

49. Rink LD, Feigenbaum H, Godley RW et al. Echocardiographic detection of left main coronary artery obstruction. *Circulation* 1982; **65**:719–24.

50. Maxted WC Jr, Swanson ST, Huntley M et al. Location of stents in the left anterior descending coronary artery using three dimensionally acquired, two dimensionally displayed transthoracic echocardiography. *Am J Cardiol* 1998; **82**:1434–6, A9.

51. Gradus-Pizlo I, Segar DS, Sawada SG, Hull S, Feigenbaum H. Detection of coronary atherosclerosis using high-resolution, two-dimensional transthoracic echocardiography. *J Am Coll Cardiol* 1999; **33**(2 (Suppl A)):484A.

52. McPherson DD, Hiratzka LF, Lamberth WC et al. Delineation of the extent of coronary atherosclerosis by high-frequency epicardial echocardiography. *N Engl J Med* 1987; **316**:304–9.

53. Gradus-Pizlo I, Bigelow B, Mahomed Y et al. Left anterior descending coronary artery wall thickness measured by high-frequency transthoracic and epicardial echocardiography includes adventitia. *Am J Cardiol* 2003; **91**:27–32.

54. Fitzgerald PJ, St Goar FG, Connolly AJ et al. Intravascular ultrasound imaging of coronary arteries. Is three layers the norm? *Circulation* 1992; **86**:154–8.

55. Velican D, Velican C. Comparative study on age-related changes and atherosclerotic involvement of the coronary arteries of male and female subjects up to 40 years of age. *Atherosclerosis* 1981; **38**:39–50.

119

56. Hatsukami TS, Ferguson MS, Beach KW et al. Carotid plaque morphology and clinical events. *Stroke* 1997; **28**:95–100.

57. Comerota AJ, Katz ML, White JV, Grosh JD. The preoperative diagnosis of the ulcerated carotid atheroma. *J Vasc Surg* 1990; **11**:505–10.

58. Glagov S, Zarins C, Giddens DP, Ku DN. Hemodynamics and atherosclerosis. Insights and perspectives gained from studies of human arteries. *Arch Pathol Lab Med* 1988; **112**:1018–31.

59. Yuan C, Mitsumori LM, Beach KW, Maravilla KR. Carotid atherosclerotic plaque: noninvasive MR characterization and identification of vulnerable lesions. *Radiology* 2001; **221**:285–99.

60. Fayad ZA, Fuster V. The human high-risk plaque and its detection by magnetic resonance imaging. *Am J Cardiol* 2001; **88**:42E–45E.

61. Hatsukami TS, Ross R, Polissar NL, Yuan C. Visualization of fibrous cap thickness and rupture in human atherosclerotic carotid plaque in vivo with high-resolution magnetic resonance imaging. *Circulation* 2000; **102**:959–64.

62. Hayes CE, Mathis CM, Yuan C. Surface coil phased arrays for high-resolution imaging of the carotid arteries. *J Magn Reson Imaging* 1996; **6**:109–12.

63. Yuan C, Mitsumori LM, Ferguson MS et al. In vivo accuracy of multispectral magnetic resonance imaging for identifying lipid-rich necrotic cores and intraplaque hemorrhage in advanced human carotid plaques. *Circulation* 2001; **104**:2051–6.

64. Estes JM, Quist WC, Lo Gerfo FW, Costello P. Noninvasive characterization of plaque morphology using helical computed tomography. *J Cardiovasc Surg (Torino)* 1998; **39**:527–34.

65. Porsche C, Walker L, Mendelow AD, Birchall D. Assessment of vessel wall thickness in carotid atherosclerosis using spiral CT angiography. *Eur J Vasc Endovasc Surg* 2002; **23**:437–40.

66. Fazio GP, Redberg RF, Winslow T, Schiller NB. Transesophageal echocardiographically detected atherosclerotic aortic plaque is a marker for coronary artery disease. *J Am Coll Cardiol* 1993; **21**:144–50.

67. Solberg LA, Strong JP. Risk factors and atherosclerotic lesions. A review of autopsy studies. *Arteriosclerosis* 1983; **3**:187–98.

68. Tunick PA, Kronzon I. Atheromas of the thoracic aorta: clinical and therapeutic update. *J Am Coll Cardiol* 2000; **35**:545–54.

69. The French study of aortic plaques in stroke group. Atherosclerotic disease of the aortic arch as a risk factor for recurrent ischemic stroke. *N Engl J Med* 1996; **334**:1216–21.

70. Fayad ZA, Nahar T, Fallon JT et al. In vivo magnetic resonance evaluation of atherosclerotic plaques in the human thoracic aorta: a comparison with transesophageal echocardiography. *Circulation* 2000; **101**:2503–9.

71. Jaffer FA, O'Donnell CJ, Larson MG et al. Age and sex distribution of subclinical aortic atherosclerosis: a magnetic resonance imaging examination of the Framingham Heart Study. *Arterioscler Thromb Vasc Biol* 2002; **22**:849–54.

72. Prince MR, Narasimham DL, Jacoby WT et al. Three-dimensional gadolinium-enhanced MR angiography of the thoracic aorta. *AJR Am J Roentgenol* 1996; **166**:1387–97.

73. Shunk KA, Garot J, Atalar E, Lima JA. Transesophageal magnetic resonance imaging of the aortic arch and descending thoracic aorta in patients with aortic atherosclerosis. *J Am Coll Cardiol* 2001; **37**:2031–5.

74. Takasu J, Takanashi K, Naito S et al. Evaluation of morphological changes of the atherosclerotic aorta by enhanced computed tomography. *Atherosclerosis* 1992; **97**:107–21.

75. Takasu J, Masuda Y, Watanabe S et al. Progression and regression of atherosclerotic findings in the descending thoracic aorta detected by enhanced computed tomography. *Atherosclerosis* 1994; **110**:175–84.

76. Tenenbaum A, Garniek A, Shemesh J et al. Dual-helical CT for detecting aortic atheromas as a source of stroke: comparison with transesophageal echocardiography. *Radiology* 1998; **208**:153–8.

77. Parthenakis F, Skalidis E, Simantirakis E et al. Absence of atherosclerotic lesions in the thoracic aorta indicates absence of significant coronary artery disease. *Am J Cardiol* 1996; **77**:1118–21.

78. Weinberger J. Noninvasive imaging of atherosclerotic plaque in the arch of the aorta with transcutaneous B-mode ultrasonography. *Neuroimaging Clin North Am* 2002; **12**:373–83.

79. Schar M, Kim WY, Stuber M et al. The impact of spatial resolution and respiratory motion on MR imaging of atherosclerotic plaque. *J Magn Reson Imaging* 2003; **17**:538–44.

80. Toussaint JF, Southern JF, Fuster V, Kantor HL. Water diffusion properties of human atherosclerosis and thrombosis measured by pulse field gradient nuclear magnetic resonance. *Arterioscler Thromb Vasc Biol* 1997; **17**:542–6.

81. Coombs BD, Rapp JH, Ursell PC, Reilly LM, Saloner D. Structure of plaque at carotid bifurcation: high-resolution MRI with histological correlation. *Stroke* 2001; **32**:2516–21.

82. Yuan C, Kerwin WS, Ferguson MS et al. Contrast-enhanced high resolution MRI for atherosclerotic carotid artery tissue characterization. *J Magn Reson Imaging* 2002; **15**:62–7.

83. Ruehm SG, Corot C, Vogt P, Kolb S, Debatin JF. Magnetic resonance imaging of atherosclerotic plaque with ultrasmall superparamagnetic particles of iron oxide in hyperlipidemic rabbits. *Circulation* 2001; **103**:415–22.

84. Flacke S, Fischer S, Scott MJ et al. Novel MRI contrast agent for molecular imaging of fibrin: implications for detecting vulnerable plaques. *Circulation* 2001; **104**:1280–5.

85. Yu X, Song SK, Chen J et al. High-resolution MRI characterization of human thrombus using a novel fibrin-targeted paramagnetic nanoparticle contrast agent. *Magn Reson Med* 2000; **44**:867–72.

86. McConnell MV, Aikawa M, Maier SE et al. MRI of rabbit atherosclerosis in response to dietary cholesterol lowering. *Arterioscler Thromb Vasc Biol* 1999; **19**:1956–9.

87. Helft G, Worthley SG, Fuster V et al. Progression and regression of atherosclerotic lesions: monitoring with serial noninvasive magnetic resonance imaging. *Circulation* 2002; **105**:993–8.

88. Corti R, Fayad ZA, Fuster V et al. Effects of lipid-lowering by simvastatin on human atherosclerotic lesions: a longitudinal study by high-resolution, noninvasive magnetic resonance imaging. *Circulation* 2001; **104**:249–52.

89. Zhao XQ, Yuan C, Hatsukami TS et al. Effects of prolonged intensive lipid-lowering therapy on the characteristics of carotid atherosclerotic plaques in vivo by MRI: a case–control study. *Arterioscler Thromb Vasc Biol* 2001; **21**:1623–9.

90. Halliburton SS, Stillman AE, Flohr T et al. Do segmented reconstruction algorithms for cardiac multi-slice computed tomography improve image quality? *Herz* 2003; **28**:20–31.

91. Flohr T, Kuttner A, Bruder H et al. Performance evaluation of a multi-slice CT system with 16-slice detector and increased gantry rotation speed for isotropic submillimeter imaging of the heart. *Herz* 2003; **28**:7–19.

92. Choudhury RP, Fuster V, Badimon JJ, Fisher EA, Fayad ZA. Magnetic resonance imaging and characterization of atherosclerotic plaque: emerging applications and molecular imaging. *Arterioscler Thromb Vasc Biol* 2002; **22**:1065–74.

93. Weissleder R, Mahmood U. Molecular imaging. *Radiology* 2001; **219**:316–33.

94. Wickline SA, Lanza GM. Nanotechnology for molecular imaging and targeted therapy. *Circulation* 2003; **107**:1092–5.

95. Wickline SA, Lanza GM. Molecular imaging, targeted therapeutics, and nanoscience. *J Cell Biochem Suppl* 2002; **39**:90–7.

96. Rudin M, Weissleder R. Molecular imaging in drug discovery and development. *Nat Rev Drug Discov* 2003; **2**:123–31.

97. Vallabhajosula S, Fuster V. Atherosclerosis: imaging techniques and the evolving role of nuclear medicine. *J Nucl Med* 1997; **38**:1788–96.

98. Iuliano L, Signore A, Vallabhajosula S et al. Preparation and biodistribution of 99m technetium labelled oxidized LDL in man. *Atherosclerosis* 1996; **126**:131–41.

99. Iuliano L, Mauriello A, Sbarigia E, Spagnoli LG, Violi F. Radiolabeled native low-density lipoprotein injected into patients with carotid stenosis accumulates in macrophages of atherosclerotic plaque: effect of vitamin E supplementation. *Circulation* 2000; **101**:1249–54.

100. Hardoff R, Braegelmann F, Zanzonico P et al. External imaging of atherosclerosis in rabbits using an ^{123}I-labeled synthetic peptide fragment. *J Clin Pharmacol* 1993; **33**:1039–47.

101. Tsimikas S, Palinski W, Halpern SE et al. Radiolabeled MDA2, an oxidation-specific, monoclonal antibody, identifies native atherosclerotic lesions in vivo. *J Nucl Cardiol* 1999; **6(1 Pt 1)**:41–53.

102. Rudd JH, Warburton EA, Fryer TD et al. Imaging atherosclerotic plaque inflammation with [^{18}F]-fluorodeoxyglucose positron emission tomography. *Circulation* 2002; **105**:2708–11.

103. Sharma V, Luker GD, Piwnica-Worms D. Molecular imaging of gene expression and protein function in vivo with PET and SPECT. *J Magn Reson Imaging* 2002; **16**:336–51.

104. Helft G, Worthley SG, Zhang ZY et al. Non-invasive in vivo imaging of atherosclerotic lesions using Fluorine-18 Deoxyglucose (18-FDG) PET correlates with macrophage content in a rabbit model. *Circulation* 1999; **100**:I-311.

105. Aime S, Cabella C, Colombatto S et al. Insights into the use of paramagnetic Gd(III) complexes in MR-molecular imaging investigations. *J Magn Reson Imaging* 2002; **16**:394–406.

106. Moreno PR, Falk E, Palacios IF et al. Macrophage infiltration in acute coronary syndromes. Implications for plaque rupture. *Circulation* 1994; **90**:775–8.

107. Schmitz SA, Coupland SE, Gust R et al. Superparamagnetic iron oxide-enhanced MRI of atherosclerotic plaques in Watanabe hereditable hyperlipidemic rabbits. *Invest Radiol* 2000; **35**:460–71.

108. Schmitz SA, Taupitz M, Wagner S et al. Magnetic resonance imaging of atherosclerotic plaques using superparamagnetic iron oxide particles. *J Magn Reson Imaging* 2001; **14**:355–61.

109. Kooi ME, Cappendijk VC, Cleutjens KB et al. Accumulation of ultrasmall superparamagnetic particles of iron oxide in human atherosclerotic plaques can be detected by in vivo magnetic resonance imaging. *Circulation* 2003; **107**:2453–8.

110. Foster-Gareau P, Heyn C, Alejski A, Rutt BK. Imaging single mammalian cells with a 1.5 T clinical MRI scanner. *Magn Reson Med* 2003; **49**:968–71.

111. Hinds KA, Hill JM, Shapiro EM et al. Highly efficient endosomal labeling of progenitor and stem cells with large magnetic particles allows magnetic resonance imaging of single cells. *Blood* 2003; **102**:867–72.

112. Louie AY, Huber MM, Ahrens ET et al. In vivo visualization of gene expression using magnetic resonance imaging. *Nat Biotechnol* 2000; **18**:321–5.

113. Davies MJ, Gordon JL, Gearing AJ et al. The expression of the adhesion molecules ICAM-1, VCAM-1, PECAM, and E-selectin in human atherosclerosis. *J Pathol* 1993; **171**:223–9.

114. Wood KM, Cadogan MD, Ramshaw AL, Parums DV. The distribution of adhesion molecules in human atherosclerosis. *Histopathology* 1993; **22**:437–44.

115. Nakashima Y, Raines EW, Plump AS, Breslow JL, Ross R. Upregulation of VCAM-1 and ICAM-1 at atherosclerosis-prone sites on the endothelium in the ApoE-deficient mouse. *Arterioscler Thromb Vasc Biol* 1998; **18**:842–51.

116. Sipkins DA, Gijbels K, Tropper FD et al. ICAM-1 expression in autoimmune encephalitis visualized using magnetic resonance imaging. *J Neuroimmunol* 2000; **104**:1–9.

117. Sipkins DA, Cheresh DA, Kazemi MR et al. Detection of tumor angiogenesis in vivo by alphaVbeta3-targeted magnetic resonance imaging. *Nat Med* 1998; **4**:623–6.

118. Nunn AD, Linder KE, Tweedle MF. Can receptors be imaged with MRI agents? *Q J Nucl Med* 1997; **41**:155–62.

119. Chen J, Tung CH, Mahmood U et al. In vivo imaging of proteolytic activity in atherosclerosis. *Circulation* 2002; **105**:2766–71.

120. Jaffer FA, Tung CH, Gerszten RE, Weissleder R. In vivo imaging of thrombin activity in experimental thrombi with thrombin-sensitive near-infrared molecular probe. *Arterioscler Thromb Vasc Biol* 2002; **22**:1929–35.

121. Fayad ZA, Fuster V. Characterization of atherosclerotic plaques by magnetic resonance imaging. *Ann NY Acad Sci* 2000; **902**:173–86.

7. VULNERABLE PLAQUE: DETECTION PARADIGMS FROM MOLECULES IN PERIPHERAL BLOOD

Arturo G Touchard, Antonio Bayes-Genis, John R Lesser, Giuseppe Sangiorgi, Timothy D Henry, Cheryl A Conover and Robert S Schwartz

Atherosclerosis is a ubiquitous, chronic inflammatory arterial disease and is found in even the earliest life stages. Stary found intimal foam cells in 45% of infants 8 months old and younger. These foam cells occur with lipid accumulations and scattered extracellular lipid in 65% of children between the ages of 12 and 14 years. An additional 8% of children progress beyond this early stage and develop advanced preatheroma or actual atheromatous lesions.

In a majority of healthy adults multiple advanced atheromatous plaques occur in the coronary, carotid and peripheral arteries. In many of these patients, the plaques rupture, forming occlusive or mural thrombi. The clinical consequences may be silent or may lead to acute coronary syndromes (ACS) including death. ACS typically result from arterial thrombi. In 60% of sudden death cases thrombus is found, while the remaining 40% have severe anatomic coronary artery disease (CAD) without thrombus.[1]

Cardiovascular mortality is the number one cause of death in adults 65 years and older in Western societies.[2,3] In all cardiac-related deaths, about half are sudden and unexpected. Detecting patients at risk of cardiovascular and neurologic events before they occur may now be possible, and research strategies are under intensive study by clinicians and researchers.

Vulnerable plaque: key features

The term 'vulnerable plaque' originated in 1994 and initially described plaques causing ACS.[4] Many investigators no longer use the 'vulnerable plaque' label since many different plaque morphologies may trigger thrombosis and ACS. These comprise not only the classic thin fibrous cap covering a lipid core, but also include eroded plaque and calcific nodules.[1] Moreover, additional factors other than plaque may contribute to ACS. In fact, plaques with similar characteristics may have different clinical presentations due to other factors such as blood coagulability.

The 'vulnerable patient' concept is now preferable to vulnerable plaque and denotes patients at risk for ACS. In the right context the term vulnerable plaque still is applicable – as a localized arterial region at risk for creating thrombus and acute arterial syndromes evolving from distal organ ischemia. This chapter uses the term vulnerable plaque in such a context.

Histopathology

Vulnerable plaque classically contains a thin fibrous cap (150 μm or less) covering lipid-rich regions deeper in the vessel wall.[5–7] Plaque rupture occurs with cap fracture at the border, and lipid extrusion into the lumen and thrombus on or near the lipid (Figure 7.1).

Sudden death autopsies implicate several other plaque morphologies causing acute thrombosis. The principal one among these is plaque erosion, a histopathologically distinct entity. This finding clusters in several patient subsets, each with substantially different risk factors.[1,7] Sudden death from plaque erosion typically shows thrombus on a bare, de-endothelialized surface.[8] These typically occur in younger patients, most often women without hyperlipidemia. The plaques typically do not contain lipid-rich regions[5,7–9] and the plaque surface gradually erodes allowing hemorrhage into the plaque body.

Inflammation and vulnerable plaque

Inflammation is generally present in vulnerable plaque.[10–16] Plaque inflammation typically comprises monocytes, macrophages and lymphocytes that occur not only in the cap (Figure 7.2) but also in the adventitia (Figure 7.3). Macrophages produce tissue degrading enzymes, the matrix metalloproteinases (MMPs) in response to T lymphocyte stimulation.[17–19] While the MMPs degrade collagen in

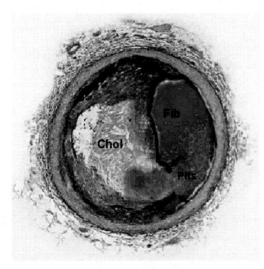

Figure 7.1 Vulnerable plaque (thin-cap atheroma) that ruptured and formed an occlusive thrombus, resulting in myocardial infarction and the unfortunate death of the patient. Note the plaque regions rich in cholesterol (Chol), the regions of cap rupture (arrows) and the occlusive thrombus that has regions rich in fibrin (Fib) and platelets (Plts). (Reproduced with permission. Photomicrograph courtesy of Dr William Edwards, Rochester, MN.)

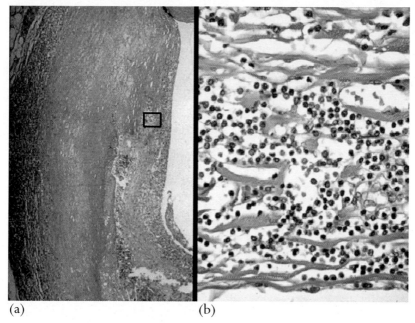

(a)   (b)

Figure 7.2 (a,b) Vulnerable plaque showing an inflammatory component present in the shoulder region of the cap. The inflammation is typically rich in lymphocytes and monocytes/macrophages. (Reproduced with permission from Dr William Edwards, MN.)

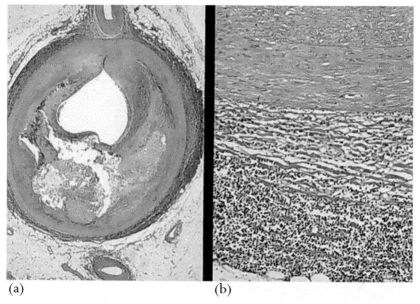

(a)   (b)

Figure 7.3 (a,b) Inflammation in a vulnerable plaque occurring in the adventitia. In this case the inflammatory response is highly lymphocytic. (Reproduced with permission. Photomicrograph courtesy of Dr William Edwards, Rochester, MN.)

127

plaque, T lymphocytes produce interferon which simultaneously inhibits collagen synthesis.

Counterbalancing these degradative processes are smooth muscle cells within plaque that produce interstitial collagen, strengthening the fibrous cap. Calcium can also be part of the vulnerable plaque, contrary to prevailing opinion that calcification occurs only with stable, older plaque (Figure 7.4). Platelet-derived growth factor (PDGF) and transforming growth factor (TGF)-β also occur in these plaques and both increase collagen production. Collagen synthesis and degradation constitute counterbalancing forces in plaque architecture. Fibrous caps that progressively thin suggest a disequilibrium in the balance between collagen and matrix synthesis, favoring degradation. This equilibrium is not yet fully characterized for atherosclerotic plaque.

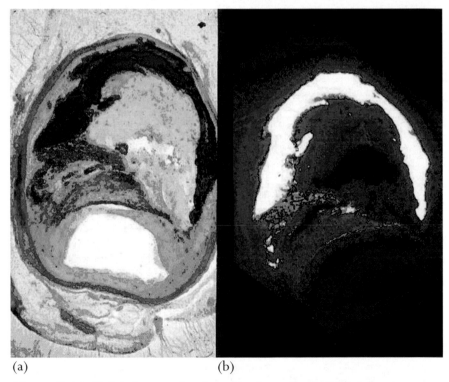

(a) (b)

Figure 7.4 (a,b) *Calcification of a plaque that has a densely lipid-rich region. Interestingly, the calcification does not encompass the luminal side of this plaque, which has a thin cap. Examples such as this dispel the view that plaque calcification necessarily implies stability. (Reproduced with permission of J Interv Cardiol 2003;16:231–42.[131])*

Detection and diagnosis of vulnerable plaque

Detecting vulnerable plaque is complicated for several reasons. Imaging and physiologically based detection modalities are under extensive evaluation and described elsewhere in this book. As we learn to reliably detect early vulnerable plaque, clinicians will soon confront problems arising from imperfect test performance and low prevalence populations. Imperfect diagnostic tests for fixed CAD include treadmill, nuclear, and echocardiographically based evaluation.[20,21] Diagnostic test performance improves proportionally to disease prevalence.[21,22] Sensitivity (true positive tests/subjects with disease) and specificity (true negatives/subjects without disease) are prevalence independent, while positive and negative predictive values (PPV, true positive tests/all positive tests; NPV, true negative tests/all negative tests) are prevalence dependent.[23] Detecting vulnerable plaque is initially complicated. The low disease prevalence of high-risk subjects in the general population amplifies the diagnostic problems for vulnerable plaque. No test as yet has high sensitivity or specificity (prevalence independent parameters), so diagnostic errors are high, with many false positives and negatives (prevalence dependent parameters). Thus identification of markers permitting highly sensitive and specific detection is needed. Such a marker is the pathophysiologic equivalent of troponin -T, troponin-I, and CK-MB (creatine kinase-myocardial band), all highly sensitive and specific for myocardial infarction (MI).

Risk stratification: the progressive Bayesian diagnostic strategy

Vulnerable plaque detection strategies may be based on tissue characterization for lipid content, or may detect plaque physiologic features such as temperature deviation caused by plaque inflammation. Although future methods may be non-invasive, current methods require physical proximity to artery and plaque. Invasive methods are time consuming, expensive, inconvenient and carry a small patient risk. These limitations make invasive screening impossible to apply to the general population, for both ethical and economic reasons.

High-risk patients should undergo catheterization for definitive invasive testing but several diagnostic steps must be applied to the general population to exclude high false positive and negative rates and derive a high-risk patient.[22] Such non-invasive tests may be applied sequentially, each test making a further decision for the next test in the sequence. This serial testing strategy, although imperfect, progressively segments the population and isolates a high-risk subset. The non-invasive Bayesian approach yields a high-risk patient group for further, invasive evaluation. The strategy concentrates cardiovascular event risk by sequential, serial test application, beginning with non-invasive examinations. Blood (or urine) measurements and non-invasive imaging such as nuclear scintigraphy, cardiac magnetic resonance (CMR) or rapid computed tomography are potential methods applicable to low-probability populations.

Detecting vulnerable plaque using peripheral blood

This chapter discusses several candidate markers, available in peripheral blood, that may singly or in combination identify healthy populations or patients at risk for new or recurrent sudden cardiovascular events. They may be useful, separately or together, to concentrate risk for vulnerable plaque, helping justify new treatment strategies for specific individuals.

The peripheral detection paradigm for vulnerable plaque finds substances that leave the plaque, enter the bloodstream and are detected peripherally. Alternatively, vulnerable plaque induces unique cell types (see below) or cytokines which appear in the peripheral blood of affected patients. Regardless, peripheral molecules may find use separately or together for identifying vulnerable plaques by a simple peripheral blood measurement.

Epidemiologic patient data are evolving using molecules in peripheral blood that elevate future events, creating the vulnerable patient. Several candidate markers are available in peripheral blood that may singly or in combination identify patients at high cardiovascular risk. 'Minor' plaque ruptures may precede or follow a clinically evident acute coronary event. ACS studies suggest circulating molecules that partially differentiate ruptured from stable plaque (unstable syndromes), stable angina and healthy controls.

LDL and oxLDL

Fewer than 50% of patients with ACS have elevated lipids. Thus, cholesterol and lipid measurement alone are poor markers to predict patients at risk of sudden vascular events.

The relation between lipids and inflammatory markers was reported by Engstrom et al who showed that high plasma cholesterol levels are associated with five separate inflammation-sensitive plasma proteins (fibrinogen, α-1 antitrypsin, haptoglobin, ceruloplasmin, and orosomucoid).[24] When elevated in hypercholesterolemic states these markers showed increased stroke and MI risk, while hypercholesterolemia without elevation of these markers showed no increased risk.[24]

While lipid oxidation is generally understood in the context of atherogenesis, the clinical importance of circulating oxidized low-density lipoprotein (oxLDL) is poorly understood. Until recently oxLDL was thought to be absent from the circulation, since no method could detect circulating oxLDL levels. Specific immunoassays now find circulating oxLDL in normal human plasma.

Many studies have demonstrated elevated oxLDL in the plasma of CAD patients.[25,26] These findings occur not only in symptomatic patients but also in subclinical atherosclerosis.[27]

Ehara and colleagues demonstrated significantly elevated plasma oxLDL levels in patients with ACS compared with control groups.[28] They also showed that oxLDL levels correlated with the severity of clinical presentation. Patients with acute MI had the highest levels, followed by those with unstable angina and finally those with stable angina. Kyoko simultaneously studied plaque pathology and circulating levels of molecules by classifying carotid plaque as macrophage-rich or macrophage-poor. Macrophage-rich plaque had higher plaque rupture rates, fibrous cap thinning, intraplaque hemorrhage, and bigger lipid cores than macrophage-poor plaque. Patients with macrophage-rich plaques had oxLDL levels significantly higher than controls. This suggested that plasma oxLDL levels correlate with macrophage infiltration and confer vulnerability and rupture in atherosclerotic lesions.

Acute phase reactants

Several molecules such as C-reactive protein (CRP), serum amyloid A, or fibrinogen are elevated in inflammation, infection, trauma, ischemia and in non-specific inflammatory disorders. They are thus sensitive inflammation molecules, but have low specificity for coronary artery inflammation.

Acute phase responses are induced by cytokines released from affected tissues. These cytokines stimulate the liver to synthesize acute phase proteins such as CRP. Since atherosclerosis is an inflammatory disease, circulating acute phase reactants are both expected and found.

C-reactive protein

CRP is a member of the pentraxin protein family, and is an acute phase reactant produced in the liver.[29] It is expressed by inflammatory macrophages in the lungs and brain.[30–32] CRP is partially regulated by interleukin (IL)-6, a cytokine also the subject of recent clinical interest.[33–35] It is a sensitive marker of inflammation and the high sensitivity C-reactive protein (hs-CRP) assay detects very low circulating CRP levels.

Atherosclerotic plaque contains CRP, generally associated with complement and macrophages or foam cells.[36] CRP was previously considered an indirect measure of vascular inflammation, with no direct involvement in the inflammatory process. Newer studies suggest CRP is directly implicated in atherosclerotic plaque formation.[10,37,38] CRP binds complement C1q, causing complement activation.[37] It co-localizes with complement membrane attack complexes in immature atherosclerotic lesions.[12] CRP stimulates macrophages to synthesize IL-6, IL-1β, and tumor necrosis factor (TNF)-α, all pro-inflammatory molecules.[39] CRP may also induce vascular cell adhesion molecule (VCAM)-1

131

and intercellular adhesion molecule (ICAM)-1 expression in endothelial cells.[40] CRP opsonization of LDL mediates LDL uptake by macrophages.[41]

Many studies now confirm CRP is an independent risk factor for atherosclerotic vascular disease (Figure 7.5).[42–46] Patients in the highest circulating hs-CRP quartile typically have a 1.5-fold or greater relative risk for symptomatic atherosclerosis compared to normals.[29,47] Baseline CRP correlates with future myocardial infarction and stroke risk.[47] Women with low serum cholesterol (LDL <130 mg/dl) but elevated CRP are at higher coronary event risk.[34,48] Other studies show comparable results for men and peripheral vascular disease.[34,49]

Although hs-CRP elevations correlate with ACS highlighting the importance of inflammation in atherosclerotic lesions, few micro-morphologic studies correlate serum CRP levels with histopathologic findings.[29,32,37,50] High hs-CRP levels suggest poor prognosis in unstable angina with more death, MI, and revascularization.[51–53]

Cell adhesion molecules

Monocyte recruitment into arteries and lesion-prone sites is regulated by the cell adhesion molecules (CAMs). These are expressed on endothelial cell surfaces in

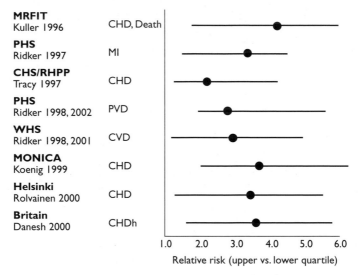

Figure 7.5 *Prospective studies of high-sensitivity C-reactive protein as a risk factor for future vascular disease. CHD, coronary heart disease; MRFIT, Multiple Risk Factor Intervention Trial; PHS, Physicians' Health Study; CHS/RHPP, Cardiovascular Health Study and the Rural Health Promotion Project; WHS, Women's Health Study; PVD, pulmonary vascular disease; CVD, cardiovascular disease; MONICA, Monitoring Trends and Determinants in Cardiovascular Disease. (Adapted with permission from Ridker.[38] See also references 127–130.)*

response to inflammatory stimuli, and CAMs play a fundamental role in both initiation and progression of atherosclerotic lesions. They may also have a role in ACS. Unstable coronary syndromes typically involve interactions between platelets, endothelium and leukocytes, with thrombus formation at atherosclerotic plaques. Soluble CAMs (sCAMs) are shed from cell surfaces and so can be studied in peripheral blood. P-selectin, E-selectin, ICAM-1 and VCAM-1 are the best known molecules of this family.

The Physicians' Health Study evaluated more than 14 000 healthy men and showed baseline sICAM-1 correlated with cardiovascular risk.[54] Subjects in the highest sICAM-1 quartile had 1.8 times the risk of those in the lowest quartile. ICAM abnormalities may occur early in atherosclerosis and in patients destined for MI as follow-up time was a key event correlate in this study. ICAM-1 also exhibited independent coronary risk in the Atherosclerosis Risk in Communities (ARIC) study.[55] Baseline VCAM-1 showed no relationship to cardiac events, suggesting that different adhesion molecules likely play diverse roles in vulnerable plaque pathogenesis and rupture.[56] This is reflected in a study examining human atherosclerotic vascular lesions finding ICAM-1 in endothelium and macrophages, but substantially fewer lesions with VCAM positivity. VCAM-1 occurred mainly in spindle cells.[57]

Soluble P-selectin predicted cardiac risk in healthy women in the Women's Health Study (WHS).[49] Mean P-selectin was elevated in women destined for cardiac events. Women in the highest P-selectin quartile had double the risk of those in the lowest quartile. This was unrelated to other cardiac risk factors.

Among the soluble adhesion molecules in studies of ACS, P-selectin is increased in patients with unstable coronary syndromes.[58–62] P-selectin is typically increased, unlike other molecules which may or may not be elevated.

Parker et al found plasma soluble P-selectin levels were independent predictors for unstable coronary syndromes and predicted adverse prognosis.[63] The basis of these results likely involves thrombin, the principal mediator of thrombus formation. Thrombin is important since it relates to a rapidly induced expression of membrane-bound P-selectin on the surface of platelet and endothelial cells. These results have been confirmed in other studies. Plasma adhesion molecules such as sICAM are increased in patients with unstable angina compared with patients with stable angina or controls.[64] Unlike P-selectin, other CAM studies found no consistent results although some demonstrate significant differences.

Monocyte chemoattractant protein-1 and macrophage colony stimulating factor

Monocyte chemoattractant protein-1 (MCP-1) and macrophage colony stimulating factor (MCSF) play important roles in recruiting and activating monocytes, and likely relate to stable and unstable atherosclerosis. Patients with unstable angina have significantly higher levels of plasma MCSF and MCP-1 than those with stable angina or control subjects, and are higher in patients with unstable angina and ischemia at rest.[65,66] Additionally, elevated macrophage colony stimulating factor levels predict worse inhospital prognosis in unstable angina.[67]

CD40 ligand

CD40 ligand (CD40L) is a transmembrane protein structurally related to TNF-α, identified on CD4+ T cells and activated platelets.[68] The interaction of both membrane-bound and soluble (s)CD40L forms with its receptor (CD40, constitutively expressed on B cells, macrophages, endothelial cells, and vascular smooth muscle cells) promotes expression of a diverse set of atherogenic molecules including cytokines, matrix metalloproteinases, adhesion molecules and tissue factor.

Elevated soluble and membrane-bound CD40L levels have been significantly elevated in unstable angina patients.[69] Soluable CD40L is also associated with increased cardiovascular risk in apparently healthy women.[70]

Interleukins

Interleukins are involved in several inflammatory processes associated with ACS. IL-1 and IL-6 are two prototypic proinflammatory cytokines: IL-1 elicits IL-6 production, increases gene expression for clotting factors and inhibitors of fibrinolysis, increases endothelial adhesion molecule expression and IL-8 production. IL-1α is expressed on the surface of activated macrophages[71,72] as a biologically active molecule, and IL-1β is released from activated platelets.[73–76] IL-6 is prominent early in focal inflammation. It has stimulatory effects on T and B lymphocytes, induces fibrinogen synthesis and is the principal initiator of hepatocyte CRP expression.[77]

The Physicians' Health Study showed higher IL-6 levels in healthy men destined for MI.[56] The risk for MI was proportional to IL-6 plasma levels, and men in the top quartile had 2.3 times the risk of the lowest quartile. CRP correlated best with IL-6 in this study (R = 0.4).

In patients with unstable angina elevated IL-1β and IL-6 serum levels were associated with poor prognosis.[65,78,79] IL-6 is an independent risk factor even after adjusting for CRP plasma level. IL-1 and IL-6 receptor upregulation measured 48 hours after hospital admission for ACS correlated with a complicated hospital course.[80] Other interleukins such as IL-18 (the interferon-γ inducing factor) are increased in patients with ACS and correlate with the severity of myocardial dysfunction.[81]

Although proinflammatory cytokines play a role in ACS few studies have directly implicated anti-inflammatory cytokines in this setting. IL-10 is an anti-inflammatory cytokine, produced by lymphocytes of the Th2 subtype and also by

134

macrophages. It is a major inhibitor of cytokine synthesis, suppressing macrophage function and inhibiting proinflammatory cytokine production. Smith et al found that patients with unstable angina had significantly lower serum IL-10 concentrations[82] than did patients with chronic stable angina.

Matrix metalloproteinases

Atherosclerotic pathophysiology is a process of continual change. While thrombus, matrix synthesis and fibrosis are building plaque volume, other processes are eroding and remodeling the plaque architecture in continuous counterbalance. Excessive extracellular matrix degradation may be a major molecular mechanism for plaque rupture, and MMPs are principal molecules responsible for this degradation. Notably, inflammatory mediators such as TNF-α and IL-1 upregulate MMP activity in macrophages, and this interaction may represent a pathogenic link between persistent immune activation and the development of plaque rupture.

The MMPs are endopeptidases that degrade virtually all extracellular matrix components.[17,19,83] Their function is not limited to degrading extracellular matrix components. Other important non-matrix MMP substrates include molecules whose biologic activity is regulated by MMP processing, such as TNF-α,[84] growth factors and their receptors,[85] plasminogen and its activators[86,87] and endothelin.[88]

MMPs comprise a large family of extracellular enzymes. Twenty-four MMPs have been characterized. These are classified in groups (Table 7.1). These enzymes have both a descriptive name (e.g. interstitial collagenase, an enzyme found in the interstitial space, degrading fibrillar collagens) and an MMP number. Although the numbering system recognizes up to MMP-24, the nomenclature does not accurately reflect the actual number of enzymes, since MMP-4, MMP-5, and MMP-6 have been eliminated as a result of duplication.

Because of their precise function, MMP activity is regulated at multiple levels. The MMP genes are transcriptionally responsive to a wide variety of oncogenes, growth factors, cytokines and hormones. MMPs are secreted proteins and are membrane-bound as inactive zymogens, although membrane type (MT)-MMPs, unlike the other members of the MMP family, are not secreted. They contain a transmembrane domain but remain attached to cell surfaces. Inactive zymogens require proteolytic processing[89] to release the catalytically active enzyme. This processing can be achieved by other MMPs (e.g. stromelysin-1 may activate procollagenase) or by other proteases (e.g. plasmin activation of prostromelysin). Also, although not all MT-MMPs are fully characterized, there is strong evidence that one function is to localize and activate secreted MMPs.

Some control mechanisms involve blocking enzyme activity. This is accomplished by interaction with one of the physiologic MMP inhibitors: the circulating general protease inhibitor α-2-macroglobulin or the tissue-localized

Table 7.1 Substrate-based classification of matrix metalloproteinases (MMPs)

MMP family	Enzyme		
	Mechanism of action	No.	Principal substrates
Collagenases	Interstitial collagenase	MMP-1	Fibrillar collagens types I, II, III
	Neutrophil collagenase	MMP-8	
	Collagenase-3	MMP-13	
	Xenopus collagenase	MMP-18	
Gelatinases	Gelatinase A	MMP-2	Non-fibrillar collagens types IV, V
	Gelatinase B	MMP-9	
Stromelysins	Stromelysin-1	MMP-3	Proteoglycans, laminin, fibronectin, non-fibrillar collagens
	Stromelysin-2	MMP-10	
	Matrilysin	MMP-7	
	Stromelysin-3	MMP-11	
Elastase	Metalloelastase	MMP-12	Serine protease inhibitors
Membrane type			
MT1-MMP		MMP-14	Elastin, non-fibrillar collagen
MT2-MMP		MMP-15	Progelatinase A, undefined
MT3-MMP		MMP-16	
MT4-MMP		MMP-17	
MT5-MMP		MMP-21	
		MMP-20	
Unclassified	Enamelysin	MMP-19	Undefined
		MMP-23	
		MMP-24	

tissue inhibitors of metalloproteinases (TIMPs). The resultant MMP–inhibitor complex is inactive and unable to bind the substrate.

All MMPs can be inhibited by a number of different TIMP proteins, and there are four known members of the TIMP family. Proteolytic activation and the potential for inhibition by TIMPs indicate that detection of MMP overexpression may not always indicate increased enzyme activity.

Several MMPs (including MT-MMPs)[90] have been identified in atherosclerotic plaque. Resident macrophage-derived foam cells have been identified as a major source of MMPs, although to a lesser extent smooth muscle and endothelial cells can also produce these. Mechanisms implicated in MMP expression are lipid ingestion, stimulation by oxLDL, cytokines (like TNF-α or IL-1),[91–95] and hemodynamic stress.[96]

Several studies have examined MMPs in human atherosclerotic plaques and compared them with the normal artery. Galis and colleagues studied interstitial collagenase (MMP-1), gelatinases A and B (MMP-2 and -9) and stromelysin-1 (MMP-3) in plaque.[19] Normal vessels stained for gelatinase, while macrophage-rich regions showed gelatinase, stromelysin, and interstitial collagenase. Because MMP overexpression does not establish their catalytic capacity, these authors also studied whether atheroma contained matrix-degradation capacity. The plaques exhibited gelatinolytic and caseinolytic activity while the normal vessel did not.

In vulnerable plaque there is strong MMP activity, principally at the plaque shoulders and sites of foam cell accumulation.[97]

Brown analyzed human coronary atherectomy specimens and revealed active MMP-9 synthesis by macrophages and smooth muscle cells in patients with unstable angina compared with stable angina, suggesting the role of this specific MMP in ACS. MMPs occur in atheromatous plaques and can be detected in peripheral blood. Thus in stable CAD significantly higher MMP-9 and TIMP-1 levels,[98] and significantly lower levels of MMP-2, MMP-3 and TIMP-2 were found compared with controls.

In patients with ACS Inokubo et al found MMP-9 and TIMP-1 levels were significantly higher than controls, although they were measured in samples from the great cardiac vein and aorta.[99] Interestingly, when measuring aortic levels no differences emerged. High peripheral blood levels of MMP-2 and MMP-9 occurred in patients with ACS compared with stable angina and controls, raising the interesting possibility of new non-invasive tests of plaque vulnerability.[100]

A new marker for vulnerable plaque: pregnancy associated plasma protein

Conover and colleagues recently identified a novel insulin-like growth factor (IGF)-dependent IGF binding protein (BP)-4 protease, and found it to be homologous with pregnancy-associated plasma protein-A (PAPP-A).[101–104] PAPP-A cleaves IGFBP-4 and releases free IGF-I. PAPP-A is an IGF-dependent IGFBP-4 protease expressed in the media and neointima of coronary arteries after experimental angioplasty.

We recently detected PAPP-A in unstable plaques from sudden cardiac death patients (Figure 7.6), and found that circulating PAPP-A levels were increased in patients suffering unstable angina and acute MI.[105,106] This study also examined free IGF-I, total IGF-I, and high sensitivity CRP and found PAPP-A expression in macrophages, smooth muscle cells and extracellular matrix in ruptured and eroded unstable coronary plaques from sudden cardiac death patients. Little to no PAPP-A occurred in stable plaques by comparison.

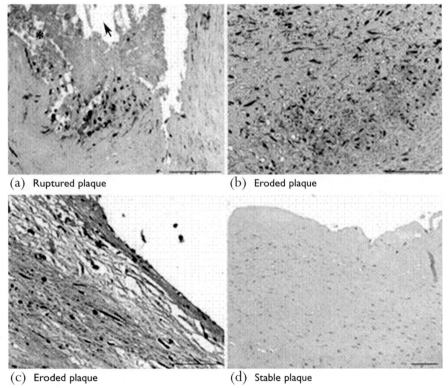

(a) Ruptured plaque   (b) Eroded plaque

(c) Eroded plaque   (d) Stable plaque

Figure 7.6 Immunohistochemical expression of pregnancy-associated plasma protein A (PAPP-A) in unstable and stable coronary atherosclerotic plaques. (a) PAPP-A expression in the inflamed shoulder region of a vulnerable plaque that ruptured. The inflammatory infiltrate is present between the cholesterol core (arrowhead) and the luminal thrombus (asterisk). (b) Immunohistochemically detectable PAPP-A within smooth muscle cells and extracellular matrix of an eroded plaque. (c) PAPP-A non-eroded endothelial cells of an eroded plaque and (d) no PAPP-A staining in a typical fibrotic region of stable plaque. (Reproduced with permission from Pidker.[38])

Circulating PAPP-A levels were significantly elevated in patients with ACS (unstable angina and acute MI). No sex differences were observed for PAPP-A among the four groups studied. Diabetic patients exhibited no differences in PAPP-A levels compared to non-diabetic patients and PAPP-A did not correlate with angiographic coronary artery disease extent. This reflects the coexistence of quiescent atherosclerotic plaques in the coronary artery tree with active, vulnerable or fissured plaques. PAPP-A in concentrations of 10 mIU/l or more was associated with ACS, at 89% sensitivity and 78% specificity.

There was also an association between PAPP-A and free IGF-I. The recent identification of PAPP-A as the digestive enzyme of IGF BP-4, an inhibitor of IGF action, suggests that PAPP-A may function to release free IGF-I, thus contributing to the progression of both coronary atherosclerosis and restenosis. The free fraction of circulating and locally synthesized IGF-I induces vascular smooth muscle cell migration, and is important for monocyte chemotaxis, activation and cytokine release within the atherosclerotic lesion.

White blood cells: detection of inflammatory processes using peripheral blood

As evident in this chapter, vulnerable plaque is associated with local and systemic activation of the immune system. This systemic activation is reflected not only by inflammatory markers. Activated peripheral cells are increased in patients with unstable coronary syndromes. Thus, such activated cells can be systematically detected,[107,108] raising the possibility that systemic inflammation may reflect and potentially drive plaque instability. Thus activated monocytes, neutrophils and lymphocytes can be detected in ACS.

Sabatine et al demonstrated elevated white blood cells in a simple blood test of patients with ACS.[109] They were associated with impaired epicardial and myocardial perfusion, more extensive CAD, and higher 6-month mortality.

Because the macrophage is integral to the inflammatory process, its activity and presence has been proposed to indicate vascular inflammation. To date, little research has focused on this strategy. Measuring monocyte membrane fluidity and soluble CD14 (a cellular activation marker), Zalai et al detected high levels of circulating activated monocytes having increased invasive capacity in patients with unstable angina.[110]

Marked neutrophil activation is observed by measuring neutrophil myeloperoxidase content,[107] and can be detected in the peripheral blood of patients with unstable angina, but not in those with stable angina, variant angina or in controls.

More work has been done evaluating peripherally detectable lymphocytes in this role. Neri Serneri et al detected a transient burst of T cell activation in patients with unstable angina.[111] Liuzzo and colleagues examined T lymphocytes and cytokine production in patients with stable or unstable angina.[112,113] T lymphocytes producing cytokines (CD4+ and CD8+) were quantified. Unstable angina patients had CD4+ and CD8+ T lymphocytes producing IFN-γ. This T cell population remained at the 12-week (3-month) time point and the study suggests that unstable angina may result from a distinct T cell population, with enhanced IFN-γ production. This is consistent with the concept that T cells promote monocyte activation and the acute phase response. IFN-γ is elevated as it is produced by CD4+ CD28(null) T cells, expanded in unstable angina patients. Patients with stable angina served as controls and had normal IFN-γ and lower CD4+ CD28(null) levels (10.8% in unstable angina versus 1.5% in controls). These studies suggest that unstable plaque contains a specific T-cell clone, and may be involved in plaque rupture and erosion from the inflammation. Unstable angina may thus have one or more monoclonal T cell populations, similar to monoclonal gammopathy of undetermined significance (MGUS).[53,112,113]

Antigenic stimulation may cause T cell activation, to date an unresolved question. Studies suggest that *Chlamydia*, herpes virus, and more recently heat shock proteins may be part of the antigenic stimulus in ACS.[114–117]

Inflammatory markers and atherosclerotic plaque burden

A serum marker for atherosclerotic disease extent does not exist. Such a marker would be useful to clinically determine whether a patient has the atherosclerotic process, and whether or not the disease is actively forming plaque. Parker et al showed soluble E-selectin level was associated with extent of atherosclerosis.[63]

Peter and colleagues showed that sICAM-1 correlated with peripheral arterial disease extent. Soluble VCAM-1 relates to atherosclerosis extent in patients with peripheral arterial disease.[118]

CRP, IL-6, sICAM-1 and sVCAM-1 were evaluated in the Rotterdam Study to determine their relationship to disease severity.[119] Of these markers, CRP and IL-6 were *inversely* related to ankle-arm indices and CRP correlated weakly with carotid intima-media thickness. Associations with markers other than CRP are less clear and have not been well studied.

The search for such a marker may be important not only to better diagnose those patients with fixed, stenotic disease, but also those who are at risk of acute clinical syndromes from arterial thrombosis.

140

Summary

The above studies suggest that non-invasive tests may some day accurately detect plaque vulnerability. Findings in both epidemiologic studies and in ACS reflect different manifestations of CAD and may also represent a new pathway or triggering of destabilization in human atheroma, though morphologic plaque studies are needed. Because no vulnerable test yet has high sensitivity or specificity, using multiple markers simultaneously may augment these.

Several molecules might be helpful as non-invasive markers of vulnerable plaque or high-risk individuals. In ACS, we could use the molecules associated with worse prognoses, to decide the next steps in the clinical evaluation.

The search to identify the vulnerable patient continues optimistically but slowly. Low prevalence of high-risk subjects in the general population amplifies the diagnostic problem. Since no test yet has high sensitivity and specificity, diagnostic errors are high, with many false positives and negatives.

Enhanced diagnostic methods will eventually permit accurate finding and treatment of vulnerable patients and their disease. Identification of substances with high sensitivity and specificity is badly needed. Such a marker, as stated before, is the pathophysiologic equivalent of troponin -T, troponin-I and CK-MB, all highly sensitive and specific for MI.

The inflammatory markers above could identify vascular lesions at risk for causing these syndromes, but much work remains to develop successful application of this strategy.

Many asymptomatic, apparently healthy adults have one or more plaques with features suggesting vulnerability. Even if we can identify such a plaque as vulnerable, we cannot yet determine if it will or will not produce clinical problems. Definitive epidemiologic studies must thus establish which plaque features carry high risk, and should define which patients should receive intervention to prevent cardiovascular catastrophies. The key diagnostic challenge will be to determine which of such plaques will be problematic.

Further studies are required to better elucidate the role of these molecules as markers of the vulnerable patient. Many questions remain open including:

1. What is the cause of these peripherally detectable molecules?

   Is it infectious disease, cardiovascular risk factors, or an autoimmune disease?

   Is it localized in the coronary tree or is it systemic?

2. What is the source and target of these peripheral molecules?

   Could they be released directly from ruptured or permeable plaques, or from ischemic injury due to damaged cell membranes (either acutely or after reperfusion) or even remote non-atherosclerotic inflammatory sources?

The CRP plasma level is the best known gauge for risk in patients with stable or unstable angina,[52,53,122,123] long term after MI,[124] and in patients undergoing revascularization therapies.[125] One study showed the only independent cardiovascular risk indicators using multivariate, age-adjusted and traditional risk analysis were CRP and total/HDL cholesterol ratio. If CRP, IL-6, and ICAM-1 levels are added to lipid levels, risk assessment can be improved.[126]

While it is clear that elevated CRP denotes increased risk and emerging evidence suggests that there are novel therapies that result in lowering of CRP, the most important unanswered question is whether suppression of inflammation and consequent lowering of CRP will translate into a decrease in clinical events. Surprisingly, despite the importance of the question, the 'inflammation hypothesis' of CRP suppression compared with standard care has not yet been tested. Such a prospective study of patients with established cardiovascular disease and elevated baseline CRP in which incremental pharmacotherapy would be guided by reassessments of the CRP marker could allow formulation of a rational therapeutic strategy instead of an approach of 'polypharmacy' for every patient.

References

1. Virmani R, Kolodgie FD, Burke AP, Farb A, Schwartz SM. Lessons from sudden coronary death: a comprehensive morphological classification scheme for atherosclerotic lesions. *Arterioscler Thromb Vasc Biol* 2000; **20**:1262–75.

2. Yusuf S, Reddy S, Ounpuu S, Anand S. Global burden of cardiovascular diseases: part II: variations in cardiovascular disease by specific ethnic groups and geographic regions and prevention strategies. *Circulation* 2001; **104**:2855–64.

3. Yusuf S, Reddy S, Ounpuu S, Anand S. Global burden of cardiovascular diseases: part I: general considerations, the epidemiologic transition, risk factors, and impact of urbanization. *Circulation* 2001; **104**:2746–53.

4. Muller JE, Abela GS, Nesto RW, Tofler GH. Triggers, acute risk factors and vulnerable plaques: the lexicon of a new frontier. *J Am Coll Cardiol* 1994; **23**:809–13.

5. Virmani R, Burke AP, Farb A. Coronary risk factors and plaque morphology in men with coronary disease who died suddenly. *N Engl J Med* 1997; **336**:1276–82.

6. Kolodgie FD, Burke AP, Farb A et al. The thin-cap fibroatheroma: a type of vulnerable plaque: the major precursor lesion to acute coronary syndromes. *Curr Opin Cardiol* 2001; **16**:285–92.

7. Virmani R, Burke AP, Farb A, Kolodgie FD. Pathology of the unstable plaque. *Prog Cardiovasc Dis* 2002; **44**:349–56.

8. Farb A, Burke AP, Tang AL et al. Coronary plaque erosion without rupture into a lipid core: a frequent cause of coronary thrombosis in sudden coronary death. *Circulation* 1996; **93**:1354–63.

9. Burke AP, Kolodgie FD, Farb A, Weber D, Virmani R. Morphological predictors of arterial remodeling in coronary atherosclerosis. *Circulation* 2002; **105**:297–303.

10. Blake GJ and Ridker PM. Novel clinical markers of vascular wall inflammation. *Circ Res* 2001; **89**:763–71.

11. Chae CU, Lee RT, Rifai N, Ridker PM. Blood pressure and inflammation in apparently healthy men. *Hypertension* 2001; **38**:399–403.

12. Blake GJ, Ridker PM. Inflammatory mechanisms in atherosclerosis: from laboratory evidence to clinical application. *Ital Heart J* 2001; **2**:796–800.

13. Ridker PM. Inflammation, atherosclerosis, and cardiovascular risk: an epidemiologic view. *Blood Coagul Fibrinolysis* 1999; **10(Suppl 1)**:S9–12.

14. Mulvihill NT, Foley JB. Inflammation in acute coronary syndromes. *Heart* 2002; **87**:201–4.

15. Libby P, Ridker PM, Maseri A. Inflammation and atherosclerosis. *Circulation* 2002; **105**:1135–43.

16. Glurich I, Grossi S, Albini B et al. Systemic inflammation in cardiovascular and periodontal disease: comparative study. *Clin Diagn Lab Immunol* 2002; **9**:425–32.

17. Celentano DC, Frishman WH. Matrix metalloproteinases and coronary artery disease: a novel therapeutic target. *J Clin Pharmacol* 1997; **37**:991–1000.

18. Shah PK, Falk E, Badimon JJ et al. Human monocyte-derived macrophages induce collagen breakdown in fibrous caps of atherosclerotic plaques. Potential role of matrix-degrading metalloproteinases and implications for plaque rupture. *Circulation* 1995; **92**:1565–9.

19. Galis ZS, Sukhova GK, Lark MW, Libby P. Increased expression of matrix metalloproteinases and matrix degrading activity in vulnerable regions of human atherosclerotic plaques. *J Clin Invest* 1994; **94**:2493–503.

20. Diamond GA. Reverend Bayes' silent majority. An alternative factor affecting sensitivity and specificity of exercise electrocardiography. *Am J Cardiol* 1986; **57**:1175–80.

21. Morise AP, Diamond GA. Comparison of the sensitivity and specificity of exercise electrocardiography in biased and unbiased populations of men and women. *Am Heart J* 1995; **130**:741–7.

22. Hachamovitch R, Berman DS, Shaw LJ et al. Incremental prognostic value of myocardial perfusion single photon emission computed tomography for the prediction of cardiac death: differential stratification for risk of cardiac death and myocardial infarction. *Circulation* 1998; **97**:535–43.

23. Schwartz RS, Jackson WG, Celio PV, Richardson LA, Hickman JR Jr. Accuracy of exercise 201Tl myocardial scintigraphy in asymptomatic young men. *Circulation* 1993; **87**:165–72.

24. Engstrom G, Lind P, Hedblad B et al. Effects of cholesterol and inflammation-sensitive plasma proteins on incidence of myocardial infarction and stroke in men. *Circulation* 2002; **105**:2632–7.

25. Holvoet P, Vanhaecke J, Janssens S, Van de Werf F, Collen D. Oxidized LDL and malondialdehyde-modified LDL in patients with acute coronary syndromes and stable coronary artery disease. *Circulation* 1998; **98**:1487–94.

26. Toshima S, Hasegawa A, Kurabayashi M et al. Circulating oxidized low density lipoprotein levels. A biochemical risk marker for coronary heart disease. *Arterioscler Thromb Vasc Biol* 2000; **20**:2243–7.

27. Hulthe J, Fagerberg B. Circulating oxidized LDL is associated with subclinical atherosclerosis development and inflammatory cytokines (AIR Study). *Arterioscler Thromb Vasc Biol* 2002; **22**:1162.

28. Ehara S, Ueda M, Naruko T et al. Elevated levels of oxidized low density lipoprotein show a positive correlation with the severity of acute coronary syndromes. *Circulation* 2001; **103**:1955–60.

29. Westhuyzen J, Healy H. Review: biology and relevance of C-reactive protein in cardiovascular and renal disease. *Ann Clin Lab Sci* 2000; **30**:133–43.

30. Dong Q, Wright J. Expression of C-reactive protein by alveolar macrophages. *J Immunol* 1996; **156**:4815–20.

31. Gould JM, Weiser JN. Expression of C-reactive protein in the human respiratory *Infect Immun* 2001; **69**:1747–54.

32. Yasojima K, Schwab C, McGeer EG, McGeer PL. Generation of C-reactive protein and complement components in atherosclerotic plaques. *Am J Pathol* 2001; **158**:1039–51.

33. Stenvinkel P, Barany P, Heimburger O, Pecoits-Filho R, Lindholm B. Mortality, malnutrition, and atherosclerosis in ESRD: What is the role of interleukin-6? *Kidney Int* 2002; **61 (Suppl 80)**:103–8.

34. Rifai N, Buring JE, Lee IM, Manson JE, Ridker PM. Is C-reactive protein specific for vascular disease in women? *Ann Intern Med* 2002; **136**:529–33.

35. Reuben DB, Ferrucci L, Wallace R et al. The prognostic value of serum albumin in healthy older persons with low and high serum interleukin-6 (IL-6) levels. *J Am Geriatr Soc* 2000; **48**:1404–7.

36. Torzewski M, Rist C, Mortensen RF et al. C-reactive protein in the arterial intima: role of C-reactive protein receptor-dependent monocyte recruitment in atherogenesis. *Arterioscler Thromb Vasc Biol* 2000; **20**:2094–9.

37. Burke AP, Tracy RP, Kolodgie F et al. Elevated C-reactive protein values and atherosclerosis in sudden coronary death: association with different pathologies. *Circulation* 2002; **105**:2019–23.

38. Ridker PM. High-sensitivity C-reactive protein: potential adjunct for global risk assessment in the primary prevention of cardiovascular disease. *Circulation* 2001; **103**:1813–18.

39. Torzewski J, Torzewski M, Bowyer DE et al. C-Reactive protein frequently colocalizes with the terminal complement complex in the intima of early atherosclerotic lesions of human coronary arteries. *Arterioscler Thromb Vasc Biol* 1998; **18**:1386–92.

40. Pasceri V, Willerson JT, Yeh ETH. Direct proinflammatory effect of C-reactive protein on human endothelial cells. *Circulation* 2000, **102**:2165–8.

41. Zwaka TP, Hombach V, Torzewski J. C-reactive protein-mediated low density lipoprotein uptake by macrophages: implications for atherosclerosis. *Circulation* 2001; **103**:1194–7.

42. Zebrack JS, Muhlestein JB, Horne BD, Anderson JL, Intermountain Heart Collaboration Study Group. C-reactive protein and angiographic coronary artery disease: independent and additive predictors of risk in subjects with angina. *J Am Coll Cardiol* 2002; **39**:632–7.

43. Morrow DA, Ridker PM. C-reactive protein, inflammation, and coronary risk. *Med Clin North Am* 2000; **84**:149–61, ix.

44. Haverkate F, Thompson SG, Pyke SD, Gallimore JR, Pepys MB. Production of C-reactive protein and risk of coronary events in stable and unstable angina. European Concerted Action on Thrombosis and Disabilities Angina Pectoris Study Group. *Lancet* 1997; **349**:462–6.

45. Koenig W, Sund M, Frohlich M et al. C-reactive protein, a sensitive marker of inflammation, predicts future risk of coronary heart disease in initially healthy middle-aged men: results from the MONICA (Monitoring Trends and Determinants in Cardiovascular Disease) Augsburg Cohort Study 1984 to 1992. *Circulation* 1999; **99**:237–42.

46. Tracy RP, Lemaitre RN, Psaty BM et al. Relationship of C-reactive protein to risk of cardiovascular disease in the elderly: results from the Cardiovascular Health Study and the Rural Health Promotion Project. *Atheriscler Thromb Vasc Biol* 1997; **17**:1121–7.

47. Ridker PM, Cushman M, Stampfer MJ, Tracy RP, Hennekens CH. Inflammation, aspirin, and the risk of cardiovascular disease in apparently healthy men. *N Engl J Med* 1997; **336**:973–9.

48. Koh KK, Schenke WH, Waclawiw MA, Csako G, Cannon RO 3rd. Statin attenuates increase in C-reactive protein during estrogen replacement therapy in postmenopausal women. *Circulation* 2002; **105**:1531–3.

49. Albert MA, Rifai N, Ridker PM. Plasma levels of cystatin-C and mannose binding protein are not associated with risk of developing systemic atherosclerosis. *Vasc Med* 2001; **6**:145–9.

50. Ridker PM, Cushman M, Stampfer MJ, Tracy RP, Hennekens CH. Plasma concentration of C-reactive protein and risk of developing peripheral vascular disease. *Circulation* 1998; **97**:425–8.

51. Tomoda H, Aoki N. Prognostic value of C-reactive protein levels within six hours after the onset of acute myocardial infarction. *Am Heart J* 2000; **140**:324–8.

52. Heeschen C, Hamm CW, Bruemmer J, Simoons ML. Predictive value of C-reactive protein and troponin T in patients with unstable angina: a comparative analysis. CAPTURE Investigators. Chimeric c7E3 AntiPlatelet Therapy in Unstable angina REfractory to standard treatment trial. *J Am Coll Cardiol* 2000; **35**:1535–42.

53. Liuzzo G, Biasucci LM, Gallimore JR et al. The prognostic value of C-reactive protein and serum amyloid A protein in severe unstable angina. *N Engl J Med* 1994; **331**:417–24.

54. Ridker PM, Rifai N, Stampfer MJ, Hennekens CH. Plasma concentration of interleukin-6 and the risk of future myocardial infarction among apparently healthy men. *Circulation* 2000; **101**:1767–72.

55. Hwang SJ, Ballantyne CM, Sharrett AR et al. Circulating adhesion molecules VCAM-1, ICAM-1, and E-selectin in carotid atherosclerosis and incident coronary heart disease cases: the Atherosclerosis Risk In Communities (ARIC) Study. *Circulation* 1997; **96**:4219–25.

56. de Lemos JA, Hennekens CH, Ridker PM. Plasma concentration of soluble vascular cell adhesion molecule-1 and subsequent cardiovascular risk. *J Am Coll Cardiol* 2000; **36**:423–6.

57. Davies MJ, Gordon JL, Gearing AJ et al. The expression of the adhesion molecules ICAM-1, VCAM-1, PECAM, and E-selectin in human atherosclerosis. *J Pathol* 1993; **171**:223–9.

58. Shyu KG, Chang H, Lin CC, Kuan P. Circulating intercellular adhesion molecule-1 and E-selectin in patients with acute coronary syndrome. *Chest* 1996; **109**:1627–30.

59. Galvani M, Ferrini D, Ottani F et al. Soluble E-selectin is not a marker of unstable coronary plaque in serum of patients with ischemic heart disease. *J Thromb Thrombolysis* 2000; **9**:53–60.

60. Ogawa HYH, Miyao Y et al. Plasma soluble intercellular adhesion molecule-1 levels in coronary circulation in patients with unstable angina. *Am J Cardiol* 1999; **83**:38–42.

61. Ghaisas NK, S C, Foley B et al. Elevated levels of circulating soluble adhesion molecules in peripheral blood of patients with unstable angina. *Am J Cardiol* 1997; **80**:617–9.

62. Ikeda H, Takajo Y, Ichiki K et al. Increased soluble form of P-selectin in patients with unstable angina. *Circulation* 1995; **92**:1693–6.

63. Parker C III, Vita JA, Freedman JE. Soluble adhesion molecules and unstable coronary artery disease. *Atherosclerosis* 2001; **156**:417–24.

64. Atalar E, Aytemir K, Haznedaroglu I et al.Increased plasma levels of soluble selectins in patients with unstable angina. *Int J Cardiol* 2001; **78**:69–73.

65. Hojo Y, Ikeda U, Takahashi M, Shimada K. Increased levels of monocyte-related cytokines in patients with unstable angina. *Atherosclerosis* 2002; **161**:403–8.

66. Mazzone A, De Servi S, Mazzucchelli I et al. Increased concentrations of inflammatory mediators in unstable angina: correlation with serum troponin T. *Heart* 2001; **85**:571–5.

67. Rallidis LS, Thomaidis KP, Zolindaki MG, Velissaridou AH, Papasteriadis EG. Elevated concentrations of macrophage colony stimulating factor predict worse in-hospital prognosis in unstable angina. *Heart* 2001; **86**:92.

68. Henn V, Slupsky JR, Grafe M et al. CD40 ligand on activated platelets triggers an inflammatory reaction of endothelial cells. *Nature* 1998; **391**:591–4.

69. Aukrust P, Muller F, Ueland T et al. Enhanced levels of soluble and membrane-bound CD40 ligand in patients with unstable angina. Possible reflection of T lymphocyte and platelet involvement in the pathogenesis of acute coronary syndromes. *Circulation* 1999; **100**:614–20.

70. Schonbeck U, Varo N, Libby P, Buring J, Ridker PM. Soluble CD-40L and cardiovascular risk in women. *Circulation* 2001; **104**:2266–8.

71. Brody DT, Durum SK. Membrane IL-1: IL-1 alpha precursor binds to the plasma membrane via a lectin-like interaction. *J Immunol* 1989; **143**:1183–7.

72. Kurt-Jones EA, Beller DI, Mizel SB, Unanue ER. Identification of a membrane-associated interleukin 1 in macrophages. *Proc Natl Acad Sci USA* 1985, **82**.204–8.

73. Kaplanski G, Porat R, Aiura K et al. Activated platelets induce endothelial secretion of interleukin-8 in vitro via an interleukin-1-mediated event. *Blood* 1993; **81**:2492–5.

74. Hawrylowicz CM, Santoro SA, Platt FM, Unanue ER. Activated platelets express IL-1 activity. *J Immunol* 1989; **143**:4015–18.

75. Hawrylowicz CM, Howells GL, Feldmann M. Platelet-derived interleukin 1 induces human endothelial adhesion molecule expression and cytokine production. *J Exp Med* 1991; **174**:785–90.

76. Dinarello CA. Biologic basis for interleukin-1 in disease. *Blood* 1996; **87**:2095–147.

77. Heinrich PC, Castell JV, Andus T. Interleukin-6 and the acute phase response. *Biochem J* 1990; **265**:621–36.

78. Simon AD, Yazdani S, Wang W, Schwartz A, Rabbani LE. Circulating levels of IL-1beta, a prothrombotic cytokine, are elevated in unstable angina versus stable angina. *J Thromb Thrombolysis* 2000; **9**:217–22.

79. Biasucci LM, Vitelli A, Liuzzo G et al. Elevated levels of interleukin-6 in unstable angina. *Circulation* 1996; **94**:874–7.

80. Biasucci LM, Liuzzo G, Fantuzzi G et al. Increasing levels of interleukin (IL)-1Ra and IL-6 during the first 2 days of hospitalization in unstable angina are associated with increased risk of in-hospital coronary events. *Circulation* 1999; **99**:2079–84.

81. Mallat Z, Henry P, Fressonnet R et al. Increased plasma concentrations of interleukin-18 in acute coronary syndromes. *Heart* 2002; **88**:467–9.

82. Smith DA, Irving SD, Sheldon J, Cole D, Kaski JC. Serum levels of the antiinflammatory cytokine interleukin-10 are decreased in patients with unstable angina. *Circulation* 2001; **104**:746–9.

83. Nagase H. Activation mechanisms of matrix metalloproteinases. *Biol Chem* 1997; **378**:151–60.

84. Gearing AJ, Beckett P, Christodoulou M et al. Matrix metalloproteinases and processing of pro-TNF-alpha. *J Leukoc Biol* 1995; **57**:774–7.

85. Levi E, Fridman R, Miao HQ et al. Matrix metalloproteinase 2 releases active soluble ectodomain of fibroblast growth factor receptor 1. *Proc Natl Acad Sci USA* 1996; **93**:7069–74.

86. Lijnen HR, Ugwu F, Bini A, Collen D. Generation of an angiostatin-like fragment from plasminogen by stromelysin-1 (MMP-3). *Biochemistry* 1998; **37**:4699–702.

87. Ugwu F, Van Hoef B, Bini A, Collen D, Lijnen HR. Proteolytic cleavage of urokinase-type plasminogen activator by stromelysin-1 (MMP-3). *Biochemistry* 1998; **1998**:7231–6.

88. Fernandez-Patron C, Radomski MW, Davidge ST. Vascular matrix metalloproteinase-2 cleaves big endothelin-1 yielding a novel vasoconstrictor. *Circ Res* 1999; **85**:906–11.

89. Knauper V, Murphy G. Membrane-type matrix metalloproteinases and cell surface-associated activation cascades for matrix metalloproteinases. In: Parks W, Mecham R eds. *Matrix Metalloproteinases*. San Diego, CA: Academic Press, 1998; 199–218.

90. Uzui HM, Harpf A, Liu M et al. Increased expression of membrane type 3-matrix metalloproteinase in human atherosclerotic plaque. Role of activated macrophages and inflammatory cytokines. *Circulation* 2002; **106**:3024.

91. Galis ZS, Sukhova GK, Kranzhofer R, Clark S, Libby P. Macrophage foam cells from experimental atheroma constitutively produce matrix-degrading proteinases. *Proc Natl Acad Sci USA* 1995; **92**:402–6.

92. Xu XP, Meisel SR, Ong JM et al. Oxidized low-density lipoprotein regulates matrix metalloproteinase-9 and its tissue inhibitor in human monocyte-derived macrophages. *Circulation* 1999; **99**:993–8.

93. Rajavashisth TB, Liao JK, Galis ZS et al. Inflammatory cytokines and oxidized low density lipoproteins increase endothelial cell expression of membrane type 1-matrix metalloproteinase. *J Biol Chem* 1999; **274**:11924–9.

94. Galis ZS, Muszynski M, Sukhova GK et al. Cytokine-stimulated human vascular smooth muscle cells synthesize a complement of enzymes required for extracellular matrix digestion. *Circ Res* 1994; **75**:181–9.

95. Lee RT, Schoen FJ, Loree HM, Lark MW, Libby P. Circumferential stress and matrix metalloproteinase 1 in human coronary atherosclerosis: implications for plaque rupture. *Arterioscler Thromb Vasc Biol* 1996; **16**:1070–3.

96. Saren P, Welgus HG, Kovanen PT. TNF- and IL-1β selectively induce expression of 92-kDa gelatinase by human macrophages. *J Immunol* 1996; **157**:4159–65.

97. Galis ZS, Sukhova GK, Lark MW, Libby P. Increased expression of matrix metalloproteases and matrix degrading activity in vulnerable regions of human atherosclerotic plaques. *J Clin Invest* 1994; **94**:2493–503.

98. Noji Y, Kajinami K, Kawashiri MA et al. Circulating matrix metalloproteinases and their inhibitors in premature coronary atherosclerosis. *Clin Chem Lab Med* 2001; **39**:380–4.

99. Inokubo Y, Hanada H, Ishizaka H et al. Plasma levels of matrix metalloproteinase-9 and tissue inhibitor of metalloproteinase-1 are increased in the coronary circulation in patients with acute coronary syndrome. *Am Heart J* 2001; **141**:211–7.

100. Kai H, Ikeda H, Yasukawa H et al. Peripheral blood levels of matrix metalloproteases-2 and -9 are elevated in patients with acute coronary syndromes. *J Am Coll Cardiol* 1998; **32**:368–72.

101. Laursen LS, Overgaard MT, Soe R et al. Pregnancy associated plasma protein-A (PAPP-A) cleaves insulin-like growth factor binding protein (IGFBP)-5 independent of IGF: implications for the mechanism of IGFBP-4 proteolysis by PAPP-A. *FEBS Lett* 2001; **504**:36–40.

102. Chen BK, Overgaard MT, Bale LK et al. Molecular regulation of the IGF-binding protein-4 protease system in human fibroblasts: identification of a novel inducible inhibitor. *Endocrinology* 2002; **143**:1199–205.

103. Soe R, Overgaard MT, Thomsen AR et al. Expression of recombinant murine pregnancy-associated plasma protein-A (PAPP-A) and a novel variant (PAPP-Ai) with differential proteolytic activity. *Eur J Biochem* 2002; **269**:2247–56.

104. Giudice LC, Conover CA, Bale L et al. Identification and regulation of the IGFBP-4 protease and its physiological inhibitor in human trophoblasts and endometrial stroma: evidence for paracrine regulation of IGF-II bioavailability in the placental bed during human implantation. *J Clin Endocrinol Metab* 2002; **87**:2359–66.

105. Bayes-Genis A, Conover CA, Overgaard MT et al. Pregnancy-associated plasma protein A as a marker of acute coronary syndromes. *N Engl J Med* 2001; **345**:1022–9.

106. Bayes-Genis A, Schwartz RS, Lewis DA et al. Insulin-like growth factor binding protein-4 protease produced by smooth muscle cells increases in the coronary artery after angioplasty. *Arterioscler Thromb Vasc Biol* 2001; **21**:335–41.

107. Biasucci LM, D'Onofrio G, Liuzzo G et al. Intracellular neutrophil myeloperoxidase is reduced in unstable angina and myocardial infarction, but its reduction is not related to ischemia. *J Am Coll Cardiol* 1996; **27**:611–6.

108. Dinerman JL, Mehta JL, Saldeen TG et al. Increased neutrophil elastase release in unstable angina pectoris and acute myocardial infarction. *J Am Coll Cardiol* 1990; **15**:1559–63.

109. Sabatine MS, Cannon CP, Murphy SA et al. Relationship between baseline white blood cell count and degree of coronary artery disease and mortality in patients with acute coronary syndromes. A TACTICS-TIMI 18 substudy. *J Am Coll Cardiol* 2002; **40**:1761–8.

110. Zalai CV, Kolodziejczyk M, Pilarski L et al. Increased circulating monocyte activation in patients with unstable coronary syndromes. *J Am Coll Cardiol* 2001; **38**:1340–7.

111. Neri Serneri GG, Prisco D, Martini F et al. Acute T-cell activation is detectable in unstable angina. *Circulation* 1997; **95**:1806–12.

112. Liuzzo G, Goronzy JJ, Yang H et al. Monoclonal T-cell proliferation and plaque instability in acute coronary syndromes. *Circulation* 2000; **101**:2883–8.

113. Liuzzo G, Kopecky SL, Frye RL et al. Perturbation of the T-cell repertoire in patients with unstable angina. *Circulation* 1999; **100**:2135–9.

114. Bobryshev YV, Lord RS. Expression of heat shock protein-70 by dendritic cells in the arterial intima and its potential significance in atherogenesis. *J Vasc Surg* 2002; **35**:368–75.

115. Ciervo A, Visca P, Petrucca A et al. Antibodies to 60-kilodalton heat shock protein and outer membrane protein 2 of *Chlamydia pneumoniae* in patients with coronary heart disease. *Clin Diagn Lab Immunol* 2002; **9**:66–74.

116. Kanwar RK, Kanwar JR, Wang D, Ormrod DJ, Krissansen GW. Temporal expression of heat shock proteins 60 and 70 at lesion-prone sites during atherogenesis in ApoE-deficient mice. *Arterioscler Thromb Vasc Biol* 2001; **21**:1991–7.

117. Wick G, Perschinka H, Millonig G. Atherosclerosis as an autoimmune disease: an update. *Trends Immunol* 2001; **22**:665–9.

118. Peter K, Nawroth P, Conradt C et al. Circulating vascular cell adhesion molecule-1 correlates with the extent of human atherosclerosis in contrast to circulating intercellular adhesion molecule-1, E-selectin, P-selectin, and thrombomodulin. *Arterioscler Thromb Vasc Biol* 1997; **17**:505–12.

119. van der Meer IM, de Maat MP, Bots ML et al. Inflammatory mediators and cell adhesion molecules as indicators of severity of atherosclerosis: the Rotterdam Study. *Arterioscler Thromb Vasc Biol* 2002; **22**:838–42.

120. Sabatine MS, Morrow DA, de Lemos JA et al. Multimarker approach to risk stratification in non-ST elevation acute coronary syndromes: simultaneous assessment of troponin I, C-reactive protein, and B-type natriuretic peptide. *Circulation* 2002; **105**:1760–3.

121. Morrow DA, Rifai N, Antman EM et al. C-reactive protein is a potent predictor of mortality independently of and in combination with troponin T in acute coronary syndromes: a TIMI 11A substudy. Thrombolysis in Myocardial Infarction. *J Am Coll Cardiol* 1998; **31**:1460–5.

122. Biasucci LM, Liuzzo G, Grillo RL et al. Elevated levels of C-reactive protein at discharge in patients with unstable angina predict recurrent instability. *Circulation* 1999; **99**:855–60.

123. Toss H, Lindahl B, Siegbahn A, Wallentin L. Prognostic influence of increased fibrinogen and C-reactive protein levels in unstable coronary artery disease. *Circulation* 1997; **96**:4204–10.

124. Ridker PM, Rifai N, Pfeffer MA et al. Inflammation, pravastatin, and the risk of coronary events after myocardial infarction in patients with average cholesterol levels. *Circulation* 1998; **98**:839–44.

125. Chew DP, Bhatt DL, Robbins MA et al. Incremental prognostic value of elevated baseline C-reactive protein among established markers of risk in percutaneous coronary intervention. *Circulation* 2001; **104**:992–7.

126. Ridker PM, Stampfer MJ, Rifai N. et al. Novel risk factors for systemic atherosclerosis: a comparison of C-reactive protein, fibrinogen, homocysteine, lipoprotein(a), and standard cholesterol screening as predictors of peripheral arterial disease. *JAMA* 2001; **285**:2481–5.

127. Kuller LH, Tracy RP, Shaten J, Meilahn EN. Relation of C-reactive protein and coronary heart disease in the MRFIT nested case–control study. Multiple Risk Factor Intervention Trial. *Am J Epidemiol* 1996; **144**:537–47.

128. Danesh J, Whincup P, Walker M et al. Low grade inflammation and coronary heart disease: prospective study and updated meta-analyses. *BMJ* 2000; **321**:199–204.

129. Roivainen M, Viik-Kajander M, Palosuo T et al. Infections, inflammation, and the risk of coronary heart disease. *Circulation* 2000; **101**:252–7.

130. Mendall MA, Patel P, Ballam L, Strachan D, Northfield TC. C Reactive protein and its relation to cardiovascular risk factors: a population based cross sectional study. *BMJ* 1996; **312**:1061–5.

131. Schwartz RS, Bayes-Genis A, Lesser JR et al. Detecting vulnerable plaque using peripheral blood: inflammatory and cellular markers. *J Interv Cardiol* 2003; **16**:231–42.

8. EMERGING ANIMAL MODELS OF THE VULNERABLE PLAQUE

Andrew J Carter and Wei Wei

Urgent demand for vulnerable plaque animal models

Plaque rupture is now recognized as a critical aspect of atherosclerosis progression inciting fatal acute myocardial infarctions (MIs) and/or sudden cardiac deaths,[1-6] the most fearful complications of coronary artery disease. As a result, investigations of mechanisms underlying plaque rupture and acute coronary syndromes have shifted toward plaque composition, vulnerability and thrombogenicity rather than plaque size and stenosis severity, thus defining the components of the vulnerable atherosclerotic plaque.[1-5] Because of the significant clinical importance, vulnerable plaque remains a critical target for investigation to identify effective diagnostic and therapeutic strategies to prevent plaque rupture.

An understanding of critical biologic events responsible for the transition from an asymptomatic stable atheroma to ruptured plaque is essential to develop effective strategies to prevent a potentially fatal acute coronary syndrome (ACS). Human clinical observations provide rich soil for making hypotheses, but for obvious ethical reasons our ability to investigate plaque biology in man is very limited. Cell culture is a convenient way to address specific questions, but it lacks complexity of a disease substrate thus limiting the scope of testable hypotheses. Experimental models may offer the opportunity to evaluate the complexities of atheroma progression in a controlled setting. Traditional animal models of atherosclerosis recapitulate initial lesion formation and progression, but only a few exhibit the features of plaque erosion/rupture and thrombosis commonly observed in human coronary atherosclerosis. The ideal animal model of vulnerable plaque should be representative of a human disease and at the same time be easy to manipulate. The purpose of this chapter is to review the emerging models of plaque rupture with particular attention to its relevance in human coronary atheroma progression.

What is vulnerable plaque?

The results from recent studies have proposed the following histopathologic (Figure 8.1) and clinical criteria for the definition of vulnerable plaque:

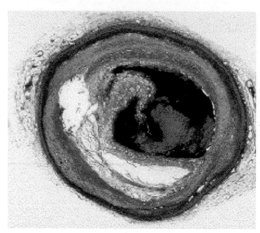

Figure 8.1 *Photomicrograph of plaque rupture of the epicardial coronary artery, demonstrating a rupture of the shoulder region of the plaque with a luminal thrombus. (Adapted with permission from AP Burke et al.* N Engl J Med *1997; 336:1276–82.[2])*

Major criteria
- Active inflammation (monocyte/macrophage infiltration).[6]
- Thin cap with large lipid core (these plaques have a cap thickness of <100 μ and a lipid core that accounts for >40% of the plaque's total area (volume).[7]
- Endothelial denudation with superficial platelet aggregation.[1]
- Fissured/wounded plaque.[1]

Minor criteria
- Superficial calcified nodule.[1]
- Yellow color (on angioscopy) – yellowish plaques.[8]
- Intraplaque hemorrhage.[1,2]
- Critical stenosis.[9]
- Endothelial dysfunction.[10]

Proposed standards for a vulnerable plaque animal model
1. The model simulates human coronary artery disease (CAD) with components of plaque progression, i.e. erosion, rupture, thrombosis.
2. The model is readily accessible, reproducible and amenable to phenotypic manipulation of the experimental system.
3. The model provides new insight into pathogenic mechanisms.[11]
4. The model facilitates translation of new insights of mechanisms/therapies into clinically relevant strategies.[11]

Limitation of traditional atherosclerosis models

Atherosclerotic plaque was traditionally induced by a high-cholesterol diet or by mechanical balloon injury of the artery, or by a combination of the two.[12–17] The main disadvantages of the traditional atherosclerotic model are (i) the low yield of triggering of plaque rupture and thrombosis, and (ii) most of the lesions in the model do not pathologically simulate the features of vulnerable plaque in humans. Instead, the plaque was relatively stable and intact (Figure 8.2 and Table 8.1).

Several investigators have attempted to develop mechanical or pharmacologic triggers for plaque rupture in rabbit models of accelerated atherosclerosis. In a rabbit model, hypercholesterolemia and mechanical arterial wall injury can produce plaques vulnerable to disruption and thrombosis by potent vasoactive substances such as Russell's viper venom and histamine (Figure 8.3), whereas

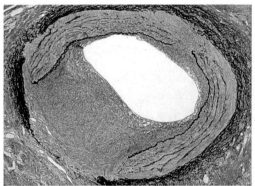

Figure 8.2 *Representative stable, intact plaque in an animal model. The plaque is characterized by a dense collection of smooth muscle cells and matrix protein with a layer of endothelial cells. This fibrocellular plaque lacks lipid accumulation, collagen cap, thrombosis and intraplaque hemorrhage.*

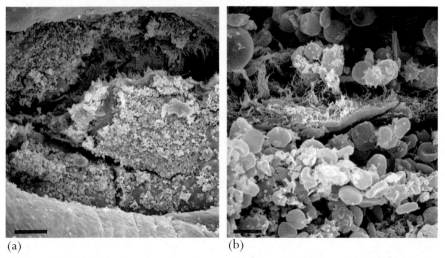

(a)   (b)

Figure 8.3 *(a) Scanning electron micrograph of ulcerated lesion at iliac bifurcation, with a small amount of thrombotic material forming at the ulcer base, from a rabbit treated with Russell viper venom (bar represents 50 μm). (b) Scanning electron micrograph at higher magnification of the same lesion, showing further detail of thrombus with red blood cells attached to fibrin strands organizing in the base of the ulcer (bar represents 10 μm). (Adapted with permission from GS Abela et al.* Circulation *1995;* **91**:*776–84.*[13]*)*

Table 8.1 Limitations of traditional atherosclerosis (AS) animal model for evaluation of vulnerable plaque

Model	Artery	Mode of AS induction	Limitation
Porcine[14,15]	Coronary	Balloon injury/high-cholesterol diet	Stable plaque; no thrombosis; no lipid accumulation in the plaque; devoid of fibrin
Porcine[18]	Peripheral (iliac/femoral)	High-cholesterol diet + balloon injury	Homogeneous stable plaque type, no calcified material
Rabbit[12,13]	Aorta/iliac/femoral	High-cholesterol diet/balloon injury	No fissured collagen cap; intact plaque, low yield of triggering; long preparatory period (8 months)
Primate[16,17]	Coronary	High-cholesterol diet	No plaque rupture, ulceration, hemorrhage, or thrombosis

Table 8.2 Comparison of rabbit vulnerable plaque models

	Plaque rupture inducer	Rupture triggering rate	Thrombosis	Endothelium denudation	Plaque fissure	Treatment period	Neoangiogenesis
Pharmacologic[12,13]	Intraplaque balloon	Low	+	(–)	(–)	Long (8 months)	(–)
Mechanical[19]	RVV + histamine	High, at will	+	+	+	Short (1 month)	+

+, reported/detected as present; (–), reported as not detected; RVV, Russell's viper venom.

normal arteries were relatively resistant to triggering. Histamine is an arterial vasoconstrictor in rabbits that induces spasm. Russell's viper venom contains proteases that activate factors V and X and is a direct endothelial toxin.[12] In the situation of Russell's viper venom administration, the endothelial function is compromised in its role as a thrombosis-resistant surface over a long period (Table 8.2).

Despite the limitation, the traditional atherosclerotic model may be adapted to evaluate the biology of vulnerable plaque by administration of potent vasoactive substances that triggers plaque rupture and formation of platelet-rich thrombi. Given the important role of inflammation in vulnerable plaque formation, the extrinsic use of an endothelial toxin such as Russell's viper venom can be potential for future model studies of systemic or local therapies to prevent plaque rupture.

Modern vulnerable plaque models

Recently emerging animal models produced by transgenic techniques combined with new concepts about the vulnerable plaque are available to reproduce almost all features of human atherosclerosis in various metabolic milieu such as hypercholesterolemia, diabetes, hypertension, insulin resistance, etc.

Mouse model

ApoE−/− mouse

The apolipoprotein E knockout (ApoE−/−) mouse is an established model of hypercholesterolemia and atherosclerotic lesion development.[20–24] Until recently, the incidence of plaque rupture had been noticed in brachiocephalic artery in ApoE−/− mice with long periods of high-fat feeding (Table 8.3).[20–24] Johnson and Jackson characterized the histologic features of atheroma formation in C57:129 homozygous ApoE knockout mice on a diet supplemented with 21% lard, 0.15% cholesterol implemented at 6–8 weeks of age.[22] The detailed histopathologic analysis (Figure 8.4) of atheroma formation in these ApoE knockout mice is summarized below.

Similarity between the ApoE−/− mouse and humans

Lipid core: An increase in lipid core size has been linked to vulnerability of human plaques.[1–3] Davies[4] and Davies and Thomas[5] reported an average core fractional volume of 56.7% in acutely ruptured plaques associated with thrombosis. In the ApoE knockout mouse model,[22] ruptured plaques in brachiocephalic arteries had a lipid content of 50.7±2.2%, which was significantly greater than the 35.9±3.0% lipid content of intact plaques.

Fibrous cap: Loss of the fibrous cap correlates with plaque rupture in human lesions.[1] Similarly, thinning and loss of the fibrous cap occurs frequently in the

Table 8.3 Summary of vulnerable plaque characteristics in ApoE knockout (ApoE–/–) mice

Model	Active Inflammation	Thin cap with large lipid core	Endothelial denudation with superficial platelet aggregation	Fissured/wounded plaque	Comments
ApoE–/– [22-24]	NR	++	(–)	++	No platelet-rich fibrin thrombi; long treatment period >6 months
ApoE–/–/ LDLR–/– [25]	NR	+++	(–)	+++	Slightly ↑ LDL cholesterol; low rate of triggering.
ApoE–/–/SR-BI–/– [26]	NR	++++	++	++++	↑VLDL; fibrin deposit; repetitive MI; severe cardiac dysfunction; short preparatory time
ApoE–/–/p53 transgenic [27]	NR	++++	+++	++++	Apoptosis of VSMCs; little fibrin-rich platelet clots
ApoE–/–/Gulo–/– [28]	NR	++++	(–)	+++	↓ Neovascularization

+, reported/detected as present; (–), reported as not detected; NR, not reported; LDL, low-density lipoprotein; VLDL, very-low density lipoprotein; MI, myocardial infarction; VSMC, vascular smooth muscle cell; ApoE, apolipoprotein E.

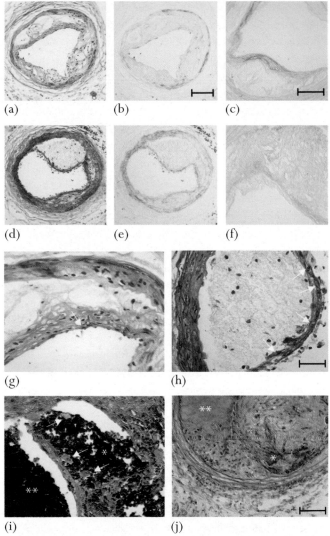

Figure 8.4 *Representative vulnerable plaque in the carotid artery of ApoE−/−/p53 gene transfer mice. Anti-α smooth muscle actin (brown) and Masson's trichrome (collagen=blue) were applied for plaque staining. Compared to the control Ad5-CMV.lacZ (a, b, c, h and g), Ad5-CMV.p53-treated plaques reveal a thinner cap because of decreased collagen content (d); a paradoxical increase of α-smooth muscle actin staining (e); and a significantly decreased cap collagen content confirmed by picrosirius red staining (f, × 200 and g, × 400). Plaque disruption was observed in Ad5-CMV.p53-incubated plaques: (i) Spontaneous cap rupture, leading to intraplaque hemorrhage (*), lumen occlusion by thrombosis (**), and phagocytosis of erythrocytes by macrophages (arrows), (j) intraplaque hemorrhage (*) and thrombosis (**) after injection of phenylephrine. (Adapted with permission from von der Thüsen et al. Circulation 2002; **105**:2064.[46])*

vulnerable plaque compared to the intact plaque in the ApoE knockout mouse model.[23] Johnson and Jackson reported a mean fibrous cap thickness $2.0\pm0.3\,\mu m$ in ruptured lesions.[22] It is noteworthy that the cap thickness observed in the ApoE knockout mouse model is much less than the $23\pm19\,\mu m$ reported for human ruptured coronary artery lesions.[1] These data identify the challenges to compare directly across species because of differences in arterial lumen size and wall thickness and, hence, the tension exerted on the cap. Human coronary arteries are typically 2.4 mm in radius with a wall thickness of 0.76 mm,[29] whereas the mouse brachiocephalic artery is approximately 0.36 mm in radius with a wall thickness of 0.04 mm. Assuming equal arterial blood pressures, it appears that fibrous caps in mouse brachiocephalic artery plaques, as well as being thinner than those overlying human coronary plaques, are subject to stresses that are greater than those encountered by rupturing human coronary artery plaques. This may account for the high frequency of plaque rupture in mouse brachiocephalic arteries.

Plaque development − buried caps: The major finding in a recent study by Williams et al was a significant increase in the number of buried caps in ruptured compared with unruptured lesions,[24] indicating previous rupture in the same plaque. Whether predisposition to frequent rupture is a risk factor for coronary artery disease in humans is not known, but healed ruptures are more frequent in patients who have survived an MI.[30] Animals with shorter inter-rupture intervals would presumably have larger plaques through the process of thrombus incorporation, and they may have thinner caps because the time available for matrix synthesis within the cap is reduced.

Luminal occlusion: The degree of occlusion of the vessel lumen was significantly greater in the arteries with evidence for plaque rupture.[22–24] This is again similar to the situation in human plaques, in which the degree of occlusion of the vessel is greater in acute ruptures than at the site of healed ruptures.[30] In addition, the data from the ApoE knockout mouse[22,23] also suggest that the fibro-fatty nodules may be the result of healing after one or more than one episode of hemorrhage. Lesions of this sort (fibrocalcific nodules) are seen in about 5% of cases of sudden death in humans. The fibrocalcific nodule, like the nodule described in the mouse, can extend completely to the surface. Intriguingly, this lesion in humans is correlated with a loss of lumen caliber.[1,2]

Layered phenotype: Layered lesions could be seen as early as 42 weeks and in most of the 60-week-old animals suggesting multiple events of plaque rupture, stabilization and progression.[22,23] Such layered lesions may be the result of confluence of lateral lesions with the central mass. The layered appearance of the brachiocephalic artery plaques has also been observed in human coronary arteries.[1,30]

Intramural hemorrhage: Up to 75% of all animals aged 30–60 weeks showed intraplaque hemorrhage.[23] The disruption appeared to occur predominantly within the lateral xanthoma and is consistent with similar plaque rupture along the lateral margins in humans. However, it is noted that the presence of intraplaque microvessels may be another possible source of intraplaque hemorrhage.[31]

Dissimilarity between the ApoE−/− mouse and humans

Sudden death: Histological analysis[22,23] shows that the incidence of brachiocephalic artery plaque rupture does not differ between animals that died suddenly (Figure 8.5) and those whose life was terminated at scheduled time points. This suggests that the occurrence of plaque rupture in this vessel is not the cause of sudden death. This is in contrast to the rupture of an atherosclerotic plaque in humans, which is a primary cause of sudden cardiac death, accounting for 60% of all cases of sudden cardiac deaths with thrombosis.[1–5] The cause of sudden death in the ApoE knockout mouse is as yet unknown but could be related to plaque instability in the coronary and/or cerebral circulations. There may be many reasons for this, such as a superior mouse circle of Willis (preventing major stroke) and a lack of involvement (or different behavior) of coronary arteries. In addition, local thrombosis in the plaque may not translate to vessel occlusion due to species-specific rheological factors or regulation of blood coagulation.[32]

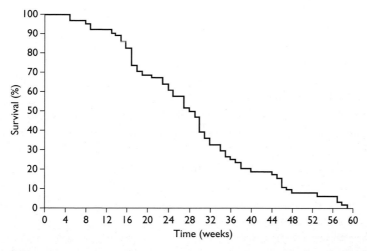

Figure 8.5 *Sudden death in ApoE−/− mice. ApoE−/− mice were fed a high-fat diet (21% lard, 0.15% cholesterol) for up to 14 months. The graph is a survival curve for those animals that died suddenly. Of the 98 mice in the study, 64 died suddenly. (Adapted from Williams et al.* Arterioscler Thromb Vasc Biol *2002; 22:788–92.[24])*

Thrombosis and coagulation within the plaque or at its surface: Occlusive thrombi within the lumen as well as intraplaque thrombi are hallmarks of advanced human lesions.[1–5] Light and electron microscopy failed to demonstrate platelet aggregates or fibrin clots in any of the mice.[32] The lack of thrombosis is surprising in this model, given previous observations that ApoE inhibits platelet aggregation in vitro in response to a variety of agonists[24] and that this effect appears to be receptor-mediated.[25]

Fibrous scarring: Fibrous scarring was seen universally in the brachiocephalic arteries from these mice by 60 weeks of age.[23] The most worrisome difference between the pathology in the mouse and the pathology of human disease is the absence of fibrin formation either within the lesion or within the lumen. The reasons for the paucity of fibrin despite the presence of fibrinogen are not known. However, if fibrin is being formed, it may be removed rapidly by fibrinolysis.[33]

It is also noted that the genetic background of the mice is a possible key determinant of susceptibility to rupture. The extent of atherosclerosis was seven- to nine-fold greater in C57BL/6 mice than in FVB, despite lower total plasma cholesterol levels.[34] Furthermore, 129Sv mice absorb dietary cholesterol more effectively than C57BL/6 mice. Possibly an even more telling difference between these strains is the platelet content of transforming growth factor-β1 (TGF-β1), which is four-fold higher in C57BL/6 mice than in 129Sv mice.[35] It is possible that TGF-β1 protects against rupture by increasing matrix synthesis and decreasing the degree of inflammation within the plaque, and indeed, inhibition of TGF-β1 at the level of its receptor produces an unstable phenotype in the lesions of ApoE knockout mice on a C57BL/6 background.

In summary, in the ApoE–/– mice model, atherosclerotic plaques exhibit many of the features of vulnerable plaque in humans, i.e. such plaques exhibit high lipid volumes, high inflammatory cell and low smooth muscle cell contents, with a relatively thin fibrous cap. The differences in features of the vulnerable plaque between the mouse and humans may be explained by the obvious reasons, e.g. the pathology of a lesion in a 0.3-mm mouse vessel would be different from the pathology of lesions in a 3-mm human coronary artery. The ApoE–/– mouse has demonstrated the most reminiscent of changes of plaque rupture in human vessels in at least three important aspects: (i) the formation of an acellular necrotic core; (ii) the erosion of that mass through to the lumen with its exposure to the lumen; and (iii) the appearance of intraplaque hemorrhage. It is confirmed that the fat-fed ApoE–/– mouse is a reliable and reproducible model of atherosclerotic plaque rupture and that the lesion characteristics in the brachiocephalic artery are similar to those associated with plaque instability in humans.

ApoE−/−/LDLR−/− mouse

The lipoproteins of the ApoE-null mice are unlike those seen in most human atherosclerosis, in which low-density lipoprotein (LDL) elevation is probably the most important contributor to the atherosclerosis. In addition, lipoprotein metabolism in ApoE−/− mice does not closely mirror that of humans with hypercholesterolemia.[20,36] In humans, mutations in the LDL receptor gene cause familial hypercholesterolemia, which in the homozygous form is characterized by markedly elevated total and LDL cholesterol levels and severe, premature atherosclerosis.[37]

In recent studies, LDL receptor knockout (LDLR−/−) mice and ApoE/LDLR double knockout (ApoE−/−/LDLR−/−) mice have been produced as vulnerable plaque models. Despite the characteristics described before, it is noted that the frequency for ApoE−/−/LDLR−/− mice to develop plaque rupture is not significantly higher than the single ApoE−/− mice, e.g. only 3/82 mice developed aortic plaque rupture in Calara et al's recent study.[25] It is assumed that the intrinsic differences in the lipoprotein metabolism of mice and humans limit the relevance and usefulness of these models. For example, in chow-fed mice deficent for LDLR−/−, the levels of LDL cholesterol in the plasma are only slightly elevated and considerable atherosclerotic lesions do not develop.[37]

SR-BI−/−/ApoE−/− mouse

The HDL receptor scavenger receptor class B, type I (SR-BI) genes and ApoE double knockout (SR-BI−/−/ApoE−/−) normally play critical roles in lipoprotein metabolism and can protect mice from atherosclerosis.[20–23,26,38–40] ApoE apparently influences atherosclerosis by mechanisms both independent of, as well as dependent on, its effects on plasma lipoprotein structure and abundance.[26,38,39] Hepatic expression of the high-density lipoprotein (HDL) receptor SR-BI controls HDL structure and metabolism and plays an important role in reverse cholesterol transport (RCT), the transport via HDL of cholesterol from peripheral tissues (including atheromatous plaques) to the liver for recycling or biliary excretion.[38] SR-BI can also mediate cholesterol efflux from cells. SR-BI deficiency doubles plasma cholesterol levels and decreases biliary cholesterol secretion.[39] Combined deficiencies of SR-BI and ApoE profoundly alter lipoprotein metabolism,[39] resulting in decreased biliary cholesterol and increased plasma cholesterol in very low density lipoproteins (VLDL)-sized and in abnormally large HDL-like particles.[39]

Both SR-BI and ApoE mice exhibit morphologic and functional defects with similarities to those seen in human coronary atherosclerosis. When fed a standard chow diet, these hypercholesterolemic animals developed significant atherosclerotic lesions in the aortic sinus as early as 4–5 weeks after birth. It is noted that they also exhibited extensive lipid-rich coronary artery occlusions and spontaneously developed multiple MIs and cardiac dysfunction (e.g. enlarged hearts, reduced ejection fraction and contractility, and ECG abnormalities).[26] The coronary arterial lesions exhibited evidence of cholesterol clefts and extensive fibrin deposition, indicating hemorrhage and clotting, which were strikingly similar to human atherosclerotic plaques. All of the SR-BI−/−/ApoE−/− mice died by 8 weeks of age (50% mortality at 6 weeks). It is a very striking advantage compared to the ApoE−/−/LDLR−/− mice, in which plaque rupture is seen at a later age, more than 42 weeks old in the study by Rosenfeld et al[23] or 9–20 months in the study by Calara et al.[25] Thus, the SR-BI−/−/ApoE−/− mice may be more optimal for vulnerable plaque in a model of acute, synchronous and reproducible rupture in a large proportion of animals.

ApoE−/−/p53 transgenic mouse

The tumor suppressor protein p53 is involved in both cell proliferation and apoptosis.[40,41] p53 is upregulated by various inducers of cellular stress known to be present in an atheromatous setting, including DNA damage, nitric oxide, hypoxia, oxidative stress, and oxidized lipoproteins.[40,41] p53 expression is increased in human atherosclerotic lesions, both in lipid-laden macrophages and vascular smooth muscle cells (VSMCs).[41] Interestingly, VSMCs isolated from atherosclerotic plaques are more susceptible to p53-mediated apoptosis than normal VSMCs. Serum from patients with ACS display a proapoptotic effect on human endothelial cells.[42]

In a study,[27] Ad5-CMV.p53-treated plaques were seen to acquire a phenotype that has been associated with increased vulnerability to rupture. Spontaneous rupture of these predisposed lesions was rare, but administration of a vasopressor compound resulted in evidence of plaque disruption in 40% of the Ad5-CMV.p53-treated vessels. p53-mediated apoptosis likely contributed to plaque rupture by reducing plaque cell number. Alternatively, p53 may induce plaque vulnerability via a decrease in cellular proliferation. The reduction in plaque cellularity is believed to be primarily responsible for the destabilization of the fibrous cap through a proportional decrease in collagen production by cap VSMCs. In addition, p53 may exert a destabilizing effect by selectively eliminating synthetic VSMCs or promoting smooth muscle cell differentiation[41,42] and thus inducing the transition of cap smooth muscle cells from a synthetic to a contractile phenotype. Both processes may lead to the tendency toward a selective elimination of VSMCs or a net increase in (re)differentiated VSMCs.

It is to be noted that the lesions described by von der Thüsen et al[48] evidently exhibited little or no fibrin formation or development of fibrin-rich platelet clots. In that respect, they resemble the unstable lesions in ApoE−/− mice described by Rosenfeld et al[23] and Johnson and Jackson[22] but not those characteristic of ruptured human vulnerable plaques. In addition, due to the complex technique used, this model may be not readily amenable to high-throughput screens.

164

Despite these differences, the ApoE−/−/p53 transgenic mice exhibit substantial similarities to human vulnerable plaque and may provide valuable insights of modulating specific factors influencing plaque stability.[1,2] These transgenic models represent an important advance toward the goal for an efficient and reproducible mouse model of atherosclerosis that exhibits the salient features of spontaneous human plaque rupture.

ApoE−/−/Gulo−/− mouse

Decreased collagen content is associated with the plaque instability.[1–5] L-gulonolactone-γ-oxidase (Gulo) gene knockout (Gulo−/−) mice are dependent on dietary vitamin C. The crossed Gulo−/− mice with ApoE−/− (ApoE−/−/Gulo−/− mice) develop advanced atherosclerotic lesions spontaneously.[20,22,23] Maeda and Nakata's recent study shows that vitamin C deficiency does not alter the initiation or volume of the atherosclerotic plaques but significantly reduces their collagen content, giving them a potentially more vulnerable plaque morphology.[28]

Whether the morphologic features induced by chronic vitamin C deficiency in the Gulo−/−/ApoE−/− mice are sufficient to cause plaque rupture is yet to be determined. Additional changes, such as hemodynamic factors, may well be necessary for even a vulnerable plaque to enter a clinically significant stage. In addition, current clinical and experimental evidence suggest that the best way to influence favorably the balance of collagen synthesis and degradation in atheroma is lipid lowering, not vitamin C.[43] Nevertheless, the vitamin C deficient Gulo−/−/ApoE−/− mice will allow study of genetic and environmental factors that trigger the rupture of plaques that have a high-risk phenotype.

Rat model

Tg[hCETP]DS rat

Epidemiologic studies have demonstrated increased risk of coronary heart disease and its various clinical manifestations with increasing severity of hypertension. The acceleration of atherosclerosis by polygenic (essential) hypertension is well characterized in humans; however, the lack of an animal model that simulates human disease hinders the elucidation of pathogenic mechanisms.

Recently, Herrera et al[44] reported a transgenic atherosclerosis–polygenic hypertension model in Dahl salt-sensitive hypertensive rats that overexpress the human cholesteryl ester transfer protein (Tg[hCETP]DS). It is demonstrated that Tg[hCETP]DS rats have hypertriglyceridemia, hypercholesterolemia and decreased HDL levels when fed regular rat chow; all of these worsen with age. Male Tg[hCETP]DS rats fed regular rat chow showed age-dependent severe combined hyperlipidemia, atherosclerotic lesions, myocardial infarctions and decreased survival, simulating human coronary heart disease. At 6 months of age, early lesions in the coronary artery are eccentric, non-occlusive foam cell and inflammatory-rich lesions. These eccentric lesions progress to culprit plaques at endstage (experimental equivalent of overt CAD) exhibiting features which simulate human 'culprit' plaques of ACS: foam cell rich, thin fibrous caps, paucity of smooth muscle cells, intraplaque hemorrhage, microthrombi, plaque erosion, plaque rupture in macrophage rich areas and occlusive thrombus. Lesion heterogeneity is also observed at endstage, as seen in humans. In addition, in the Tg[hCETP]DS rat model, both VCAM-1 and MCP-1 expression are increased. As VCAM-1 is a potent adhesion molecule in atherosclerosis[6] preceding lesion formation[10] and MCP-1 is an inducer of procoagulant tissue factor in atherosclerosis,[6] persisting endothelial activation through resultant proinflammatory and prothrombotic 'cross-talk' may underlie the exacerbation of atherosclerosis by hypertension. This is consistent with the present hypotheses of ACS in man.[45]

The robust combined hyperlipidemia–coronary heart disease phenotype in Tg[hCETP]DS rats indicates a genetic model that simulates the complexities of hypertension and atherosclerosis in humans. However, critical questions can be addressed in Tg[hCETP]DS rat model, which are not possible in other animal models simply because of its robust CAD phenotype. Therefore, further studies to test whether this model is ideal for vulnerable plaque research is necessary.

JCR:LA-cp rat

Profound insulin resistance is regarded as one of the independent risk factors for CAD. The JCR:LA-cp rat[46] is one of a number of strains that carry the mutant autosomal recessive cp gene. Animals of all strains, that are homozygous for the gene (cp/cp) become obese, insulin resistant, and hypertriglyceridemic. Heterozygous or homozygous normal rats (+/+) are lean and metabolically normal. JCR:LA-cp rats with cp/cp are sensitive to cholesterol in the diet and highly prone to atherosclerosis. The hypertriglyceridemia of the cp/cp rat is due to a marked hepatic hypersecretion of VLDL, but without any increase in the secretion of HDL.

JCR:LA-cp rat[46] shows many similarities to human atherosclerosis such as occluded thrombus, necrotic foam cells, intimal vascular lesions, macrophages adherent to the endothelial surface and increased plasma concentration of plasminogen activator inhibitor-1. Thus, the JCR:LA-cp rat shows the elements of the metabolic syndrome in a very pronounced form. The use of animal models for complex diseases, such as the metabolic syndrome and its pathophysiologic sequelae, is an essential step to unraveling the underlying mechanisms and multiple causative factors. Animal models like the JCR:LA-cp rat may be useful for the study of vulnerable plaque and are also very valuable tools for the development of new pharmaceutical or dietary approaches to prevention and treatment of human disease.

Rabbit model

Recently, a rabbit model in which an atherosclerotic plaque can be ruptured at will was established.[19] An inflatable balloon becomes embedded into the plaque (Figure 8.6). The pressure needed to inflate the plaque-covered balloon was reflected as an index of overall plaque mechanical strength. The thoracic aorta of hypercholesterolemic rabbits underwent mechanical removal of endothelial cells, and then a specially designed balloon catheter was introduced into the lumen of the thoracic aorta. As early as 1 month after catheter placement, atherosclerotic plaque formed around the indwelling balloon (see Table 8.2).

The balloon-associated lesion in the rabbit model is reminiscent of human atherosclerotic plaques[1-6] in terms of architecture (presence of an acellular core and a fibrous cap), cellular composition (smooth muscle cells, macrophages, T cells), growth characteristics (cell proliferation, collagen synthesis) and patterns of lipid accumulation. Morphologic features of disrupted lesions are also suggestive of human atherosclerotic plaque in that the fissures are localized in the shoulder region, associated with the presence of macrophage and smooth muscle cell depletion, and associated with thrombus formation after in vivo disruption. Moreover, neoangiogenesis, an important feature of advanced human lesions relevant to plaque rupture, was observed.

However, the presence of an inflatable balloon within atherosclerotic plaque may comprise the core of this model for examination of events that lead to plaque rupture. Nonetheless, this model may be helpful in accurate imaging and identification of fibrous cap fissures, as well as serial examinations of events after rupture, i.e. thrombus formation and organization.

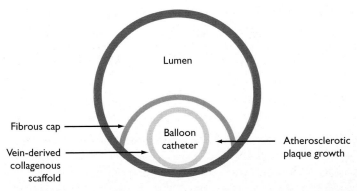

Figure 8.6 *Diagram of the Rekhter-Ryan mechanical plaque rupture model of rabbit thoracic aorta.*

Pig model

Currently, there is no genetic pig model available for vulnerable plaque study. However, due to the similarity of coronary artery size, access, and injury response to human vessels, the pig remains the potential optimal vulnerable plaque model.[18,47] In addition, with the maturation techniques to produce vulnerable plaque in other small animals such as mice and rat, it is optimistic to expect the quick advent of the pig model to better meet the goal to evaluate the detection of vulnerable plaque and pharmacologic intervention.

Summary

The animal model for vulnerable plaque may be the toughest model to mimic the human condition. However, a plethora of experimental approaches are available for growing atherosclerotic lesions in various animal species. Prevention of heart attack depends on detection of vulnerable plaques and development of plaque-stabilizing therapies. In turn, progress in diagnostics and treatment is contingent on our understanding of molecular mechanisms of plaque vulnerability. Hence, it is essential and necessary to develop the proper animal model which will provide such an ideal scaffold for future studies in better understanding of the pathophysiology of plaque vulnerability and rupture, developing new diagnostic methods and therapies.

References

1. Virmani R, Kolodgie FD, Burke AP, Farb A, Schwartz SM. Lessons from sudden coronary death: a comprehensive morphological classification scheme for atherosclerotic lesions. *Arterioscler Thromb Vasc Biol* 2000; **20**:1262–75.

2. Burke AP, Farb A, Malcom GT et al. Coronary risk factors and plaque morphology in men with coronary disease who died suddenly. *N Engl J Med* 1997; **336**:1276–82.

3. Falk E, Shah PK, Fuster V. Coronary plaque disruption. *Circulation* 1995; **92**:657–71.

4. Davies MJ. A macro and micro view of coronary vascular insult in ischemic heart disease. *Circulation* 1990; **82**:II38–46.

5. Davies MJ, Thomas AC. Plaque fissuring: the cause of acute myocardial infarction, sudden ischaemic death, and crescendo angina. *Br Heart J* 1985; **53**:363–73.

6. Shah PK, Falk E, Badimon JJ et al. Human monocyte-derived macrophages induce collagen breakdown in fibrous caps of atherosclerotic plaques. Potential role of matrix-degrading metalloproteinases and implications for plaque rupture. *Circulation* 1995; **92**:1565–9.

7. Kolodgie FD, Burke AP, Farb A et al. The thin-cap fibroatheroma: a type of vulnerable plaque: the major precursor lesion to acute coronary syndromes. *Curr Opin Cardiol* 2001; **16**:285–92.

8. Takano M, Mizuno K, Okamatsu K et al. Mechanical and structural characteristics of vulnerable plaques: analysis by coronary angioscopy and intravascular ultrasound. *J Am Coll Cardiol* 2001; **38**:99–104.

9. Goldstein JA, Demetriou D, Grines CL et al. Multiple complex coronary plaques in patients with acute myocardial infarction. *N Engl J Med* 2000; **343**:915–22.

10. Libby P. Molecular bases of the acute coronary syndromes. *Circulation* 1995; **91**:2844–50.

11. Rekhter MD. How to evaluate plaque vulnerability in animal models of atherosclerosis? *Cardiovasc Res* 2002; **54**:36–41.

12. Constantinides P, Chakravarti RN. Rabbit arterial thrombosis production by systemic procedures. *Arch Pathol* 1961; **72**:197–208.

13. Abela GS, Picon PD, Friedl SE et al. Triggering of plaque disruption and arterial thrombosis in an atherosclerotic rabbit model. *Circulation* 1995; **91**:776–84.

14. Mihaylov D, van Luyn MJ, Rakhorst G. Development of an animal model of selective coronary atherosclerosis. *Coron Artery Dis* 2000; **11**:145–9.

15. Reddick RL, Read MS, Brinkhous KM et al. Coronary atherosclerosis in the pig. Induced plaque injury and platelet response. *Arteriosclerosis* 1990; **10**:541–50.

16. Weingand KW. Atherosclerosis research in cynomolgus monkeys (*Macaca fascicularis*). *Exp Mol Pathol* 1989; **50**:1–15.

17. Stevenson SC, Sawyer JK, Rudel LL. Role of apolipoprotein E on cholesteryl ester-enriched low density lipoprotein particles in coronary artery atherosclerosis of hypercholesterolemic nonhuman primates. *Arterioscler Thromb* 1992; **12**:28–40.

18. de Korte CL, Sierevogel MJ, Mastik F et al. Identification of atherosclerotic plaque components with intravascular ultrasound elastography in vivo: a Yucatan pig study. *Circulation* 2002; **105**:1627–30.

19. Rekhter MD, Hicks GW, Brammer DW et al. Animal model that mimics atherosclerotic plaque rupture. *Circ Res* 1998; **83**:705–13.

20. Zhang SH, Reddick RL, Piedrahita JA, Maeda N. Spontaneous hypercholesterolemia and arterial lesions in mice lacking apolipoprotein E. *Science* 1992; **258**:468–71.

21. Nakashima Y, Plump AS, Raines EW, Breslow JL, Ross R. ApoE deficient mice develop lesions of all phases of atherosclerosis throughout the arterial tree. *Arterioscler Thromb Vasc Biol* 1994; **14**:133–140.

22. Johnson JL, Jackson CL. Atherosclerotic plaque rupture in the apolipoprotein E knockout mouse. *Atherosclerosis* 2001; **154**:399–406.

23. Rosenfeld ME, Polinsky P, Virmani R et al. Advanced atherosclerotic lesions in the innominate artery of the ApoE knockout mouse. *Arterioscler Thromb Vasc Biol* 2000; **20**:2587–92.

24. Williams H, Johnson JL, Carson KGS, Jackson CL. Characteristics of intact and ruptured atherosclerotic plaques in brachiocephalic arteries of apolipoprotein E knockout mice. *Arterioscler Thromb Vasc Biol* 2002; **22**:788–92.

25. Calara F, Silvestre M, Casanada F et al. Spontaneous plaque rupture and secondary thrombosis in apolipoprotein E-deficient and LDL receptor-deficient mice. *J Pathol* 2001; **195**:257–63.

26. Braun A, Trigatti BL, Post MJ et al. Loss of SR-BI expression leads to the early onset of occlusive atherosclerotic coronary artery disease, spontaneous myocardial infarctions, severe cardiac dysfunction, and premature death in apolipoprotein E-deficient mice. *Circ Res* 2002; **90**:270–6.

27. Bennett MR, Littlewood TD, Schwartz SM et al. Increased sensitivity of human vascular smooth muscle cells from atherosclerotic plaques to p53-mediated apoptosis. *Circ Res* 1997; **81**:591–9.

28. Nakata Y, Maeda N. Vulnerable atherosclerotic plaque morphology in apolipoprotein E-deficient mice unable to make ascorbic acid. *Circulation* 2002; **105**:1485–90.

29. Kornowski R, Lansky AJ, Mintz GS et al. Comparison of men versus women in cross-sectional area luminal narrowing, quantity of plaque, presence of calcium in plaque, and lumen location in coronary arteries by intravascular ultrasound in patients with stable angina pectoris. *Am J Cardiol* 1997; **79**:1601–5.

30. Burke AP, Kolodgie FD, Farb A et al. Healed plaque ruptures and sudden coronary death: evidence that subclinical rupture has a role in plaque progression. *Circulation* 2001; **103**:934–40.

31. Moulton KS, Heller E, Konerding MA et al. Angiogenesis inhibitors endostatin or TNP-470 reduce intimal neovascularization and plaque growth in apolipoprotein E-deficient mice. *Circulation* 1999; **99**:1726–32.

32. Bennett MR. Breaking the plaque: evidence for plaque rupture in animal models of atherosclerosis. *Arterioscler Thromb Vasc Biol* 2002; **22**:713–14.

33. Courtman DW, Schwartz SM, Hart CE. Sequential injury of the rabbit abdominal aorta induces intramural coagulation and luminal narrowing independent of intimal mass: extrinsic pathway inhibition eliminates luminal narrowing. *Circ Res* 1998; **82**:996–1006.

34. Dansky HM, Charlton SA, Sikes JL et al. Genetic background determines the extent of atherosclerosis in ApoE-deficient mice. *Arterioscler Thromb Vasc Biol* 1999; **19**:1960–8.

35. Abdelouahed M, Ludlow A, Brunner G, Lawler J. Activation of platelet transforming growth factor β-1 in the absence of thrombospondin-1. *J Biol Chem* 2000; **275**:17933–6.

36. Plump AS, Smith JD, Hayek T et al. Severe hypercholesterolemia and atherosclerosis in apolipoprotein E-deficient mice created by homologous recombination in ES cells. *Cell* 1992; **71**:343–53.

37. Powell-Braxton L, Veniant M, Latvala RD et al. A mouse model of human familial hypercholesterolemia: markedly elevated low density lipoprotein cholesterol levels and severe atherosclerosis on a low-fat chow diet. *Nat Med* 1998; **4**:934–8.

38. Kozarsky KF, Donahee MH, Rigotti A et al. Overexpression of the HDL receptor SR-BI alters plasma HDL and bile cholesterol levels. *Nature* 1997; **387**:414–17.

39. Trigatti B, Rayburn H, Vinals M et al. Influence of the high density lipoprotein receptor SR-BI on reproductive and cardiovascular pathophysiology. *Proc Natl Acad Sci USA* 1999; **96**:9322–7.

40. Ko LJ, Prives C. p53: puzzle and paradigm. *Genes Dev* 1996; **10**:1054–72.

41. Ihling C, Menzel G, Wellens E et al. Topographical association between the cyclin-dependent kinases inhibitor P21, p53 accumulation, and cellular proliferation in human atherosclerotic tissue. *Arterioscler Thromb Vasc Biol* 1997; **17**:2218–24.

42. Valgimigli M, Agnoletti L, Curello S et al. Serum from patients with acute coronary syndromes displays a proapoptotic effect on human endothelial cells: a possible link to pan-coronary syndromes. *Circulation* 2003; **107**:264–70.

43. Libby P, Aikawa M. Vitamin C, collagen, and cracks in the plaque. *Circulation* 2002; **105**:1396–8.

44. Herrera VL, Makrides SC, Xie HX et al. Spontaneous combined hyperlipidemia, coronary heart disease and decreased survival in Dahl salt-sensitive hypertensive rats transgenic for human cholesteryl ester transfer protein. *Nat Med* 1999; **5**:1383–9.

45. Lee RT, Libby P. The unstable atheroma. *Arterioscler Throm Vasc Biol* 1997; **17**:1859–67.

46. Russell JC, Graham SE, Richardson M. Cardiovascular disease in the JCR:LA-cp rat. *Mol Cell Biochem* 1998; **188**:113–26.

47. Fernandez-Ortiz A, Badimon JJ, Falk E et al. Characterization of the relative thrombogenicity of atherosclerotic plaque components: implications for consequences of plaque rupture. *J Am Coll Cardiol* 1994; **23**:1562–9.

48. von der Thusen JH, van Vlijmen BJ, Hoeben R et al. Induction of atherosclerotic plaque rupture in apolipoprotein E−/− mice after adenovirus-mediated transfer of p53. *Circulation* 2002; **105**:2064–70.

9. INTRAVASCULAR THERMOGRAPHY FOR THE DETECTION OF VULNERABLE PLAQUE: SOME LIKE IT HOT!

Mohammad Madjid, Morteza Naghavi, Silvio Litovsky,
S Ward Casscells and James T Willerson[*]

Cardiovascular disease is the principal cause of death in the United States (US) and Europe[1] despite the advent of numerous measures for prevention and control. By 2010, cardiovascular disease will become the leading cause of death throughout the entire world.[2]

The major underlying cause of coronary artery disease (CAD), stroke, and sudden cardiac death is atherosclerosis, which results from a series of complicated, highly specific cellular and molecular responses that can best be described as an inflammatory process.[3] High plasma concentrations of cholesterol, particularly of low-density lipoprotein (LDL) cholesterol, play an important role in atherogenesis. Therefore, this process was long considered to be a degenerative one, largely involving the accumulation of lipids within the arterial wall and the gradual progression of stenosis. Eventually, blood flow would be severely reduced, and a thrombotic event would culminate in an acute coronary syndrome (ACS).

In contrast, the current response-to-injury theory of atherogenesis, developed initially by Virchow[4] and more recently expanded by Ross and Glomset,[5] maintains that inflammation plays a major role in both the initiation and the progression of atherosclerosis, as well as the development of acute clinical complications. According to this theory, atherosclerotic lesions result from an excessive inflammatory-fibroproliferative response to injury of the endothelium and smooth muscle cells of the arterial wall; a large number of growth factors, cytokines, and vasoregulatory molecules contribute to the disease process.[3]

*Potential conflict of interest: Drs Madjid, Naghavi, Casscells and Willerson are shareholders in Volcano Therapeutics, Inc. (Rancho Cordova, CA), a company that develops diagnostic and therapeutic modalities for managing vulnerable plaque.

Anybody may have atherosclerosis

Atherosclerosis begins during the very early years of life. In fact, oxidation of LDL cholesterol and formation of fatty streaks has even been observed at the fetal stage.[6] Enos and associates demonstrated the presence of CAD in young US soldiers (18–25 years old) killed in the Korean War.[7] Similar findings were later observed during autopsies of young soldiers killed in Vietnam.[8] These findings have been confirmed in a number of studies, including the Pathobiological Determinants of Atherosclerosis in Youth (PDAY) study, which showed that atherosclerosis originates in childhood and that the prevalence and extent of fatty streaks and fibrous plaques increase rapidly between the ages of 15 and 34 years.[9]

Tuzcu and coworkers[10] used intravascular ultrasound (IVUS) to study 262 hearts from asymptomatic young transplant donors. Coronary atheromas were found in 17% of the donors younger than 20 years, 37% of those aged 20–29 years, and 60% of those aged 30–39 years; in contrast, angiographic results were negative for CAD in 97% of these individuals. The prevalence of atherosclerosis increased to 85% in IVUS subjects older than 50 years.

Importance of detecting vulnerable plaques

Despite the high prevalence of atherosclerotic disease in adults, a relatively small fraction of these individuals develop cardiovascular complications. Most atherosclerotic plaques follow a subclinical course for years. Nevertheless, some plaques suddenly become ulcerated or develop surface fissures, which are believed to lead to thrombosis and rapid disease progression. As previously mentioned, until the mid 1980s, the natural progression of atherosclerotic lesions was thought to involve a continuous growth of plaque, which would eventually lead to a marked reduction in blood flow. Physicians believed that plaques would not cause a problem unless they blocked the lumen enough to cause hemodynamic irregularities. In 1988, however, several research teams[11–13] showed that about 70% of myocardial infarctions (MIs) involve non-obstructive lesions that are not hemodynamically significant. Later studies confirmed these findings.[14,15] These small, hemodynamically insignificant, yet 'high-risk', lesions were named 'vulnerable plaques'.[16]

In a series of autopsy studies, various research groups[17–21] demonstrated that vulnerable plaques develop at sites of local inflammation in the arterial wall. The plaques undergo rupture and erosion, leading to ACS and sudden cardiac death. These findings confirmed the earlier, pioneering work of Friedman (Friedman and Van Den Bovenkamp[17]) and Constantinides.[22] Vulnerable plaques are usually characterized by the presence of a lipid pool, a necrotic core, a thin fibrous cap (<65 μm), and macrophage infiltration.

Plaque rupture/erosion is known to occur in areas of macrophage infiltration. The increased macrophage activity results in secretion of matrix metalloproteinases (MMPs) (and possibly other proteases) and softening of the plaque cap, leading to a breakdown of collagen in the fibrous cap, which becomes prone to rupture and erosion.[21,23–25]

It is important to know which lesions, in which patients, are at risk for rupture leading to ACS. Unfortunately, current diagnostic methods are unable to predict the risk associated with a particular lesion. The shortcomings of angiography in predicting the site of rupture have already been discussed.[11–15,26] White and colleagues,[27] as well as Kern and associates,[28] have demonstrated that the percentage of diameter stenosis is a poor indicator of ischemia. Using myocardial scintigraphy, Naqvi and coworkers[29] showed that a reversible perfusion abnormality could be detected in only 60% of segments that would be culprit sites for future acute MIs.

Knowing that inflammation plays a crucial part in the pathogenesis of ACS, investigators concluded that detection of inflammatory loci in blood vessels could help locate future culprit lesions and target appropriate therapy.

Detection of inflammation in coronary arteries

Ex vivo studies

In 1996, Casscells and coworkers[30] sought to determine whether heat (as one of the four cardinal signs of inflammation) might indicate inflammation in the arterial wall. Casscells et al[30] postulated that the heat released by activated macrophages in atherosclerotic plaques might predict acute coronary events.

Macrophages are known to be metabolically active and to have a high turnover rate of total adenosine triphosphate (ATP).[31] The high metabolic rate of atherosclerotic plaques is also suggested by their high concentrations of oxygen, ATP and lactate, and their high glucose uptake.[32,33] This high metabolic rate leads to increased heat production in areas of macrophage accumulation; such heat production is not observed in areas of smooth muscle cell accumulation in the absence of inflammatory cell infiltrates (foam cells consume three times more oxygen than smooth muscle cells).[34] Kockx and coauthors[35] have shown that macrophages in atherosclerotic plaques strongly express mitochondrial uncoupling proteins (UCP) 2 and 3. These proteins are homologs of thermogenin (UCP-1), which is responsible for thermogenesis in brown fat tissue.

To test their hypothesis, Casscells and coworkers[30] measured the intimal surface temperatures of 50 carotid artery plaque samples obtained from 48 endarterectomy patients (Figure 9.1). These researchers used a thermistor to measure the temperature at 20 sites on each plaque sample. In multiple regions, the surface temperature varied reproducibly by 0.2–0.3 °C. In 37% of the

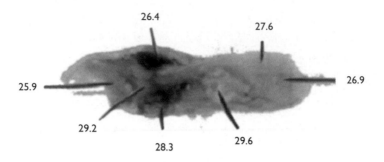

Figure 9.1 *Endarterectomized carotid plaques show temperature heterogeneity.*
Temperatures shown are °C. (Reprinted with permission from M Madjid et al. In:
Fuster V, ed. Assessing and Modifying the Vulnerable Atherosclerotic Plaque.
Armonk, NY: Futura Publishing Company, Inc. 2002.[36])

plaques, some regions were substantially (0.4–2.2 °C) warmer than others.
Despite being very close to each other (<1 mm apart), sites with substantially
different temperatures could not be distinguished from one another with the
naked eye. The temperature correlated positively with cell density (mostly
macrophages) (R = 0.68; P = 0.0001) and inversely with the distance of the cell
clusters from the luminal surface (R = –0.38; P = 0.0006) (Figure 9.2). Although
the temperature correlated with the density of macrophages/monocytes (which
have a high metabolic rate), it did not correlate with the density of smooth muscle
cells (which have a lower metabolic rate). Infrared thermographic images also
revealed a heterogeneity in temperature among the plaques.

Later, the same group showed that, whereas the temperature correlated
positively with the density of the macrophages, (R = 0.66; P = 0.0001) (Figure
9.3a), it correlated inversely with the density of the smooth muscle cells (R =
–0.41; P = 0.0001) (Figure 9.3b).[37] Using the genus-specific monoclonal
antibody CF-2 against *Chlamydia pneumoniae*, the researchers found no significant
association between temperature heterogeneity and the presence of *C. pneumoniae*
in human atherosclerotic carotid plaques. The gross color of the luminal surface
could not indicate the underlying temperature.[37] Incubation of plaques with
indomethacin (1 mg/ml) caused a gradual decrease in plaque heat production over
a 5-hour period, suggesting that heat production in atherosclerotic plaques has an
inflammatory origin.[37]

In another series of studies, Naghavi and colleagues[38] showed that, in inflamed
areas of human carotid plaques (obtained at endarterectomy), atherosclerotic
rabbit aortas, and apolipoprotein E (ApoE)-deficient mice aortas, a lower pH was
associated with a higher temperature (R = 0.7; P<0.0001); areas with a large

176

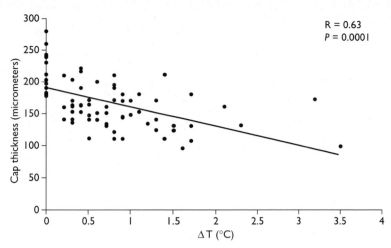

Figure 9.2 *There is an inverse relation between temperature measured at the surface of the plaque with the thickness of the fibrous cap. (Reproduced with permission from M Madjid et al. In: Fuster V, ed.* Assessing and Modifying the Vulnerable Atherosclerotic Plaque. *Armonk, NY: Futura Publishing Company, Inc. 2002.*[36]*)*

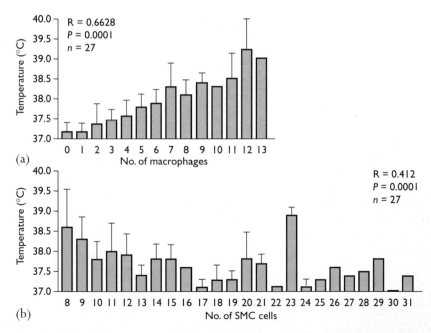

Figure 9.3 *(a) Close correlation between surface temperature (intimal surface temperatures of carotid artery plaques taken at endarterectomy) and the density of monocyte-macrophages. (b) Inverse relation between temperature and the density of the smooth muscle cells (SMC). (Reproduced with permission from M Madjid et al.* Am J Cardiol *2002;* **90**:*36L–39L.*[37]*)*

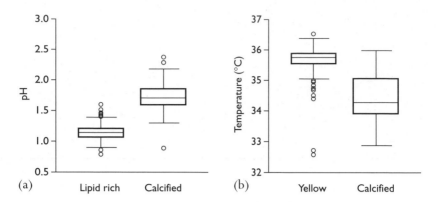

Figure 9.4. *Comparison of mean pH (a) and temperature (°C) (b) between yellow (lipid-rich) and calcified areas. (Reproduced with permission from M Madjid et al. In: Fuster V, ed.* Assessing and Modifying the Vulnerable Atherosclerotic Plaque. *Armonk, NY: Futura Publishing Company, Inc., 2002.[36])*

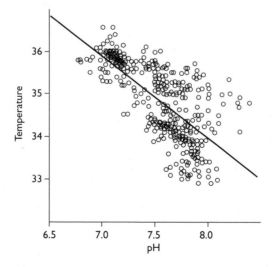

Figure 9.5 *Inverse correlation of pH and temperature (°C) in human carotid artery plaques. (Reproduced with permission from M Madjid et al. In: Fuster V, ed.* Assessing and Modifying the Vulnerable Atherosclerotic Plaque. *Armonk, NY: Futura Publishing Company, Inc., 2002.[36])*

lipid core had a lower pH and a higher temperature, but calcified regions had a higher pH and a lower temperature (Figure 9.4). pH heterogeneity is believed to result from inflammation, which is accompanied by macrophage accumulation. This phenomenon, along with low oxygen diffusion related to the thickness of plaque, causes the atherosclerotic lesion to have an anaerobic metabolism and a

178

lowered pH.[31,34] Fluorescent microscopic imaging confirmed pH heterogeneity in both humans and rabbits but not in human umbilical artery samples, which served as control samples.[38] An inverse relationship existed between the temperature and the pH (R = 0.94; $P<0.001$) (Figure 9.5).

These studies, which were the first to show thermal heterogeneity in atherosclerotic plaques, suggested that thermography could be used to identify plaques at high risk of rupture or thrombosis.

In vivo thermography: animal studies

Several methods may be used for in vivo thermal imaging. Infrared photography has been used to detect a heterogeneous pattern of heat emission over the atherosclerotic coronary arteries of dogs.[36] Infrared imaging has also been used to detect thermal heterogeneity over areas of skin that covered arteriovenous grafts in patients undergoing hemodialysis for chronic renal failure; thermal heterogeneity was correlated with graft blood flow ($\dot{Q}B_{max}$) and venous resistance at $\dot{Q}B_{250}$ (VR_{250}).[36]

Naghavi and associates[39] developed a 'thermo-basket' catheter for measuring the temperature over the arterial wall. This thermocouple-based catheter comprises a nitinol system loaded with small, flexible thermocouples; a 3-F catheter with an expandable, externally controllable basket, consisting of four highly flexible wires with built-in thermocouples; a personal computer, equipped with a computer board that has special digital transistors for high-speed sampling; and customized software that allows real-time data acquisition, tracking and thermographic imaging. A circulating microbath is used for automatic thermal calibration. Each basket wire has one sensor located at the point of maximum curvature, allowing temperature monitoring upon wire expansion and contact with the plaque. Each basket catheter also has a central wire that is equipped with a thermal sensor to permit simultaneous monitoring of the blood temperature. The real-time data acquisition software supports digital transmitters for each channel, with a thermal resolution of $0.02\,°C$ and a sampling rate of 20 readings per second. This software displays a circumferential and longitudinal thermal map of the vascular wall. In a phantom model, featuring simulated blood vessels and hot plaques, the basket catheter had a temperature resolution of $0.02\,°C$ and was able to detect temperature heterogeneity at various blood flows, plaque temperatures and degrees of luminal stenosis. When this system was tested in five inbred atherosclerotic dogs (Figure 9.6) and ten Watanabe rabbits, it detected temperature heterogeneity on atherosclerotic lesions in the femoral arteries of the dogs and the aortas of the rabbits.[36,39]

In another approach for measuring vascular wall temperature, Naghavi and colleagues[40] designed and built an infrared angiothermography catheter small enough (4 Fr) for use in the coronary system. This side-viewing fiberoptic catheter

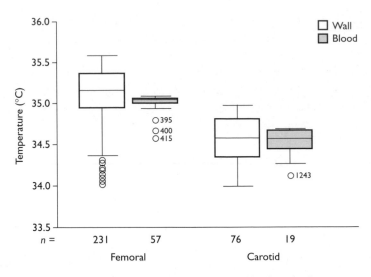

Figure 9.6 *Studies with thermobasket catheter showed higher absolute temperature as well as temperature heterogeneity in femoral arteries of atherosclerotic dogs compared to their carotid arteries which are free of disease. (Reproduced with permission from M Madjid et al. In: Fuster V, ed.* Assessing and Modifying the Vulnerable Atherosclerotic Plaque. *Armonk, NY: Futura Publishing Company, Inc., 2002.[36])*

uses a 180° scope to measure the temperature of the vascular wall. Nineteen chalcogenide fibers, each measuring 100 μm in diameter, are bundled hexagonally within the catheter, whose tip features a 1-mm wide, wedge-shaped mirror assembly made of zinc selenide. The mirror is transparent to infrared radiation, and heat is reflected onto it from the side of the catheter. A lumen through the fiber bundle allows passage of a guidewire. The catheter is connected to a focal plane array cooled infrared camera. The system has a thermal resolution of 0.01 °C and a spatial resolution of 100 μm. Real-time image reconstruction software continuously records the linear images and processes them into two-dimensional and virtual longitudinal, color-coded thermographic images. The catheter was tested in a phantom model that uses a continuous flow of normal saline in a silicone tube to simulate blood vessels and hot plaques. When multiple 'hot spots' were created, the catheter was able to detect temperature heterogeneity along the side of the tube.[40]

Verheye and associates[41] have shown that temperature heterogeneity is determined by plaque composition and macrophage mass. These researchers used an over-the-wire thermography catheter with four thermistors and a retractable covering sheath. They randomized 20 New Zealand rabbits to receive 6 months of either a normal diet ($n = 10$) or a cholesterol-rich (0.3%) diet ($n = 10$). At 6 months, 10 control rabbits and five hypercholesterolemic rabbits were sacrificed, and the five remaining rabbits were put on a normal diet for 3 months. The aortas were studied with IVUS and a thermography catheter (Figure 9.7). In the hypercholesterolemic rabbits, marked temperature heterogeneity (up to >1°C) was observed at sites of thick plaques with a high macrophage content, but no temperature heterogeneity was seen in plaques with a low macrophage content. Interestingly, in rabbits who received 3 months of a low cholesterol diet, plaque thickness remained unchanged, but the macrophage content decreased significantly. In ex vivo studies, these same researchers showed a relationship between the local temperature and the local total macrophage mass.

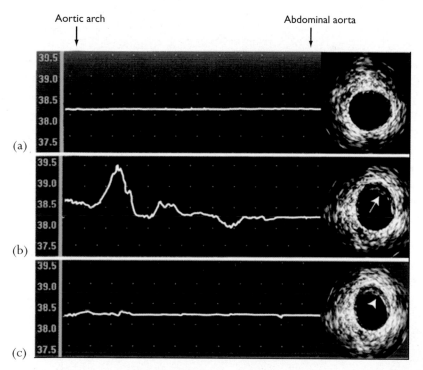

Figure 9.7 In vivo temperature measurements of the endoaortic surface in rabbits. (a) In control rabbits at 6 months, temperature differences are absent along the aortic wall. Intravascular ultrasound (IVUS) image illustrates the absence of plaque formation. (b) In atherosclerotic rabbits at 6 months, marked temperature variations up to >1 °C are apparent along the endoluminal surface of the aortic wall. IVUS demonstrates plaque formation at the level of the proximal descending aorta just distal from the arch (arrow). (c) In atherosclerotic rabbits after 3 months of dietary cholesterol lowering, temperature heterogeneity is absent, although IVUS (taken at the same level as in (b) demonstrates the presence of a similar plaque (arrowhead). (Reproduced with permission from S Verheye et al. Circulation 2002; 105:1596–601.[41])

181

In vivo thermography: human studies

The first in vivo human thermographic studies were performed in 1999 by Stefanadis and colleagues,[42] of Athens, who used a single-channel, thermistor-based catheter to demonstrate thermal heterogeneity in human atherosclerotic coronary arteries. Temperature differences (ΔT) between atherosclerotic plaque and healthy vascular wall increased progressively, being lowest in patients with stable angina (ΔT: 0.106±0.110 °C) and highest in those with unstable angina (ΔT: 0.683±0.347 °C) and acute MI (ΔT: 1.472±0.691 °C) (Figure 9.8). Intraplaque temperature heterogeneity was found in 20%, 40% and 67% of the patients with stable angina, unstable angina and acute MI, respectively, but no such temperature heterogeneity was found in the control subjects. Thermal heterogeneity was not correlated with the degree of stenosis.

Lesser degrees of temperature heterogeneity have been observed by Webster et al,[43] Verheye et al,[44] and Erbel and coworkers (R Erbel, 2003, personal communication). These findings may have been related to the fact that many more of their patients were taking aspirin and/or statins; moreover, the thermography techniques used by these investigators did not obstruct flow, but the larger thermistor used by Stefanadis often 'wedged' the lesion.[42] In addition, blood flow can attenuate the measured temperature heterogeneity over the atherosclerotic plaque (see Limitations of intravascular thermography later).

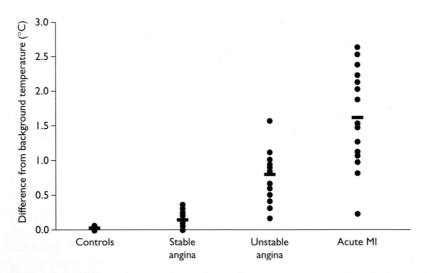

Figure 9.8 *Differences in maximum region of interest temperature from background temperature in four study groups. Temperature differences increase progressively from stable angina to acute myocardial infarction (MI) patients. (Reproduced with permission from C Stefanadis et al. Circulation 1999; 99:1965–71.[42])*

Stefanadis and colleagues[45] studied 60 patients with CAD, including stable angina (20 patients), unstable angina (20 patients) and acute MI (20 patients), as well as 20 sex and age-matched control subjects without CAD. These researchers found that C-reactive protein (CRP) and serum amyloid A levels were strongly correlated with ΔTs.

Pooling of the two small series recently reported by Webster and colleagues[43] and by Erbel and coworkers (R Erbel, 2003, personal communication) (six patients with unstable angina and 14 patients with stable angina) and use of a cutoff temperature of ≥0.1 °C yields 10 patients with no temperature heterogeneity, four patients with a single hot spot, three patients with two hot spots and three patients with three hot spots. Alternatively, if a cutoff temperature of ≥0.2 °C is used, only two of 17 patients had a hot spot, and one patient had two such lesions. Notably, most patients had a normal CRP level, and the number of hot spots did not correlate well with the percentage of diameter stenosis or the CRP level. These findings differ from those of Stefanadis, whose patients probably used more statins and anti-inflammatory medications.

Toutouzas and coauthors[46] reported a high correlation between the coronary remodeling index (defined as the ratio of the external elastic membrane area at the lesion to that at the proximal site, as determined by intracoronary ultrasound) and the ΔT between the atherosclerotic plaque and healthy vascular wall in patients with ACS. The investigators also showed that the serum MMP-9 concentration is correlated with these ΔTs.[47]

In another study, in which Stefanadis and coworkers[48] followed 86 patients for 17±7 months after successful percutaneous intervention, ΔT was a strong predictor of adverse cardiac events during the follow-up period. The risk of an adverse cardiac event significantly increased when the ΔT was >0.5 °C. The risk of an adverse cardiac event was 41% in patients with a ΔT of ≥0.5 °C, compared with 7% in those with a ΔT of <0.5 °C (Figure 9.9).

In a stratified, randomized study involving 72 patients, these same researchers[49] found that the use of statins decreased the ΔT in patients with stable angina, unstable angina and acute MI (mean ΔT: 0.29±0.33 in treated vs 0.56±0.41 °C in non-treated groups). Interestingly, ΔT was not correlated with the cholesterol level at hospital admission. This finding confirms the results of animal studies showing that statins reduce the number of inflammatory cells in plaques.[50]

To detect bladder and lung cancers, Stefanadis's group has begun to use thermography catheters to measure temperatures in peripheral arteries and at non-vascular sites.[51–53] In addition, when they used a thermography catheter to measure the coronary sinus temperature in 60 patients, these researchers found that the ΔT between the coronary sinus and the right atrium was increased in patients who had significant left anterior descending coronary artery lesions but not in subjects who lacked lesions. These researchers concluded that coronary

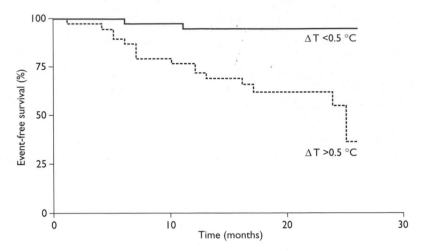

Figure 9.9 *Estimated survival among the study group according to temperature difference (ΔT). The risk of an adverse cardiac event in patients with ΔT >0.5 °C is significantly increased, as compared with that in patients with ΔT <0.5 °C. (Reproduced with permission from the American College of Cardiology. C. Stefanadis et al.* J Am Coll Cardiol *2001; 37:1277–83.[48])*

sinus thermography may be a measure of inflamed atherosclerotic plaques in the left anterior descending artery.[54] The reproducibility of this technique and the clinical implications of the study remain to be confirmed in further trials.

Limitations of intravascular thermography

Although the surface temperature of arterial plaque has been correlated with the number of macrophages near the plaque cap, investigators are not certain to what extent macrophages deep within the plaque contribute to the heat measured at the plaque surface.

In vivo coronary temperature measurements are influenced by coronary flow, which has a 'cooling effect'. Complete interruption of blood flow significantly increases the degree of detected temperature heterogeneity (up to 60% in patients with trivial temperature heterogeneity at baseline and up to 76% in patients without temperature heterogeneity at baseline).[55] Proximal balloon occlusion can overcome this problem, but this method is not desirable because it interrupts coronary blood flow.

Although the clinical use of thermography is not yet established, it is supported by evidence from the controlled, prospective studies that are currently underway. Clinical studies must show not only the safety, feasibility, and reproducibility of the procedure, but also the therapeutic benefits to be gained from it. A cost–benefit analysis will be the next step before the clinical use of thermography can be advocated. However, once this method is proved to be beneficial, mass production of catheters and related devices will markedly reduce its cost.

Future implications

Intravascular thermography is an emerging, rapidly evolving approach for detecting vulnerable plaques and evaluating them functionally. If human clinical trials prove that this approach is safe, reproducible and beneficial, it may find a place in the detection of vulnerable plaques and the risk stratification of vulnerable lesions and patients, as well as in clinical decision making and prediction of a specific patient's clinical course and prognosis.

On the basis of current developments involving different techniques for detecting vulnerable plaques, we can predict that a major improvement in this area will be achieved by combining anatomic imaging methods (e.g. IVUS, elastography, optical coherence tomography) with functional imaging methods, such as thermography, thereby obtaining maximal insight into the structure and activity of plaques.[56] This combined approach will greatly enhance our ability to determine which plaques are vulnerable and to choose the intervention most suitable for treating a particular lesion in a specific patient.

Acknowledgment

This work was supported in part by DOD Grant #DAMD 17-01-2-0047.

References

1. American Heart Association. *2001 Heart and Stroke Statistical Update*. Dallas, Texas: American Heart Association, 2001.

2. Murray C, Lopez A. *The Global Burden of Disease. A comprehensive assessment of mortality and disability from diseases, injuries, and risk factors in 1990 and projected to 2020*. World Health Organization; Cambridge, MS: Harvard University Press, 1996.

3. Ross R. Atherosclerosis – an inflammatory disease. *N Engl J Med* 1999; **340**:115–26.

4. Virchow R. *Phlogose und Thrombose in Getissystem, Gesanmelte Unhandlungen zur Wissensehaftlichen Medlein*. Frankfurt-am-Main, Germany: Meidinger Sohn, 1856:458.

5. Ross R, Glomset JA. The pathogenesis of atherosclerosis (first of two parts). *N Engl J Med* 1976; **295**:369–77.

6. Napoli C, D'Armiento FP, Mancini FP et al. Fatty streak formation occurs in human fetal aortas and is greatly enhanced by maternal hypercholesterolemia. Intimal accumulation of low density lipoprotein and its oxidation precede monocyte recruitment into early atherosclerotic lesions. *J Clin Invest* 1997; **100**:2680–90.

185

7. Enos WF, Holmes RH, Beyer J. Landmark article, July 18, 1953: Coronary disease among United States soldiers killed in action in Korea. Preliminary report. *JAMA* 1986; **256**:2859–62.

8. McNamara JJ, Molot MA, Stremple JF, Cutting RT. Coronary artery disease in combat casualties in Vietnam. *JAMA* 1971; **216**:1185–7.

9. Pathobiological Determinants of Atherosclerosis in Youth (PDAY) Research Group. Natural history of aortic and coronary atherosclerotic lesions in youth. Findings from the PDAY Study. *Arterioscler Thromb* 1993; **13**:1291–8.

10. Tuzcu EM, Kapadia SR, Tutar E et al. High prevalence of coronary atherosclerosis in asymptomatic teenagers and young adults: evidence from intravascular ultrasound. *Circulation* 2001; **103**:2705–10.

11. Ambrose JA, Tannenbaum MA, Alexopoulos D et al. Angiographic progression of coronary artery disease and the development of myocardial infarction. *J Am Coll Cardiol* 1988; **12**:56–62.

12. Little WC, Constantinescu M, Applegate RJ et al. Can coronary angiography predict the site of a subsequent myocardial infarction in patients with mild-to-moderate coronary artery disease? *Circulation* 1988; **78**:1157–66.

13. Hackett D, Davies G, Maseri A. Pre-existing coronary stenoses in patients with first myocardial infarction are not necessarily severe. *Eur Heart J* 1988; **9**:1317–23.

14. Lichtlen PR, Nikutta P, Jost S et al. Anatomical progression of coronary artery disease in humans as seen by prospective, repeated, quantitated coronary angiography. Relation to clinical events and risk factors. The INTACT Study Group. *Circulation* 1992; **86**:828–38.

15. Giroud D, Li JM, Urban P, Meier B, Rutishauer W. Relation of the site of acute myocardial infarction to the most severe coronary arterial stenosis at prior angiography. *Am J Cardiol* 1992; **69**:729–32.

16. Muller JE, Tofler GH, Stone PH. Circadian variation and triggers of onset of acute cardiovascular disease. *Circulation* 1989; **79**:733–43.

17. Friedman M, Van Den Bovenkamp GJ. The pathogenesis of a coronary thrombus. *Am J Pathol* 1966; **48**:19–44.

18. Farb A, Tang AL, Burke AP et al. Sudden coronary death. Frequency of active coronary lesions, inactive coronary lesions, and myocardial infarction. *Circulation* 1995; **92**:1701–9.

19. Falk E. Morphologic features of unstable atherothrombotic plaques underlying acute coronary syndromes. *Am J Cardiol* 1989; **63**:114E–120E.

20. Arbustini E, Dal Bello B, Morbini P et al. Plaque erosion is a major substrate for coronary thrombosis in acute myocardial infarction. *Heart* 1999; **82**:269–72.

21. Davies MJ, Thomas T. The pathological basis and microanatomy of occlusive thrombus formation in human coronary arteries. *Philos Trans R Soc Lond B Biol Sci* 1981; **294**:225–9.

22. Constantinides P. Plaque fissures in human coronary thrombosis. *J Atheroscler Res* 1966; **6**:1–17.

23. Lendon CL, Davies MJ, Born GV, Richardson PD. Atherosclerotic plaque caps are locally weakened when macrophages density is increased. *Atherosclerosis* 1991; **87**:87–90.

24. Buja LM, Willerson JT. Role of inflammation in coronary plaque disruption. *Circulation* 1994; **89**:503–5.

25. Libby P, Geng YJ, Aikawa M et al. Macrophages and atherosclerotic plaque stability. *Curr Opin Lipidol* 1996; **7**:330 5.

26. Haft JI, Haik BJ, Goldstein JE, Brodyn NE. Development of significant coronary artery lesions in areas of minimal disease. A common mechanism for coronary disease progression. *Chest* 1988; **94**:731 6.

27. White CW, Wright CB, Doty DB et al. Does visual interpretation of the coronary arteriogram predict the physiologic importance of a coronary stenosis? *N Engl J Med* 1984; **310**:819–24.

28. Kern MJ, Donohue TJ, Aguirre FV et al. Assessment of angiographically intermediate coronary artery stenosis using the Doppler flowire. *Am J Cardiol* 1993; **71**:26D–33D.

29. Naqvi TZ, Hachamovitch R, Berman D et al. Does the presence and site of myocardial ischemia on perfusion scintigraphy predict the occurrence and site of future myocardial infarction in patients with stable coronary artery disease? *Am J Cardiol* 1997; **79**:1521–4.

30. Casscells W, Hathorn B, David M et al. Thermal detection of cellular infiltrates in living atherosclerotic plaques: possible implications for plaque rupture and thrombosis. *Lancet* 1996; **347**:1447–51.

31. Newsholme P, Newsholme EA. Rates of utilization of glucose, glutamine and oleate and formation of end-products by mouse peritoneal macrophages in culture. *Biochem J* 1989; **261**:211–18.

32. Heinle H. Metabolite concentration gradients in the arterial wall of experimental atherosclerosis. *Exp Mol Pathol* 1987; **46**:312–20.

33. Vallabhajosula S, Fuster V. Atherosclerosis: imaging techniques and the evolving role of nuclear medicine. *J Nucl Med* 1997; **38**:1788–96.

34. Bjornheden T, Bondjers G. Oxygen consumption in aortic tissue from rabbits with diet-induced atherosclerosis. *Arteriosclerosis* 1987; **7**:238–47.

35. Kockx MK, Knaapen MWM, Martinet W et al. Expression of the uncoupling protein UCP-2 in macrophages of unstable human atherosclerotic plaques. *Circulation* 2000; **102**:II–12.

36. Madjid M, Naghavi N, Willerson JT, Casscells W. Thermography: a novel approach for identification of plaques at risk of rupture and/or thrombosis. In: Fuster V, ed. *Assessing and Modifying the Vulnerable Atherosclerotic Plaque*. Armonk, NY: Futura Publishing Company, Inc., 2002:107–27.

37. Madjid M, Naghavi M, Malik BA et al. Thermal detection of vulnerable plaque. *Am J Cardiol* 2002; **90**:36L–39L.

38. Naghavi M, John R, Naguib S et al. pH Heterogeneity of human and rabbit atherosclerotic plaques; a new insight into detection of vulnerable plaque. *Atherosclerosis* 2002; **164**:27–35.

39. Naghavi M, Madjid M, Gul K et al. Thermography basket catheter: in vivo measurement of the temperature of atherosclerotic plaques for detection of vulnerable plaques. *Catheter Cardiovasc Interv* 2003; **59**:52–9.

40. Naghavi M, Melling M, Gul K et al. First prototype of a 4 French 180 degree side-viewing infrared fiber optic catheter for thermal imaging of atherosclerotic plaque. *J Am Coll Cardiol* 2001; **37**:3A.

41. Verheye S, De Meyer GRY, Van Langenhove G, Knaapen MWM, Kockx MM. In vivo temperature heterogeneity of atherosclerotic plaques is determined by plaque composition. *Circulation* 2002; **105**:1596–601.

42. Stefanadis C, Diamantopoulos L, Vlachopoulos C et al. Thermal heterogeneity within human atherosclerotic coronary arteries detected in vivo: a new method of detection by application of a special thermography catheter. *Circulation* 1999; **99**:1965–71.

43. Webster M, Stewart J, Ruygrok P et al. Intracoronary thermography with a multiple thermocouple catheter: Initial human experience (abstract). *Am J Cardiol* 2002; **90**:24H.

44. Verheye S, Van Langenhove G, Diamantopoulos L, Serruys PW, Vermeersch P. Temperature heterogeneity is nearly absent in angiographically normal or mild atherosclerotic coronary segments: interim results from a safety study (abstract). *Am J Cardiol* 2002; **90**:24H.

45. Stefanadis C, Diamantopoulos L, Dernellis J et al. Heat production of atherosclerotic plaques and inflammation assessed by the acute phase proteins in acute coronary syndromes. *J Mol Cell Cardiol* 2000; **32**:43–52.

46. Toutouzas MK, Stefanadis CM, Vavuranakis MM et al. Arterial remodeling in acute coronary syndromes: correlation of IVUS characteristics with temperature of the culprit lesion. *Circulation* 2000; **102**:II–707.

47. Toutouzas K, Stefanadis C, Tsiamis E et al. The temperature of atherosclerotic plaques is correlated with matrix metalloproteinases concentration in patients with acute coronary syndromes. *J Am Coll Cardiol* 2001; **37**:356A.

48. Stefanadis C, Toutouzas K, Tsiamis E et al. Increased local temperature in human coronary atherosclerotic plaques: an independent predictor of clinical outcome in patients undergoing a percutaneous coronary intervention. *J Am Coll Cardiol* 2001; **37**:1277–83.

49. Stefanadis C, Toutouzas K, Vavuranakis M et al. Statin treatment is associated with reduced thermal heterogeneity in human atherosclerotic plaques. *Eur Heart J* 2002; **23**:1664–9.

50. Sukhova GK, Williams JK, Libby P. Statins reduce inflammation in atheroma of nonhuman primates independent of effects on serum cholesterol. *Arterioscler Thromb Vasc Biol* 2002; **22**:1452–8.

51. Stefanadis C, Toutouzas K, Tsiamis E et al. Thermography of human arterial system by means of new thermography catheters. *Catheter Cardiovasc Interv* 2001; **54**:51–8.

52. Stefanadis C, Chrysohoou C, Panagiotakos DB et al. Temperature differences are associated with malignancy on lung lesions: a clinical study. *BMC Cancer* 2003; **3**:1.

53. Stefanadis C, Chrysohoou C, Markou D et al. Increased temperature of malignant urinary bladder tumors in vivo: the application of a new method based on a catheter technique. *J Clin Oncol* 2001; **19**:676–81.

54. Stefanadis C, Toutouzas K, Vaina S, Vavuranakis M, Toutouzas P. Thermography of the cardiovascular system. *J Interv Cardiol* 2002; **15**:461–6.

55. Stefanadis C, Toutouzas K, Tsiamis E et al. Thermal heterogeneity in stable human coronary atherosclerotic plaques is underestimated in vivo: the 'cooling effect' of blood flow. *J Am Coll Cardiol* 2003; **41**:403–408.

56. Naghavi M, Madjid M, Khan MR et al. New developments in the detection of vulnerable plaque. *Curr Atheroscler Rep* 2001; **3**:125–35.

10. OPTICAL COHERENCE TOMOGRAPHY

Evelyn Regar, Johannes A Schaar, Eric Mont,
Renu Virmani and Patrick W Serruys

Optical coherence tomography (OCT) is a light-based imaging modality that can be used in biologic systems to study tissues in vivo with near histologic, ultra-high resolution.[1]

OCT originates from early work on white-light interferometry and optical coherence-domain reflectometry (OCDR). OCDR is a one-dimensional optical ranging technique that uses short coherence length light and interferometric detection[2] that was developed for finding faults in fiberoptic cables and network components.[3] Its potential for medical application was soon recognized.[4,5] Researchers at the Massachusetts Institute of Technology extended the technique of OCDR and developed *optical coherence tomography* in the early 1990s as a *two-dimensional*, tomographic imaging modality in biologic systems.[6] The second dimension of the two-dimensional image was created by a physical translation or rotation of a fiberoptic probe. Since then improvements of the light source, the interferometer and beam scanning optics are being continuously researched.[7–9]

Clinical application of OCT has been initiated in the field of ophthalmology, where it has become an established method for the assessment of epiretinal processes and macula pathology.[10]

Intravascular optical coherence tomography

The rationale for intravascular application of OCT is its potential for in vivo visualization of the coronary artery microstructure.

In the context of atherosclerosis research plaques at high risk for rupture have become a field of intense investigation. Several morphologic features described in autopsy series are of particular interest in these vulnerable plaques. This includes the presence of a thin fibrous cap, a necrotic lipid core[11,12] and the accumulation of macrophages.[13] Until now, there has been no validated method for the in vivo

The opinions and assertions contained herein are the private views of the authors and are not to be construed as official or reflecting the views of the United States Department of the Army or the Department of Defense.

detection of vulnerable plaque. This unique image resolution of OCT offers the potential to detect key features of vulnerable plaque in vivo.

The in vivo visualization of a *thin fibrous cap* is missed by angiography and angioscopy because these are limited to the visualization of the lumen. It is missed by intravascular ultrasound (IVUS) by its limited image resolution (axial 150–200 mm, radial 200–400 mm). An overview on image resolution of different diagnostic techniques is given in Figure 10.1. OCT allows, similar to IVUS, for real-time imaging of the arterial wall but offers 10 times higher resolution and thus the possibility to detect thin fibrous caps. Likewise, OCT might offer a much higher sensitivity for the detection of necrotic/lipid cores within coronary atheromas than IVUS, that has a relatively low sensitivity (50–83%) for detection of lipid-rich lesions.[14] Furthermore, in vitro data propose the possibility to detect macrophage accumulation within atherosclerotic plaques by OCT.[15] In theory, sophisticated signal processing or combination with other techniques such as spectroscopy might allow more detailed plaque characterization. Further applications may include the analysis of early atherosclerotic lesions in the intima and the mechanisms of progression of coronary artery disease (CAD).

Another field where OCT can be used is the pharmacologic or catheter-based intervention on plaque structure and vessel architecture. This is of interest in relation to drug eluting and new generation coronary stents. Drug eluting stents have been shown to significantly limit neointimal growth to such extent that the neointimal tissue might consist of only a few cell layers that cannot be accurately visualized with the gold standard IVUS. The high image resolution capability of OCT might offer the possibility to assess stent expansion (Figure 10.2) and the delicate interaction between vessel wall and stent strut[16] as well as neointimal growth patterns.[17]

Furthermore, the high level of device miniaturization will make OCT suitable for application in combined diagnostic and therapeutic devices in the future (e.g.

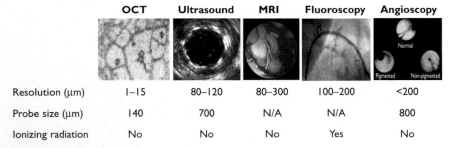

	OCT	Ultrasound	MRI	Fluoroscopy	Angioscopy
Resolution (μm)	1–15	80–120	80–300	100–200	<200
Probe size (μm)	140	700	N/A	N/A	800
Ionizing radiation	No	No	No	Yes	No

Figure 10.1 Overview of image resolution of different coronary imaging modalities. OCT, optical coherence tomography; MRI, magnetic resonance imaging; N/A, not applicable.

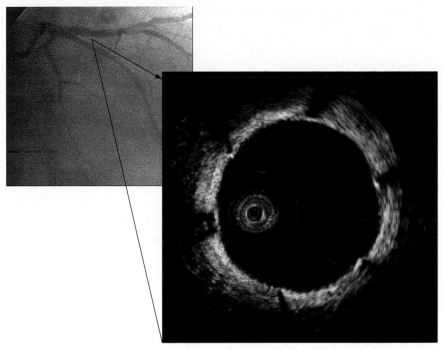

Figure 10.2 *Assessment of coronary stent deployment with intravascular optical coherence tomography, showing a circular, well expanded stent with apposition of all stent struts against the vessel wall.*

combination with tissue ablative techniques such as atherectomy or radiofrequency ablation).

Currently, two different systems for intravascular OCT are used, one utilizes a modified IVUS catheter,[18] the other system applies dedicated imaging wires or imaging catheters.[19] Both systems have been described in detail in this handbook (see Chapters 21 and 22).

The principle

The principle is analogous to pulse–echo ultrasound imaging, however, light is used rather than sound to create the image.

Low coherent near-infrared light is emitted by a superluminescent diode. A wavelength around 1300 nm is used since it minimizes the energy absorption in the light beam caused by protein, water, hemoglobin and lipids. The light waves are reflected by the internal microstructures within the biologic tissues as a result of their different optical indices. The echo time delay of reflected light waves is determined by an interferometer. The angular position of the imaged line is varied and converted into a two-dimensional spatial image. The intensity of the reflected light waves is translated into an intensity map and encoded using a gray or false color scale.

Experimental data

The first OCT imaging of a human coronary artery was described in vitro by Huang and coworkers in 1991 proving the hypothesis that OCT is able to image non-transparent tissue.[6] These findings were later confirmed by in vitro studies of human aortic segments.[20]

Comparison with histology

Intravascular OCT can reliably visualize the structure of normal and atherosclerotic coronary arteries. OCT images correlate well with the histologic specimens. OCT produces accurate images of the arterial lumen and the lumen–vessel wall interface and is able to clearly identify thin fibrous cap atheroma. Lipid-rich, necrotic plaques are visualized as low reflective structures within the artery wall, predominantly fibrous plaque shows a highly reflective, uniform pattern, calcified lesions appear as low reflective structures with relatively sharp boundaries. Normal arteries show a clear demarcation between tunica intima (high reflective), tunica media (low reflective) and tunica adventitia (high reflective) by OCT. Examples of OCT images and their corresponding histologic sections are shown in Figure 10.3.

The capability of OCT for characterizing plaque was confirmed by an in vitro study of more than 300 human atherosclerotic artery segments (aorta, carotid and

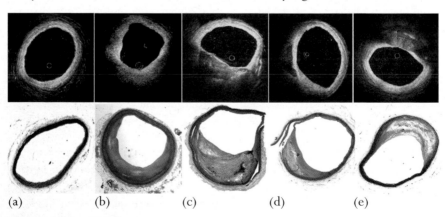

(a)   (b)   (c)   (d)   (e)

Figure 10.3 Comparison of intravascular OCT with the histology of human cadaver arteries. (a) Normal artery with clear demarcation between tunica intima, tunica media and tunica adventitia. (b) Eccentric fibrous plaque. (c) Complex plaque with multiple necrotic cores and focal calcification. (d) Fibrous cap atheromas with focal dense calcification in necrotic core. (e) Fibrous cap atheromas with thin cap and lipid-rich core.

coronary arteries).[18] Plaque types were defined by OCT as follows: fibrous plaques were characterized by homogeneous, signal-rich regions; fibrocalcific plaques by well delineated, signal-poor regions with sharp borders; and lipid-rich plaques by signal-poor regions with diffuse borders. Independent validation of these criteria by two OCT readers demonstrated high sensitivity and specificity (Table 10.1) with high interobserver and intraobserver reliability of OCT assessment (κ values of 0.88 and 0.91, respectively).[18] In vitro quantitative analysis of fibrous cap thickness in atherosclerotic specimens suggests high agreement (R = 0.91, P = 0.0001) compared to histomorphometry (Figure 10.4).[21]

Detection of macrophages in atherosclerotic plaques

Detection of macrophage accumulation by OCT is based on the hypothesis that plaques containing macrophages have high heterogeneity of optical refraction indices that exhibit strong optical scattering. Optical scattering results in a relatively high variance of the OCT signal intensity that can be expressed as normalized standard deviation (NSD) of the OCT signal.

Tearney and coworkers compared in vitro the correlation between NSD of the OCT signal and immunohistochemical detection of macrophages in 26 human atherosclerotic aortic and carotid arteries.[15] OCT was performed using an OCT microscope in a pre-set region of interest within the plaque. NSDs of the conventional, compressed (base 10 logarithm) OCT images and of the uncompressed raw OCT data images were calculated (Figure 10.5). The NSD of OCT raw data showed a high degree of positive correlation between OCT and fibrous cap macrophage density (R = 0.84, P<0.0001) (Table 10.2). Additionally, a negative correlation between OCT and histological measurements of smooth muscle actin density (R = −0.56, P<0.005) was found.

Comparison with IVUS

Intravascular OCT is analogous to IVUS. The major difference in the image quality is that the resolution of OCT is an order of magnitude higher than in commercially available IVUS imaging systems, however, the penetration depth is significantly worse.

Early descriptive in vitro studies of sections of the human abdominal aorta (n = 5 patients)[22] and coronary arteries[23] suggested superior detail resolution of plaques structures, which were close to the luminal surface, with OCT as compared with a 30 Mz IVUS system. These findings were confirmed by in vivo animal studies. These studies showed that (i) intravascular application of OCT is feasible, (ii) OCT can detect in vivo, both normal and pathologic artery structures and, (iii) OCT is superior in visualizing intimal tears and fissures. Furthermore OCT is able to penetrate calcified plaques and thus overcome a classical limitation of IVUS, that is dorsal shadowing caused by calcium.[24,25]

Table 10.1 Sensitivity and specificity of OCT criteria for plaque characterization in comparison with histology.[*]

Histopathologic diagnosis	Sensitivity	Specificity	Positive predictive value	Negative predictive value
OCT reader 1				
Fibrous (n = 77)	79 (68–88)	97 (94–99)	91 (82–97)	93 (89–96)
Fibrocalcific (n = 162)	95 (91–98)	97 (92–99)	97 (93–99)	95 (90–98)
Lipid-rich (n = 68)	90 (80–96)	92 (87–95)	75 (64–84)	97 (94–99)
OCT reader 2				
Fibrous (n = 77)	71 (60–81)	98 (96–100)	93 (84–98)	91 (87–94)
Fibrocalcific (n = 162)	96 (92–99)	97 (92–99)	97 (93–99)	96 (91–98)
Lipid-rich (n = 68)	94 (86–98)	90 (86–94)	74 (63–82)	98 (95–100)

(Adapted with permission from H. Yabushita et al. *Circulation* 2002; **106**:1640–45.[18])

[*]Data are percentages. Numbers in parentheses are 95% confidence intervals. OCT, optical coherence tomography.

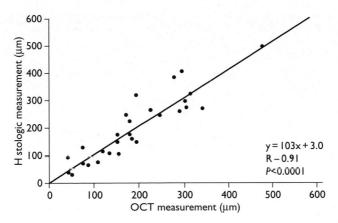

Figure 10.4 *In vitro assessment of cap thickness with optical coherence tomography. Correlation with histomorphometry. (Reproduced with permission from IK Jang, presented at the 4th Vulnerable Plaque Symposium, Chicago, IL, 2002.[21])*

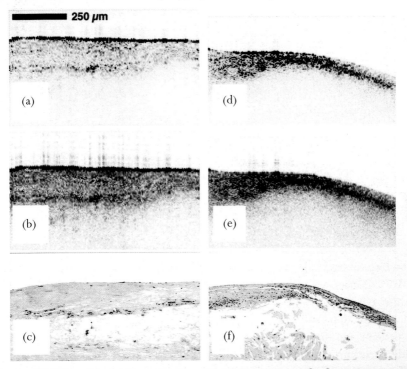

Figure 10.5 *Raw (a) and logarithm base 10 (b) OCT images of a fibroatheroma with a low density of macrophages within the fibrous cap. (c) Corresponding histology of (a) and (b). Raw (d) and logarithm base 10 (e) OCT images of a fibroatheroma with a high density of macrophages within the fibrous cap. (f) Corresponding histology of (d) and (e). All histology images: CD68 immunoperoxidase; original magnification ×100. (Adapted with permission from G. Tearney et al. Circulation. 2003; **107**:113–19.[15])*

197

Table 10.2 Summary of correlation between raw OCT data and logarithm OCT data NSD compared with CD68 percent staining.*

	Raw OCT signal	Logarithm OCT signal
Correlation (R)	0.84 (P<0.0001)	0.47 (P<0.05)
NSD cutoff (%)	6.2	7.7
Sensitivity	1.0 (0.69–1.0)	0.70 (0.35–0.93)
Specificity	1.0 (0.8–1.0)	0.75 (0.48–0.93)
Positive predictive value	1.0 (0.69–1.0)	0.64 (0.3–0.89)
Negative predictive value	1.0 (0.8–1.0)	0.80 (0.52–0.96)

(Adapted with permission from G. Tearney et al. *Circulation* 2003; **107**:113–19.[15])

*CD68 percent staining cutoff, 10%. Data in parentheses represent 95% confidence intervals. OCT, optical coherence tomography; NSD, normalized standard deviation.

Clinical experience

To date, there is only limited experience with intravascular OCT in the clinical setting. A first clinical study provided proof for the concept of in vivo intravascular OCT using a modified 3.2 Fr IVUS catheter. In 10 patients scheduled for coronary stent implantation, mild to moderate coronary lesions that were remote from the target stenosis were investigated. Most coronary structures that were detected by IVUS could also have been visualized with OCT. All fibrous plaques, macrocalcifications and echolucent regions identified by IVUS were visualized on corresponding OCT images. Intimal hyperplasia and echolucent regions, which may correspond to lipid pools, were identified more frequently by OCT than by IVUS (Table 10.3).[26]

We performed a pilot study using dedicated OCT imaging wires and catheters. Sixteen patients scheduled for percutaneous coronary intervention in a native coronary artery underwent preinterventional OCT imaging. OCT with motorized catheter pullback was successfully performed in all vessels and well tolerated in all patients. OCT analysis of the coronary artery wall was possible in all patients and the entire vessel circumference was visualized all of the time. A wide spectrum of different plaque morphologies was seen. OCT allowed for differentiation of the normal artery wall, of inhomogeneous, low reflecting plaques suggestive of predominantly fatty/fibro-fatty material and the visualization of mixed plaque with small spots of calcification. Two thin-cap fibroatheromas were seen. They consisted of inhomogeneous, low reflecting necrotic cores, covered by highly reflecting fibrous caps with a thickness of 45 and 50 μm (Figure 10.6).[19]

Table 10.3 IVUS and OCT findings for corresponding image pairs.

Feature	Identified by both OCT and IVUS*	Identified by OCT alone†
Intimal hyperplasia	3 ($n = 3$)	8 ($n = 7$)
Internal elastic lamina	NE	11 ($n = 8$)
External elastic lamina	NE	10 ($n = 7$)
Plaque	17 ($n = 10$)	0
fibrous	13 ($n = 10$)	0
calcific	4 ($n = 4$)	0
echolucent region	2 ($n = 2$)	2 ($n = 2$)

(Adapted with permission from IK Jang et al. *J Am Cardiol* 2002; **39**:604–9.[26])

*All features of the vessel wall structure identified by the IVUS reader were seen in the corresponding OCT image.
†Additional findings by OCT that were not identified by the IVUS reader
IVUS, intravascular ultrasound; NE, not evaluated; OCT, optical coherence tomography; *n*, patients.

Safety

The applied energies in intravascular OCT are relatively low (output power in the range of 5.0–8.0 mW) and are not considered to cause functional or structural damage to the tissue.

Safety issues thus mainly seem to be concerning OCT catheter design and the extend of ischemia caused by flow obstruction from the catheter itself and the displacement of blood. Representative safety data for intravascular OCT are not yet available, as there is only preliminary clinical experience in a small number of patients. These data are difficult to interpret as all patients underwent angioplasty before or after the OCT imaging procedure. In our series, the most frequent complications were transient ECG changes indicative of ischemia (58%) and chest pain (38%). In two patients (12.5%) post-stenting troponine-T elevation was seen.[19]

These data match well with large IVUS registries that reported transient coronary ischemia caused by the imaging catheter in 67% and by angina in 22% of patients.[27,28] Elevation of troponine-T is a well described phenomenon occurring in 20–30% of the angioplasty population.[29]

Limitations

Optical imaging in non-transparent biologic tissues is, in general, a difficult problem, primarily due to the scattering in the tissue. In coronary arteries blood

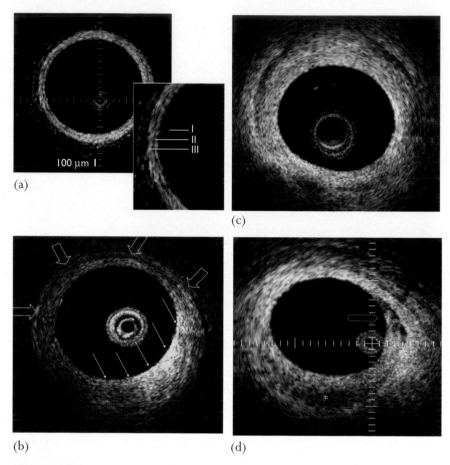

Figure 10.6. *In vivo intravascular OCT of human coronary arteries. (a) Normal artery with clear demarcation between a highly reflective intimal layer (I), a low-reflective media (II), and a highly reflective adventitial layer (III). (b) Eccentric fibrous plaque with highly reflective plaque formation from 2 o'clock to 7 o'clock (thin arrows) and intimal thickening with intact, low reflective media (thick arrows) in the remaining circumference. (c) Concentric fibrous plaque with uniform, highly reflective tissue over 360° of vessel circumference. (d) Thin fibrous cap atheroma: thin fibrous cap (thick arrow) at the transition zone between plaque and vessel segment with intact media covering a small necrotic core (*). Additional necrotic core (*) in the 6 o'clock position.*

(namely red blood cells) represents that non-transparent tissue causing multiple scattering and substantial signal attenuation. As a consequence, blood must be displaced during OCT imaging. This can be accomplished in several ways, e.g. by saline infusion through the guiding catheter, limiting blood flow by a percutaneous transluminal coronary angioplasty or a soft balloon, or continuous flushing during imaging by a dedicated OCT catheter design. These approaches have different advantages, however, all of them may cause, and are limited by, ischemia in the territory of the artery under study. Special techniques like index matching may improve imaging through blood in the future.[30]

Another limitation is the relatively low penetration depth of OCT that restricts in vivo imaging to small to medium sized coronary arteries (up to a lumen diameter of 4.0 mm) or to the visualization of the luminal vessel surface.

To date, the significance and clinical relevance of OCT findings in coronary arteries is unclear and further validation of OCT imaging is mandatory.

Summary

OCT is a new-generation imaging modality that principally allows for ultra high resolution such as visualization of the structure of living cells. It is therefore also named 'microscopy during life'. The rationale for intravascular application of OCT is its potential for in vivo visualization of the coronary artery microstructure.

Experimental studies confirmed the ability of intravascular OCT for plaque characterization and accurate assessment of vascular structures that are close to the luminal surface. Preliminary clinical experience has provided proof for the concept of in vivo intravascular OCT. To date, however, the significance and clinical relevance of OCT findings in coronary arteries is unclear and further validation of OCT imaging is mandatory.

Future application might consist of the combination of OCT with other diagnostic technologies such as spectroscopy or polarization imaging, or combination with other therapeutic modalities.

References

1. Boppart SA, Bouma BE, Pitris C et al. In vivo cellular optical coherence tomography imaging. *Nat Med* 1998; **4**:861–5.

2. Youngquist RC, Carr S, Davies DEN. Optical coherence-domain reflectometry: a new optical evaluation technique. *Opt Lett* 1987; **12**:158–60.

3. Takada K, Yokohama I, Chida K, Noda J. New measurement system for fault location in optical waveguide devices based on an interferometric technique. *Appl Opt* 1987; **26**:1603–6.

4. Fercher AF, Mengedoht K, Werner W. Eye-length measurement by interferometry with partially coherent light. *Opt Lett* 1988; **13**:186–8.

5. Huang D, Wang JP, Lin CP, Puliafito CA, Fujimoto JG. Micron-resolution ranging of cornea anterior-chamber by optical reflectometry. *Lasers Surg Med* 1991; **11**:419–25.

6. Huang D, Swanson EA, Lin CP, et al. Optical coherence tomography. *Science* 1991; 254:1178–81.

7. Tearney GJ, Brezinski ME, Bouma BE et al. In vivo endoscopic optical biopsy with optical coherence tomography. *Science* 1997; **276**:2037–9.

8. Fujimoto JG, Bouma B, Tearney GJ et al. New technology for high-speed and high-resolution optical coherence tomography. *Ann NY Acad Sci* 1998; **838**:95–107.

9. Schmitt JM. Optical coherence tomography (OPT): a review. *IEEE J Select Topics Quantum Electron* 1999; **5**:1205–15.

10. Hrynchak P, Simpson T. Optical coherence tomography: an introduction to the technique and its use. *Optom Vis Sci* 2000; **77**:347–56.

11. Falk E. Plaque rupture with severe pre-existing stenosis precipitating coronary thrombosis. Characteristics of coronary atherosclerotic plaques underlying fatal occlusive thrombi. *Br Heart J* 1983; **50**:127–34.

12. Burke AP, Farb A, Malcom GT et al. Coronary risk factors and plaque morphology in men with coronary disease who died suddenly. *N Engl J Med* 1997; **336**:1276–82.

13. Kolodgie FD, Narula J, Burke AP et al. Localization of apoptotic macrophages at the site of plaque rupture in sudden coronary death. *Am J Pathol* 2000; **157**:1259–68.

14. Hiro T, Leung CY, Russo RJ et al. Variability of a three-layered appearance in intravascular ultrasound coronary images: a comparison of morphometric measurements with four intravascular ultrasound systems. *Am J Card Imaging* 1996; **10**:219–27.

15. Tearney GJ, Yabushita H, Houser SL et al. Quantification of macrophage content in atherosclerotic plaques by optical coherence tomography. *Circulation* 2003; **107**:113–19.

16. Jang IK, Tearney G, Bouma B. Visualization of tissue prolapse between coronary stent struts by optical coherence tomography: comparison with intravascular ultrasound. *Circulation* 2001; **104**:2754.

17. Grube E, Gerckens U, Buellesfeld L, Fitzgerald PJ. Images in cardiovascular medicine. Intracoronary imaging with optical coherence tomography: a new high-resolution technology providing striking visualization in the coronary artery. *Circulation* 2002; **106**:2409–10.

18. Yabushita H, Bouma BE, Houser SL et al. Characterization of human atherosclerosis by optical coherence tomography. *Circulation* 2002; **106**:1640–45.

19. Regar E, Schaar J, van der Giessen W, van der Steen A, Serruys PW. Real-time, in-vivo optical coherence tomography of human coronary arteries using a dedicated imaging wire. *Am J Cardiol* 2002; **90(Suppl 6A)**:129H.

20. Brezinski ME, Tearney GJ, Bouma BE et al. Optical coherence tomography for optical biopsy. Properties and demonstration of vascular pathology. *Circulation* 1996; **93**:1206–13.

21. Jang IK. Cardiovascular optical coherence tomography. Ex-vivo results. The 4th Vulnerable Plaque Satellite Symposium at TCT 2002, Chicago. Association for the Eradication of Heart Attack, 2002.

22. Brezinski ME, Tearney GJ, Weissman NJ et al. Assessing atherosclerotic plaque morphology: comparison of optical coherence tomography and high frequency intravascular ultrasound. *Heart* 1997; **77**:397–403.

23. Patwari P, Weissman NJ, Boppart SA et al. Assessment of coronary plaque with optical coherence tomography and high-frequency ultrasound. *Am J Cardiol* 2000; **85**:641–4.

24. Fujimoto JG, Boppart SA, Tearney GJ et al. High resolution in vivo intra-arterial imaging with optical coherence tomography. *Heart* 1999; **82**:128–33.

25. Tearney GJ, Jang IK, Kang DH et al. Porcine coronary imaging in vivo by optical coherence tomography. *Acta Cardiol* 2000; **55**:233–7.

26. Jang IK, Bouma BE, Kang DH et al. Visualization of coronary atherosclerotic plaques in patients using optical coherence tomography: comparison with intravascular ultrasound. *J Am Coll Cardiol* 2002; **39**:604–9.

27. Hausmann D, Erbel R, Alibelli-Chemarin MJ *et al*. The safety of intracoronary ultrasound. A multicenter survey of 2207 examinations. *Circulation* 1995; **91**:623–30.

28. Batkoff BW, Linker DT. Safety of intracoronary ultrasound: data from a Multicenter European Registry. *Cathet Cardiovasc Diagn* 1996; **38**:238–41.

29. Shyu KG, Kuan PL, Cheng JJ, Hung CR. Cardiac troponin T, creatine kinase, and its isoform release after successful percutaneous transluminal coronary angioplasty with or without stenting. *Am Heart J* 1998; **135**:862–7.

30. Brezinski M, Saunders K, Jesser C, Li X, Fujimoto J. Index matching to improve optical coherence tomography imaging through blood. *Circulation* 2001; **103**:1999–2003.

11. Diffuse reflectance near-infrared spectroscopy as a clinical technique to detect high-risk atherosclerotic plaques

Pedro R Moreno, Barbara J Marshik and James E Muller[*]

Systemic inflammation and local variations in plaque composition are crucial pathophysiologic processes leading to plaque rupture and thrombosis. While widespread inflammation is often present and multiple sites of plaque rupture are frequently seen in patients with acute coronary events,[1,2] the majority of patients will present with a single, severe stenosis responsible for the heart attack.[3] If these culprit lesions can be identified before they become symptomatic, new prophylactic methods could be tested with the aim of aborting heart attacks. However, previous angiographic studies have shown that these potentially lethal plaques are usually non-stenotic and not detectable by currently available imaging technologies. Consequently, a clinical need exists for a method(s) capable of identifying high-risk plaques before disruption. Multiple scientific centers around the world have concentrated their efforts on developing techniques to identify high-risk, non-stenotic atherosclerotic plaques, which are now considered a *new* target in interventional cardiology.

Three different types of technologies have received the greatest attention: (i) techniques to image the plaque: high frequency intravascular ultrasound (IVUS), optical coherence tomography (OCT) and intravascular magnetic resonance imaging (MRI) are being tested with the hope that visual reconstruction of the microanatomy of the plaque will provide sufficient information to identify those that are vulnerable to disruption; (ii) techniques to measure structural and metabolic features of the plaque: elastography and thermography are being tested in patients to identify plaques with increased biomechanical weakness and temperature respectively; and (iii) techniques to measure plaque composition and higher characterization: near-infrared (NIR) reflectance spectroscopy is being tested for its ability to assess chemical composition of plaques in vivo. Several

---

[*]Drs Moreno, Marshik and Muller have financial interest in InfraReDx, a company developing near-infrared spectroscopy to detect vulnerable plaques.

forms of spectroscopy are also under study for characterization of atherosclerotic tissue. A recent review[4] summarizes the research with nuclear magnetic resonance spectroscopy, Raman NIR spectroscopy and fluorescence spectroscopy. This chapter will focus on diffuse reflectance NIR spectroscopy, which is based upon unique interactions of molecules with NIR photonic energy.

Diffuse reflectance near-infrared spectroscopy

The electromagnetic spectrum includes light or radiation with wavelength varying from 10^{-14} to 10^4 m (Figure 11.1). The NIR range consists of light of wavelength ranging from 700 to 2500 nm. Many portions of the electromagnetic spectrum such as γ–rays, x-rays, ultraviolet, infrared, microwaves, and AM and FM radiation, have been utilized to create valuable medical and commercial devices.

Definition of spectroscopy

Spectroscopy is the science of measurement of electromagnetic radiation as it is absorbed or emitted by molecules or their atoms as they move from one energy level to another. When a molecule is exposed to infrared radiation (of which NIR is a subset) the atoms absorb a portion of the light at frequencies that induce twisting, bending, rotating and vibrating atoms within the molecule. A key feature of the infrared transition is that the molecule must have a non-zero dipole

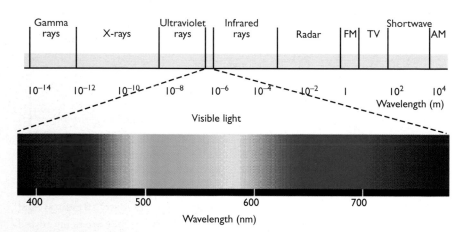

Figure 11.1 *Electromagnetic spectrum. Specific wavelength scales are given for each form of light, from γ-rays to audio/radio light (see text for details). (Reproduced with permission from P.E. Kaiser. www.yorku.ca/eye/how-to.htm[5]). Peter K Kaiser either owns the intellectual property rights in the underlying HTML, text, audio clips, video clips and other content that is made available to you on our website, or has obtained the permission of the owner of the intellectual property in such content to use the content on our website.*

moment in order for the transition to occur. For this reason linear diatomic molecules such as N_2 and H_2 are not active in the infrared region, while HCl and the functional group $C = O$ have very strong signals. A spectrometer measures the frequencies of the radiation that are absorbed by the molecule as a function of energy. The resulting group of frequencies versus absorbance is directly correlated to the characteristic vibrations of functional chemical groups. The magnitude of the absorption is related to the concentration of the species within the material being analyzed.

Understanding the interaction between photons and tissue is crucial for a variety of diagnostic and therapeutic biomedical applications of spectroscopy, which vary depending upon the wavelength of the incident light and the intrinsic optical characteristics of tissue. Combinations of carbon-hydrogen and/or carbon-oxygen functional groups, water and other components in tissue result in characteristic absorbance patterns for that particular tissue. The presence or absence of specific frequencies is the basis of sample identification and tissue characterization. Figure 11.2 shows the NIR absorbance spectra from a human aortic atherosclerotic plaque.

Interactions between light and tissue evaluated by diffuse reflectance near-infrared spectroscopy

When light meets an interface between two media, photons are either absorbed by the new medium, or transmitted through it. Light that is not absorbed will penetrate a portion of the sample. As it progresses, it may change directions,

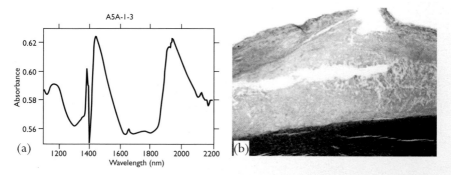

Figure 11.2 *Near-infrared spectra collected from an atheromatous, lipid-rich aortic plaque. (a) Near-infrared absorbance tracing from spectra collected with a Bran + Luebbe (Hamburg, Germany) InfraAlyzer 500 spectrophotometer. Absorbance values were collected from the 1100 to 2200 nm wavelength window at 10 nm intervals. (b) Lipid-rich aortic plaque (Elastic Trichrome staining). The spike at 1400 nm is an instrumentation artifact. (Spectra obtained at Dr Lodder's spectroscopy lab at the University of Kentucky, Lexington, KY.)*

or scatter, as it encounters another medium or particle boundary. This light scattering is a result of reflection, refraction and random diffraction at the surfaces of the various media and particles encountered. As the light continues through the sample some is absorbed while the rest continues to be scattered randomly. This process produces diffusely reflected light. Scattering and absorption occur simultaneously until the light emerges back at the entry point attenuated due to all the interactions with the medium (Figure 11.3).

Diffuse reflectance NIR spectroscopy is the analysis of the frequencies of the multiply scattered and absorbed photons of molecules excited by NIR light from 700 nm to 2500 nm. The NIR region contains absorbance bands resulting from the harmonic overtones and combinations of the fundamental vibrating and stretching bands in the mid infrared region. While absorbance intensities in the NIR region are only about 1/100 the intensity of those fundamental bands, most organic compounds still have a measurable spectrum that can be identified in the NIR region. Even though the spectral features are less intense and broader in the NIR region than the mid infrared, the application of mathematical techniques such as

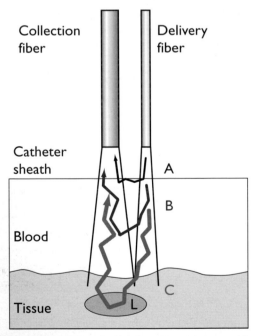

Figure 11.3 *Diagram of the path of light from the catheter and back. As the near-infrared light leaves the delivery fiber and interacts with tissue, some photons are absorbed and some are scattered or reflected by the catheter to the collection fiber in the catheter sheath (A). Blood particles (B) and tissue (C) photons may be reflected. The most valuable photons are those that interact with the lipid pool (L) within tissue and are reflected back to the catheter fiber.*

multivariate and principal component regression analysis upon the NIR spectral signals combined with the known chemical information of the system[7] has promoted the use of the NIR region as the premier region for quantitative and qualitative analysis of the chemical composition of specimens.[8] This method of analysis has been termed chemometrics.

Photons in the NIR region penetrate into tissue relatively well, providing simultaneous, multicomponent, non-destructive chemical analysis of biologic tissue with acquisition times less than one second.[9] No sample preparation is required and physical and biological properties, as well as molecular information can be derived from spectra. As a result, diffuse reflectance NIR spectroscopy has been successfully used to quantify systemic and cerebral oxygenation, and to identify multiple plasma constituents including glucose, total protein, triglycerides, cholesterol, urea, creatinine, uric acid and human metalloproteins.[10–14] In the NIR wavelength region, hemoglobin – the main chromophore in the visible region – has relatively low absorbance, making diffuse reflectance NIR an attractive technique for evaluation of plaque composition through blood.

Near-infrared atherosclerotic plaque characterization

Atherosclerotic plaque characterization using diffuse reflectance NIR was initially performed by Lodder and Cassis at the University of Kentucky using a novel NIR fiberoptic probe in the hypercholesterolemic rabbit more than a decade ago.[14] A vectorized three-dimensional cellular automaton-based algorithm using the quantile bootstrap error-adjusted single-sample theory (BEST) technique was developed to analyze the spectra in hyperspace. A NIR color imaging system was then constructed on an IBM 3090-600J parallel vector supercomputer and displayed on an IBM RS 6000 workstation. Figure 11.4 shows an example of color-reconstructed images from aortas with and without LDL accumulation.[14]

Analysis of plaque composition by diffuse reflectance NIR spectroscopy in humans was performed by Dempsey et al on carotid plaques exposed at the time of surgery.[8] After surgical exposure of the carotid bifurcation, NIR spectra were obtained from the plaque prior to endarterectomy. After surgery, the excised plaque was examined by a pathologist and frozen in liquid nitrogen for in vitro NIR scanning followed by validation of lipoprotein composition by ultracentrifugation and gel electrophoresis. Figure 11.5 shows a probability density contour map of the NIR spectra, showing regions of lipoprotein content as well as normal tissue (see Figure 11.5 legend for details).

Near-infrared spectra of high-risk atherosclerotic plaques
Our group (while at the University of Kentucky) collected spectra from 199 human aortic samples using an InfraAlyzer 500 spectrophotometer and compared

209

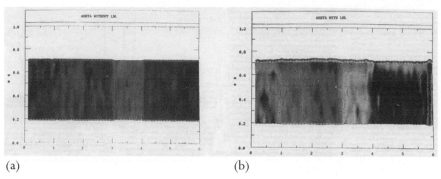

(a)   (b)

Figure 11.4 *LDL reconstructed color images from near-infrared diffuse reflectance spectra analyzed using the quantile bootstrap error-adjusted single-sample theory technique. (a) Normal rabbit aorta; (b) LDL-rich aorta from a hypercholesterolemic rabbit. (Reproduced with permission from LA Cassis et al.* Anal Chem *1993; 65:1247–56.[14])*

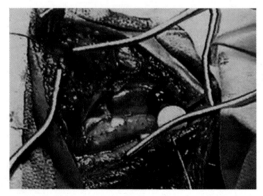

Figure 11.5 *A visible light image of a human carotid bifurcation exposed during endarterectomy. The target artery is located at about 8 o'clock relative to the white sterile reflectance standard. The top two reflectors in the black reflectance standard are the surgical lights, which are equipped with cold filters and emit little NIR light. The two smaller reflections are the tungsten sources for the NIR camera. Images are collected at each wavelength with the NIR sources on and off to enable correction for sample blackbody emission in the NIR and for other light sources in the room. (Picture and legend reproduced with permission from RJ Dempsey et al.* Appl Spectroscopy *1996; 50:18A–34A.[8])*

the results with histologic findings associated with high-risk atherosclerotic plaques. A chemometric algorithm of principal component regression was used to construct a prediction model using 50% of the samples as a calibration set, and the others as a validation set to predict high-risk features as determined by histology. Sensitivity and specificity as determined by the NIR method were 90%

and 93% for lipid pool, 77% and 93% for thin cap, and 84% and 91% for inflammatory cells, respectively.[15] These findings were consistent with data obtained by Jarros et al in their study using human aortic plaque tissue.[16] They found a high correlation coefficient of 0.96 between the cholesterol content determined by NIR spectroscopy compared with that determined by reversed-phase, high-pressure liquid chromatography. In addition, Wang et al. also found a high correlation between direct ex vivo measurements of lipid/protein ratios in human carotid plaques and results obtained using an NIR spectrometer fitted with a fiberoptic probe.[17] The same promising results have also been obtained by our group in studying human coronary autopsy specimens ex vivo.[18] However, in all of the experiments listed above involving human tissue measurements the results were obtained without the presence of blood, which would be encountered in the clinical setting. In most cases the tissue samples had been frozen or even fixed in formalin or paraffin prior to the acquisition of the NIR spectra.

Simulating in vivo detection of vulnerable plaques in an ex vivo setting

A significant challenge for detection of vulnerable plaques in patients is the development of an ex vivo method that will simulate in vivo performance. At this time, no animal model has been shown to have the same optical properties of diseased and normal human coronary tissue, so results on an animal model could not test all components of an NIR system designed to identify vulnerable plaques in living patients. Our group (at Cambridge, MA) has used human autopsy material to develop algorithms that discriminate high-risk atheromas from all other tissue types (such as fibrotic, calcific and normal) in ex vivo conditions. We elected to use fresh human ex vivo tissue because it has the same variety of chemical composition and morphology as in vivo tissue. We also believe that the simulated in vivo system will be of much greater value if the analysis is performed through blood, so the studies were performed through varying depths of blood. Even though the absorbance of hemoglobin from the blood stream is low within some portions of the NIR wavelength region, other NIR regions are obscured by the absorbance of water. Another contributing factor that strongly affects the NIR spectra is the scatter of the incident light as it penetrates and bounces off particles (e.g. red blood cells) within the blood stream.

A Foss NIRSystems (Hamburg, Germany) Model 6500 equipped with a 1 cm fiber optic probe (SmartProbe™) was used to acquire NIR spectra of 751 specimens from 78 fresh human aortic tissue samples. Specimens were pinned to a $5 \times 5 \times 0.5$ cm black rubber sheet and immersed in bovine blood prewarmed to 37 ± 1 °C. NIR spectra were subsequently acquired at various probe-to-tissue separations of 0.0, 0.25, 0.5, 1.0, 1.5, 2.0, 2.5 and 3.0 mm with blood intervening (Figure 11.6). Specimens were then classified by histology into normal, lipid-rich, fibrotic, and calcific tissue as shown in Figure 11.7. The solid

211

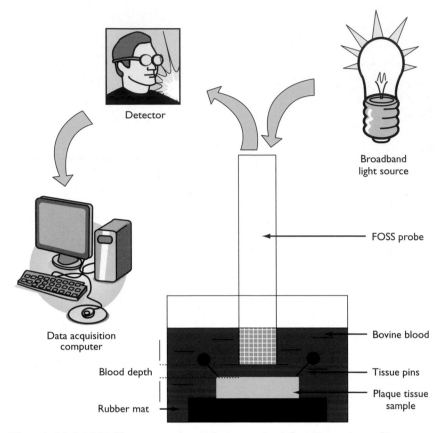

Figure 11.6 *FOSS fiberoptic probe configuration used for NIR analysis of human aortic tissue conducted through varying depths of blood. The FOSS probe was connected to a micrometer fixed to the Z-axis staging for moving the probe up and down.*

lines demonstrating the spectra recorded near the surface of the tissue reveal visible differences between the various types of plaques. As the probe-to-tissue separation was increased, the NIR signal over plaques and normal tissue looked much more like the spectrum of blood, as seen by the overlapping signals of the dashed lines showing measurements taken at 3.0 mm from the sample in Figure 11.8. However, chemometric methods can detect differences that are not identifiable by simple visual inspection.

The chemometric method of partial least squares discriminate analysis (PLS-DA) fortified with bootstrapping[19] was used to create a discrimination model that distinguishes the plaques containing large lipid pools regardless of plaque cap thickness from all of the other tissue types. The PLS-DA method creates a mathematical model based upon the spectral information from the two separate populations for which discernment is sought. The specimens used to build and test

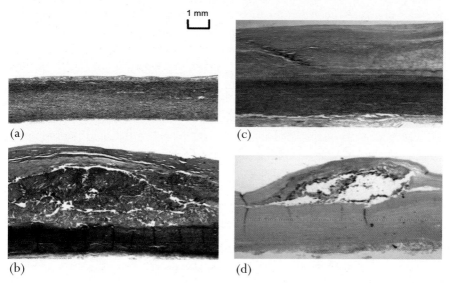

Figure 11.7 *Examples of the classifications used in the human aortic tissue NIR study with the FOSS probe. The probe illumination spot was estimated as 1.0 cm. Normal tissue (a), large lipid pool with a thick fibrous cap (b), large fibrotic plaque (c) and large calcific plaque (d).*

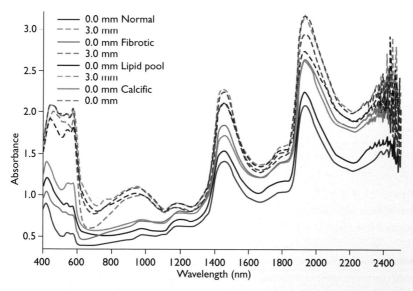

Figure 11.8 *Plot of NIR spectra of human aortic tissue specimens under a layer of bovine blood just above the sample (solid lines – 0.0 mm), and at 3.0 mm above the sample (dashed lines). The normal specimens are plotted in magenta, the fibrotic in green, the lipid pool in blue and the calcific in orange. Differences between spectra of various tissue types become less visible in the presence of 3 mm of blood.*

the discrimination algorithm for each of the types of plaques were selected by maximizing the amount of one constituent (lipid pool, fibrotic or calcific tissue) over all of the others. In the initial study a discrimination threshold was set to distinguish fibrotic tissue samples from lipid pool samples (Figure 11.9). The best model separating the lipid pool samples from the fibrotic samples was used to produce a blinded discrimination of lipid pool against other plaque tissue compositions (normal, calcific and fibrotic), also shown in Figure 11.9.

The separation of the resultant prediction scores of the lipid pool samples shown as sensitivity (SENS) from all other tissue types (fibrotic, calcific and normal) expressed as specificity (SPEC), using the best discrimination model, is displayed in Figure 11.10 at varying probe-to-tissue separations (blood depth) from 0.0 mm up to 3.0 mm. Table 11.1 summarizes the actual prediction values expressed as sensitivity of the model to identify the lipid pool samples as lipid

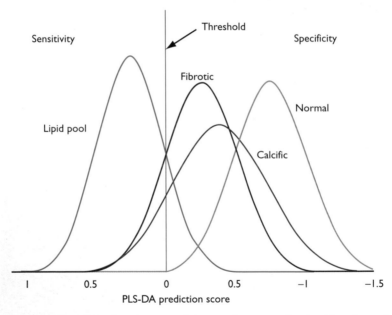

Figure 11.9 *Plot of the distributions of the populations used to build and test the partial lease squares discriminate analysis (PLD-DA) prediction algorithm. The model assigns a score from 1 to −1.5 for each NIR spectrum for all four types of atherosclerotic tissue studied. The separation of scores between the lipid pool samples (green) was maximized with respect to the fibrotic samples (blue) and a threshold for predictions was applied (red line). The distributions of the resultant predictions for the discrimination of the other populations for calcific samples (magenta) and normal samples (orange) are also displayed. Values to the left of the model threshold line (red line) indicate a prediction that the sample contains lipid pool and indicate the method sensitivity. Values to the right of the line indicate a prediction that the sample contains no lipid pool and indicate the method specificity.*

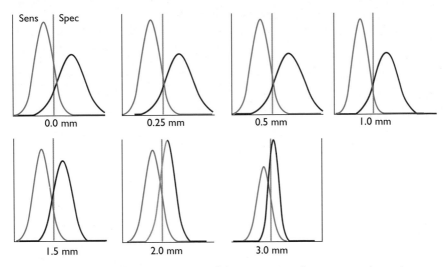

Figure 11.10 Plot of the distribution of the PLS-DA prediction scores (x-axis) as a function of sensitivity (SENS) of the lipid pool (green line) versus specificity (SPEC) with respect to all other tissue types (blue line) as a function of the probe-to-tissue separation and blood depth from 0.0 mm up to 3.0 mm.

Table 11.1 PLS-DA lipid pool model (SENS) predicted against all other tissue types (SPEC)

	0 mm	0.25 mm	0.5 mm	1.0 mm	1.5 mm	2.0 mm	2.5 mm	3.0 mm
SENS (%)	86	92	92	94	92	83	81	86
SPEC (%)	88	87	87	90	87	85	77	72

PLS-DA, partial lease squares discriminate analysis; SENS, sensitivity; SPEC, specificity

pools and as specificity of the model to discriminate all other tissue types from lipid pool. As seen in the results, the PLS-DA model was able to distinguish between lipid pool and other tissue samples through up to 3 mm of blood with at least 86% sensitivity and 72% specificity.

This study proved that an algorithm can be developed that is insensitive to blood thickness using NIR spectra of both diseased and normal samples of fresh human tissue through blood correlated to histology.[20] This is a key development for the use of an in vivo diagnostic tool, since the data indicate that it is possible to acquire spectral information from a catheter regardless of its position within the coronary artery. These very promising results were obtained under two conditions that were more difficult than those that will be encountered in the eventual clinical application: first the probe illumination area was quite large (around 1 cm in diameter) resulting in very heterogeneous plaques as determined by histology, creating some degree of misclassification. Second, the data set did not contain many lipid pools with thin fibrous caps. Such specimens, which are the clinical goal, should give a stronger lipid signal than lipid pools with thick (>300 µm) fibrous caps.

In vivo catheter-based vulnerable plaque system

An in vivo coronary catheter has been developed for the measurement of intracoronary NIR spectra in living patients. Initial safety studies were successfully performed in the coronary arteries of six normal swine using an over-the-wire, 3.2 Fr, NIR-catheter (MedVenture, Louisville, KY). Microscopic histologic evaluation showed no evidence of dissection, thrombus or perforation in any of the coronary vessels studied. This first-generation catheter was then tested in six patients previously scheduled for percutaneous coronary intervention for stable angina pectoris at the Lahey Clinic in Burlington, MA under the guidance of Dr Richard Nesto. Substantial motion artifact was observed due to the 2.5-second acquisition time of the system, which guided the development of a second-generation NIR catheter system. On the basis of these extensive data obtained in the preliminary autopsy and clinical studies, it is considered highly likely that a NIR system can be developed. Such a system will be capable of identifying the chemical composition of coronary plaques in patients already undergoing coronary angiography.

The future

Multiple technologies are under development that will provide the interventional cardiologist information about the composition and other features of plaques in the coronary arteries of living patients. The clinical significance of this information, however, must be determined through clinical trials. Such trials will determine if it is possible to identify a plaque that is 'vulnerable' or at high-risk of disruption and thrombosis. This will help to identify 'vulnerable' or high-risk patients likely to develop symptomatic coronary thrombosis and/or an acute coronary event. The trials will determine a 'vulnerability index' based on both plaque composition and clinical markers.

If localized, high-risk areas of an artery can be detected, both systemic and local therapy might be required. Local therapy with drug-eluting stents is an attractive option, though it may not be sufficient in patients with extensive, diffuse disease. Stenting is associated with significant reductions in total plaque and lipid core areas, increased collagen type III, and most importantly, with a dramatic increase in fibrous cap thickness.[21] While drug-eluting stents offer promise for the treatment of non-stenotic, high-risk plaques,[22,23] such therapy should not be adopted until proven to be safe and effective in a randomized clinical trial. The development of technologies such as NIR spectroscopy that might prospectively identify the high-risk plaque, together with new treatment options creates the possibility that many coronary events may be prevented.

References

1. Buffon A, Biasucci LM, Liuzzo G et al. Widespread coronary inflammation in unstable angina. *N Engl J Med*. 2002; **347**:5–12.

2. Rioufol G, Finet G, Ginon I et al. Multiple atherosclerotic plaque rupture in acute coronary syndrome: a three-vessel intravascular ultrasound study. *Circulation* 2002; **106**:804–8.

3. Goldstein JA, Demetriou D, Grines CL et al. Multiple complex coronary plaques in patients with acute myocardial infarction. *N Engl J Med* 2000; **343**:915–22.

4. Moreno PR, Muller JE. Identification of high-risk atherosclerotic plaques: a survey of spectroscopic methods. *Curr Opin Cardiol* 2002; **17**:638–47.

5. Kaiser PE. The Joy of Visual Perception. (e book) www.yorku.ca/eye/how-to.htm

6. Reeves III JB. 2000. Use of near infrared reflectance spectroscopy. Chapter 9 (p.185–208). In JPF D'Mello (Ed) *Farm Animal Metabolism and Nutrition: Critical Reviews*. Oxford: CAB Publishing.

7. De Maesschalck R, Estienne F, Verdú-Andrés J et al. The development of calibration models for spectroscopic data using principal component regression. *Internet J Chem* 1999; **2**:19.

8. Dempsey RJ, Davis DG, Buice RG et al. Biological and medical applications of near-infrared spectroscopy. *Appl Spectroscopy* 1996; **50**:18A–34A.

9. McKinley BA, Marvin RG, Cocanour CS et al. Tissue hemoglobin O_2 saturation during resuscitation of traumatic shock monitored using near infrared spectrometry. *J Trauma* 2000; **48**:637–42.

10. Spielman AJ, Zhang G, Yang C et al. Intracerebral hemodynamics probed by near infrared spectroscopy in the transition between wakefulness and sleep. *Brain Res* 2000; **866**:313–25.

11. Gabriely I, Wozniak R, Mevorach M et al. Transcutaneous glucose measurement using near-infrared spectroscopy during hypoglycemia. *Diabetes Care* 1999; **12**:2026–32.

12. Shaw RA, Kotowich S, Leroux M et al. Multianalyte serum analysis using mid-infrared spectroscopy. *Ann Clin Biochem* 1998; **35**:624–32.

13. Shaw RA, Mansfield JR, Kupriyanov VV et al. In vivo optical/near-infrared spectroscopy and imaging of metalloproteins. *J Inorg Biochem* 2000; **79**:285–93.

14. Cassis LA, Lodder RA. Near-IR imaging of atheromas in living arterial tissue. *Anal Chem* 1993; **65**:1247–56.

15. Moreno PR, Lodder RA, Purushothaman KR et al. Detection of lipid pool, thin fibrous cap, and inflammatory cells in human aortic atherosclerotic plaques by near-infrared spectroscopy. *Circulation* 2002; **105**:923–7.

16. Jarros W, Neumeister V, Lattke P et al. Determination of cholesterol in atherosclerotic plaques using near infrared diffuse reflection spectroscopy. *Atherosclerosis* 1999; **147**:327–337.

17. Wang J, Geng YJ, Guo B et al. Near-infrared spectroscopic characterization of human advanced atherosclerotic plaques. *J Am Coll Cardiol* 2002; **39**:1305–13.

18. Moreno PR, Eric Ryan S, Hopkins D et al. Identification of lipid-rich plaques in human coronary artery autopsy specimens by near-infrared spectroscopy. *J Am Coll Cardiol* 2001; **37**:1219–90.

19. Martens H, Martens M. Eds. *Multivariate Analysis of Quality: An Introduction.* John Wiley and Sons, 2000.

20. Marshik D, Tan H, Tang J et al. Discrimination of lipid-rich plaques in human aorta specimens with NIR spectroscopy through blood. *Am J Cardiol* 2002: **90**:129H.

21. Moreno PR, Kilpatrick D, Purushothaman KR, Coleman L, O'Connor WN. Stenting vulnerable plaque improves fibrous cap thickness and reduces lipid content: understanding alternatives for plaque stabilization. *Am J Cardiol* 2002: **90**:50H

22. Echeverri D, Purushothaman KR, Moreno PR. Evaluating vascular healing after metallic, polymer, beta-estradiol and everolimus-eluting stents on thin cap fibroatheroma: strut per strut analysis. *Vulnerable Plaque Meeting Symposium Proceedings,* March 2003 (in press).

23. Echeverri D, Purushothaman KR, Moreno PR. Fibrous cap rupture after metallic, beta-estradiol and everolimus eluting stents on thin cap fibroatheroma: potential implications for stent deployment in high-risk, non-stenotic plaques. *Vulnerable Plaque Meeting Symposium Proceedings,* March 2003 (in press).

12. INTRAVASCULAR ULTRASOUND AND TISSUE CHARACTERIZATION

Brian K Courtney and Peter J Fitzgerald

Since its introduction in 1988, intravascular ultrasound (IVUS) has become a pivotal imaging technology in cardiovascular medicine, having developed a significant track record in both clinical and research applications. IVUS has provided significant insights into biologically mediated processes of the vasculature such as restenosis, transplant rejection, the extent of plaque burden and vascular remodeling.[1] Furthermore, it has been an extremely useful tool in the evaluation and validation of several interventional techniques and devices including conventional stenting and angioplasty,[2] cutting balloons,[3] debulking techniques,[4] brachytherapy[5] and most recently, drug eluting stents.[6] It also has played a role in the development of provisional stenting strategies[7] and in identifying factors, such as embolic potential and plaque burden, that are associated with less favorable peri-interventional outcomes.[8] Improvements in core IVUS technology have allowed for higher resolution images, greater operator convenience and more powerful analysis tools such as three-dimensional analysis packages. The identification of vulnerable plaques via high frequency ultrasound tissue characterization methods has been a significant area of research over the past decade. Although no particular adaptation of IVUS to date has established itself as a robust standard for vulnerable plaque detection, several important contributions have brought IVUS notably closer towards achieving that goal.

Description of conventional IVUS technology

In 1971, Bom and colleagues developed one of the first catheter-based real-time ultrasound systems for use in the cardiac system.[9] In placing a set of phased-array ultrasound transducers within the cardiac chambers, it was shown that higher frequencies could be used to produce high resolution images of cardiac structures without interference from bony structures that occurs with transthoracic ultrasound imaging. By the late 1980s, Yock et al had sufficiently miniaturized a single-transducer system to enable the placement of a transducer within the coronary arteries.[10] From these origins, two general platforms have emerged for IVUS imaging (Figure 12.1). Both platforms produce two-dimensional images by performing a series of pulse—echo sequences, or vectors, in which an acoustic

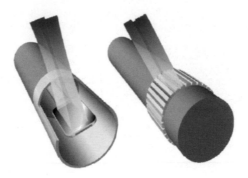

Figure 12.1 Two platforms of intravascular ultrasound catheters are commercially available. The first consists of a single transducer at the end of a mechanically rotating cable. The transducer rotates up to 30 times per second to produce cross-sectional images. A second platform consists of an array of circumferentially placed phased-array transducers, whereby the degree and relative timing of activation of the transducers are responsible for determining both the beam direction and beam shape.

pulse is emitted and the subsequent reflections from the tissue are detected. Each vector is acquired by directing the ultrasound beam from the catheter in a slightly different direction than the previous vector. The first platform directs the beam by mechanical means, in which a single transducer facing radially outwards from the catheter sheath is mounted onto the distal end of an inner torque cable. The torque cable and transducer are rotated by a motor drive unit at the proximal end of the catheter to provide two-dimensional cross-sectional images. The second platform is based on solid-state technology in which a set of several (e.g. 32 or 64) smaller transducers are arranged circumferentially around a distal portion of the catheter. These transducers are controlled electronically to produce an ultrasound beam in a direction determined by slight differences in the timing of their emitted pulses.

Image reconstruction in conventional IVUS

A grayscale IVUS image is made using all the vectors for a particular cross-section (256 vectors with most current commercial systems), with each vector acquired at a different angle of rotation. For each pulse—echo sequence, the raw ultrasound waveform, represented as an analog electric signal, is amplified and filtered. The envelope of this filtered signal is then detected. In order to compensate for the attenuation in the amplitude of the acoustic pulse that occurs as it travels through blood and tissue, a process, referred to as time-gain compensation, is performed. This process essentially amplifies each subsequent sample within a vector by an increasing amount which is defined by a curved function that the user can adjust. The same time-gain compensation curve is applied to each vector. Finally, the ultrasound signal is scan-converted from polar coordinates to cartesian

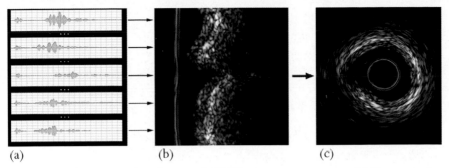

(a)   (b)   (c)

Figure 12.2 Intravascular ultrasound (IVUS) image reconstruction. (a) Five examples of the 256 vectors received in a single rotation of the transducer are shown. The pale red tracings represent the acoustic signal (recorded by radiofrequency IVUS) while the pale blue tracings represent the envelope, or magnitude of the signal. (b) A grayscale image is made, where the intensity of each pixel in a given row is based on the envelope of the signal within the corresponding vector. (c) The image (b) is transformed into cartesian co-ordinates to more closely match the true vessel anatomy.

coordinates (Figure 12.2), in order to display the ultrasound image in a manner that directly maps to the true anatomical geometry of the imaged vessel.

Effects of catheter specifications

Several clinically relevant properties of the ultrasound image, such as the resolution, depth of penetration and attenuation of the acoustic pulse by tissue are dependent on the geometric and frequency properties of the transducer.[11] A crystal transducer emits a signal which spans a range of frequencies. The higher the center frequency, the better the radial resolution, but the lower the depth of penetration. Current IVUS catheters used in the coronary arteries have center frequencies ranging from 25 to 40 MHz, providing theoretical lower limits of resolution (calculated as half the wavelength) of 31 μm and 19 μm respectively. In practice, the radial resolution is at least two to five times poorer, determined by factors such as the length of the emitted pulse and the position of the imaged structures relative to the transducer.

Three-dimensional IVUS imaging

The use of an automated pullback system combined with three-dimensional analysis and visualization software has made longitudinal and volumetric analyses possible, in addition to traditional cross-sectional analyses. ECG gating, initially thought to be fundamental to compensate for catheter motion that occurs over the many cardiac cycles that transpire during a typical pullback, is helpful but may not be necessary. Overall, three-dimensional IVUS has led to important observations regarding the longitudinal extent of plaque and about patterns of restenosis that occur with interventional technologies such as drug eluting stents[6] and brachytherapy. Main drawbacks of three-dimensional IVUS are the considerable time commitment required to perform volumetric analyses, and the absence of important vessel curvature information due to the assumption that the pullback is perfectly linear. Automated border detection algorithms are in development by several groups.[12] Bi-plane angiography is now being used in combination with IVUS to produce three-dimensional images that more accurately reflect the true longitudinal geometry of imaged vessels.[13] The association of positive remodeling with vulnerable plaques suggests that there may be utility to the application of three-dimensional IVUS analysis to the characterization of vulnerable plaques in vivo.

Correlating tissue types to acoustic properties

There are three general methods of analysis that have been employed for purposes of tissue characterization. The first employs categorizing an entire cross-section in both the histologic and IVUS images. This method, while simple for analysis and clinical reporting of vessel cross-sections, is rather poor for the purposes of establishing new techniques to characterize tissues as it suffers from poor spatial localization.

A second method employs user-defined regions of interest (as shown in Figures 12.3a and 12.3b), where regions within the image are delineated and the signal properties are measured and reported. This method provides for the

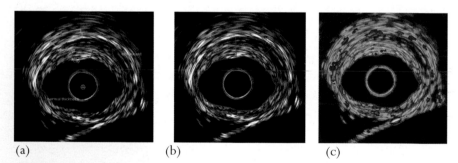

(a)   (b)   (c)

Figure 12.3 Methods of analysis. In order to match spatially localized signal properties to tissue types or vice versa, it is necessary to define regions of interest (ROIs) over which the signal's properties are measured. ROIs are typically defined by either (a) manual tracing, (b) a more regimented, but less localized manner using the lumen, the external elastic membrane and radial lines as borders or (c) over a small region of a given size surrounding a pixel. In the latter case, the value of a parameter (e.g. integrated backscatter), or a tissue type based on some pattern recognition scheme, can be color-mapped and superimposed onto the reconstructed intravascular ultrasound image to assist in locally assessing the underlying tissue composition.

opportunity to measure signal features (e.g. integrated backscatter) for a region in which a high level of confidence of knowledge of the underlying tissue type exists. However, this method also requires considerable experience to be used for the purposes of detection of certain features, and is dependent on the investigators using a standardized method of delineating the regions of interest (ROIs) in order to be reproducible. Some investigators may define ROIs by manually delineating their boundaries, while others may have fixed templates of ROI shapes that are positioned over the image. A more easily reproducible variant of this method was proposed by Stähr et al.[14] It requires the identification of the luminal border and external elastic membrane, and then divides the plaque area into sector-shaped regions by applying a template of as many as 8–12 radial lines that extend from the center of the vessel onto the image.

The third, and perhaps more favorable approach to analyze IVUS data, is to automatically define a region of interest for each pixel in the image. For example, each pixel may be associated with a small sector-shaped region centered around that pixel. Then the features of the signal calculated within that ROI can be used as inputs into a color-mapping or classification algorithm to provide an objective assessment of the cross-section based on one or more parameters. The pixel's color can then be determined by the results of the classification algorithm. Alternatively, the pixel's color can be determined as a combination of intensity and hue (as seen in Figure 12.3c),[15] where the intensity is derived directly from the conventional IVUS image, and the hue is derived from the output of the color-mapping or classification algorithm.

In order to develop a database of signal properties that match to specific histologic tissue types, Nair et al developed a method with which histologic images could be superimposed on top of an IVUS image.[16] The histologic image could be morphed so that its shape matched that of the IVUS image with a 1:1 correspondence. The tissue types assigned to each pixel in the morphed histologic images were then assigned to the automatically defined ROIs in the IVUS-RF datasets, thus allowing them to accurately correlate tissue types with acoustic properties of the tissues.

Tissue characterization and vulnerable plaque imaging

As demonstrated elsewhere in this handbook, we have learned much about the composition of vulnerable plaques in the past several years. In general, they have structural components (weak or thin fibrous cap, necrotic core, calcified nodules), inflammatory components and, in some cases, physiologic components (elevated shear stress and/or hypercoagulability). Although the current definition of vulnerable plaques encompasses several subtypes, it is illustrative to consider a set of structural features that would provide significant sensitivity in identifying the most commonly discussed subtype, that of the thin-cap fibroatheroma.[17] For example, it may be desirable to establish whether fibrous caps with a thickness of less than 100 µm and necrotic cores thicker than 200 µm could be reliably identified by IVUS-related techniques. A clinically validated criterion of the structural features of those plaques most likely to cause events, such as acute coronary syndrome, has not yet been established. As advanced methods for vascular tissue characterization continue to migrate from the in vitro setting to clinical use, the criteria and specific thresholds used to categorize lesions can be validated and/or modified, based on clinical outcomes or other appropriate measures.

Several tissue classifications by conventional IVUS for arterial tissues have been proposed. The American College of Cardiology Clinical Expert Consensus Document for IVUS Imaging discusses the general appearance of various tissue types, and broadly describes that a potentially vulnerable plaque can be expected to appear as a hypoechoic plaque, without a well-formed fibrous cap.[18] A summary of the tissue types and their appearance is provided in Table 12.1.

Some groups have proposed and made use of combinations of quantitative and qualitative measures to identify potentially vulnerable plaques. Using IVUS to identify a set of plaques that were suspect for potential instability, Yamagishi et al defined a combination of an eccentricity index as well as lipid core thickness and position to characterize plaques of interest.[19] They collected IVUS images of 114 coronary lesions with <50% stenosis from 106 patients who underwent diagnostic or interventional cardiac catheterization. During a 24-month follow-up period, those patients who developed acute coronary syndromes (ACS) were identified. All patients who experienced ACS were found to have demonstrated

Table 12.1 The most common tissue types qualitatively identifiable by intravascular ultrasound waveform

Type	Acoustic characteristics	Presumed tissue types
Soft (echolucent)	Low echogenicity	High lipid density, or necrotic zone, or thrombus
Calcified	Highly echogenic with acoustic shadowing	Calcifications
Fibrous	Intermediate echogenicity	Elastin or collagen content
Mixed	More than one acoustical subtype	Fibrocalcific, fibro-fatty
Thrombus	Variable, usually echolucent with speckling or scintillation	Acute or chronic thrombus
Intimal hyperplasia	Initially demonstrates low intraluminal echogenicity	Smooth muscle cells

eccentric plaques at the time of their previous IVUS imaging, and were more likely to have had lipid cores at a shallow position in the plaques that were identified by IVUS. The features of plaque eccentricity and lipid cores in close proximity to the luminal border are consistent with histological features of plaques that are believed to be most vulnerable to rupture. This study provided support to the notion that IVUS may play a role in identifying vulnerable plaques, but was not designed to be capable of defining criteria to identify vulnerable plaques. Techniques to objectively estimate fibrous cap thickness and to identify lipid cores based on quantitative measures of the backscattered signal had not yet been established.

Picano et al,[20] Di Mario et al[21] and others have reported on the strong dependency of the acoustic backscatter of various tissue types with respect to the angle of incidence of the ultrasound beam on the vessel. Hiro et al[22] exploited the property that fibrous tissues are more sensitive than most non-fibrous tissues to variations in the angle of incidence of the ultrasound beam. They used conventional 30 MHz IVUS technology to take images at two different positions in the same cross-section of a plaque. The changes in the backscattered intensity were combined with changes in the angle of incidence of the ultrasound beam along the luminal surface of the vessel wall to successfully identify fibrous caps in an in vitro experiment. Furthermore, they reported an ability to measure fibrous cap thicknesses with a standard deviation in error of measurement of 100 μm.

Perhaps one of the most interesting studies published to date on the use of IVUS for the purposes of evaluating the progression and regression of atherosclerosis was reported by Schartl and colleagues.[23] In essence, they compared the grayscale pixel intensity of lesions which were imaged at baseline and at 12-month follow up in a group of patients placed on statin therapy, as compared to non-statin controls. In order to account for some of the distortions in true echogenicity that occur when measuring grayscale values from conventional IVUS (c.f. with IVUS-RF, described below), a normalized intensity index of the brightness of pixels within the plaque was developed. This intensity index was defined as the grayscale value of the intraplaque pixel divided by the grayscale value of the adventitia. A hyperechogenicity index for each volume of a lesion was calculated, which identified the percentage of pixels in an intraplaque volume that had an intensity index >1. Their results demonstrated that lesions in patients on statins became relatively more echogenic compared to the non-statin group within a 12-month span, consistent with what would be expected in a lesion that either increased its fibrous content and/or reduced its lipid content.

Radiofrequency IVUS

As mentioned above, the detected ultrasound signals used to generate conventional IVUS images undergo considerable processing, such as *envelope detection, time-gain compensation and logarithmic compression*. While this processing is useful for the generation of real-time images that allow for qualitative image interpretation, these processing steps are generally believed to significantly reduce the ability to characterize imaged tissue by objective criteria of the reflected signal's properties. Time-gain compensation, logarithmic compression and the mapping of signal intensity to a grayscale pixel value make objective assessment of the echogenicity of the imaged tissue difficult to repeat and interpret quantitatively. They also make it more difficult to compare and interpret results between different studies. Perhaps most importantly, envelope detection discards a considerable amount of information in the signal, precluding the ability to use the finer details of the received acoustic wave that lie between its peaks. Radiofrequency IVUS (IVUS-RF) systems are capable of recording ultrasound waveforms at their highest level of detail, which may prove to be valuable in more precisely identifying the composition of the imaged tissue. A tabulated comparison between conventional IVUS and IVUS-RF is presented in Table 12.2.

IVUS-RF acquisition systems

Most commercial IVUS systems have an external connector that provides access to the unprocessed ultrasound signal before any envelope detection or other processing steps are performed. This signal is frequently referred to as the radiofrequency, or RF signal, as the frequency bandwidth of this signal spans a wide portion of the spectrum used for radio communications.

The signal is acquired using a digital oscilloscope, or digital signal acquisition card, that has a sampling frequency in the range of 100 MHz to 2 GHz. This hardware can either be stand-alone, or more conveniently, incorporated into a personal computer. A significant hindrance to IVUS-RF research to date has been the technical limitations in available digital acquisition systems. One of the most important specifications is the sampling frequency, which must be theoretically at least two times as high as the highest frequency detected by the transducer, and preferably three or four times higher. The second is the bit-depth, which determines the resolution of the system as it converts a continuous analog signal to one of a finite number of digital values. An 8-bit system can only represent up to 256 discrete voltages, while 12 bits allow for up to 1024 levels. Due to the large range of amplitudes of the ultrasound signal that is reflected from various tissues, such as hypoechoic lipids and hyperechoic calcium, it is difficult to acquire digital data with satisfactory resolution along the voltage axis from the full range of tissue types using an 8-bit system. Twelve-bit systems provide superior resolution, but until recently have only been available with a maximum sampling frequency of 100 MHz. A 12-bit system has been used to produce results with 30 MHz catheters,[16] but would not likely be technically satisfactory for use with 40 MHz catheters. Improvements in digital signal acquisition technology will certainly overcome these hurdles, and greatly simplify IVUS-RF imaging for both research and eventual clinical purposes.

Table 12.2 Features of conventional IVUS and radiofrequency IVUS		
Feature	*Conventional IVUS*	*Radiofrequency IVUS*
Real-time display	Yes	Not at present, although single frames can be reconstructed within seconds
Number of frames that can be acquired	Several minutes	1–10 seconds worth (each frame requires ~0.2–1.5 megabytes of physical memory)
Morphologic measurements (distances, areas, volumes etc.)	Yes	Yes
Three-dimensional analysis	Yes	Yes
Sampled signal	Envelope of acoustic waveforms	Raw waveforms
Stored signal (and units)	Reconstructed images (in grayscale intensity)	Raw waveforms (in volts)
Flexibility of post-processing (adjust filters, time-gain compensation parameters, etc)	Limited	Significant
Ability to perform measurements in frequency domain	No	Yes
Complexity	Minimal	Greater than conventional

IVUS-RF time domain analysis methods

One method that has made significant use of IVUS-RF is elastography[24], also known as palpography, and is described more thoroughly elsewhere in this handbook. Komiyama et al made use of the envelope of IVUS-RF signals to identify changes in the statistical parameters of manually drawn regions of interest for different tissue types.[25] They reported results from a small number ($n = 24$) of ROIs in which a threshold for each of the skewness, kurtosis and mean-to-standard deviation ratio (MSR) could be established to provide greater sensitivity and specificity for discriminating between ROIs containing a lipid core and those without.

227

In an animal transplantation experiment that investigated a relationship between inflammatory changes and acoustic properties of tissue, Jeremias et al were able to detect differences between the attenuation of IVUS-RF signals from aortic allografts and native aortas.[26] IVUS signals acquired from the adventitia of native segments of aorta had a much higher degree of attenuation than the transplanted segments. Although useful for the purposes of investigating transplant pathology, it should be noted that the use of attenuation measurements to identify inflammatory activity requires large regions of interest, likely making them unsuitable for detecting the focal zones of inflammation that are associated with vulnerable plaques.

IVUS-RF frequency domain analysis methods

A basic tenet of signal processing that is used widely throughout engineering and scientific disciplines is that every signal has at least two unique representations, and that one representation can be transformed uniquely into the other. Typically, the time domain representation of the signal (the representation acquired by an oscilloscope or similar instrument) can be mathematically converted into a frequency domain representation (Figure 12.4). This transformation is referred to as the Fourier Transform, and aside from its seemingly abstract and complex nature, it is one of the most useful tools available for signal analysis. In many respects, the frequency domain representation can be simpler to analyze, and provides more useful features of the signal. Furthermore, the different frequency components of acoustic waves behave differently as they travel through tissue. A prime example of this is the increase in attenuation that higher frequency components of a wave undergo through typical media, such as soft tissues.

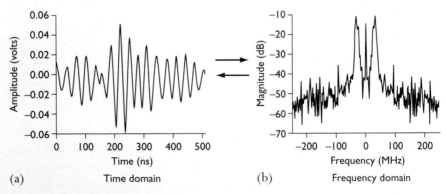

(a)   Time domain   (b)   Frequency domain

Figure 12.4 *Every time domain signal, such as a segment of a radiofrequency intravascular ultrasound waveform, as shown in (a), has a unique representation in the frequency domain (b). Note that the peak of the signal in the frequency domain lies close to 30 MHz, which is the nominal frequency for the catheter used to generate the signal in (a).*

Linker et al proposed early on in the development of IVUS that one or more frequency domain properties of backscattered ultrasound could be used to better discriminate between different tissue types than simply the grayscale pixel values for IVUS images.[27] For example, small scatterers, such as blood cells, tend to increase in their echogenicity, relative to other structures, with increases in frequency, while larger structures tend to produce more constant degrees of backscattering at higher frequencies. Due to the wideband nature of ultrasound transducers, it is possible to use frequency domain representations of the reflected signals to look at trends in the backscattered intensity over a wide range of frequencies. Figure 12.5 demonstrates several of the most studied frequency domain features used in vascular tissue characterization.

In 1998, Moore et al examined pressure perfused ex vivo specimens from autopsied human coronary arteries using an IVUS-RF system and off-line analysis.[28] They used sector-shaped ROIs that were manually positioned over a region of the IVUS-RF image data for which the underlying tissue type was known and classified as belonging to one of six subgroups. The line of best fit in the power spectrum for each ROI was calculated over the range of frequencies between 17 and 42 MHz, from which the spectral slope and y-intercept values were derived. Also calculated were the mean and maximum powers (in dB) over that same bandwidth. Lipid-rich and loose fibrotic regions were shown to have relatively flat

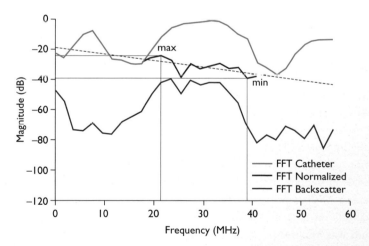

Figure 12.5 *Once a signal, or a portion thereof, has been converted to the frequency domain, many useful features can be calculated that reflect physical properties of both the transducer and the interrogated tissue. Biases caused by the transducer's frequency profile can be minimized by subtracting the power spectrum of the transducer (measured using a perfect reflector) from that of the backscattered signal from the tissue. This provides a normalized power spectrum, whose features are most useful to identify the underlying tissue type. FFT, fast fourier transform.*

spectral slopes (−0.17 and −0.06 dB/MHz respectively) which were well separated from the slopes of other plaque tissue types, such as moderately and densely fibrous tissues, as well as calcium and microcalcified regions.

Kawasaki et al performed an in vitro study of 18 arterial segments and 12 in vivo human arteries.[29] In each case, the integrated backscatter was calculated in the frequency domain for each 100 μm long window in each vector. The integrated backscatter was measured relative to the backscatter, from a steel plate, which is a commonly used reference standard. They produced color-coded images where each of five colors corresponded to ranges of integrated backscatter determined from the ex vivo arteries as belonging to one of five broad tissue categories: (i) thrombus, (ii) lipid core or intimal hyperplasia, (iii) fibrous tissue, (iv) mixed lesions and (v) calcified lesions. In the in vivo studies, angioscopy was used as a basis of comparison with the IVUS-RF color-mapped images. The thickness of the fibrous cap, as estimated from the IVUS-RF images had a notable relationship with the color of the vessel wall as seen by angioscopy. An example of a two-dimensional color-mapped image generated in a fashion similar to that used by Kawasaki is shown in Figure 12.6, alongside an image of the cross-section's histologic section. It should be mentioned that the span of intensity levels between lipid cores and calcium as reported by Kawasaki is significantly larger than that previously reported by Moore et al.[28] These differences have not been resolved, but may reflect differences in methodology of the two studies. However, the order of intensities for the various tissue types is consistent.

Stähr et al used a sector-based approach, where each ROI was defined by the luminal border, the external elastic membrane and two radial lines spaced 45° apart from each other.[14] The radial lines originated at the center of the catheter and split each vessel cross-section into eight sectors. This ex vivo experiment examined 234 ROIs in 32 autopsied coronary arteries and each ROI was defined as being either early/intermediate or advanced/complicated based on features found in the American Heart Association atheroscerotic plaques as defined originally by Stary et al.[30] Thirty MHz IVUS catheters were used with the power spectrum calculated over a 15.3–40.3 MHz range at 2.3 MHz intervals. Thresholds in the power spectrum were defined for each frequency bin in order to provide a >85% sensitivity in identifying advanced/complicated regions. Using these cutoffs on the same dataset, it was observed that the value of the power spectrum was a more specific discriminator at low frequency bins compared to higher frequencies. A possible explanation of this observation is that lower frequencies attenuate less, resulting in a more homogeneous image, but this remains yet to be supported by further studies. However, Stähr's results suggest a role for including signal analysis at relatively low frequencies (<20 MHz) in algorithms that attempt to acoustically characterize arterial tissues. This is in direct contrast to the notion that higher frequencies with higher resolution may provide a better approach to tissue characterization.

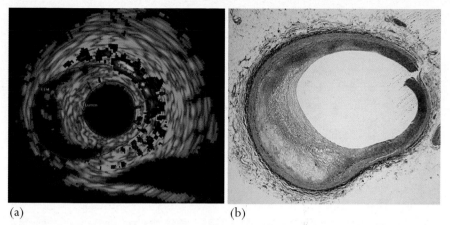

(a)   (b)

Figure 12.6 A color-mapped image demonstrates the normalized integrated backscatter of the tissue. Each color corresponds to a range of backscatter values. Other signal parameters, such as the mean-to-standard deviation ratio, can similarly be represented, as can results of tissue classification algorithms that combine one or more parameters measured in a region around each pixel to determine the most likely underlying tissue type. Note the appearance of the lipid core (re-brown hue) with a thick fibrous cap (green hue) in the lower left corner of the colour-mapped image. EEM, external elastic membrane.

Nair et al recently made a very significant step toward a robust implementation of a radiofrequency IVUS system to identify plaque components based on a multifeature classification algorithm.[31] Their algorithm accepts two borders, namely the luminal border and the media–adventitia border. For each point within these two borders, they estimate eight frequency domain features of the signal within a 480 µm window centered around that point, including the maximum power, the frequency with the maximum power, the minimum power, the frequency with the minimum power, and several other parameters. Each combination of these parameters maps to one of four histologically derived categories (fibrous, fibrolipid, calcium and calcified necrosis). Color-mapped images of vessels imaged in vitro provided reasonable agreement with histologic images of their cross-sections. The algorithm was reported to provide greater than 80% predictive accuracies for identifying all four categories of tissue.

Discussion and future directions

In the past 10–15 years, IVUS has developed into an indispensable tool for research and clinical purposes. By providing a platform for real-time, high resolution images of the vasculature, it has been possible to evaluate a wide variety of interventional devices, and develop optimal therapeutic strategies for patients with cardiovascular disease. Improvements in related technologies, such as signal digitization, computational power and three-dimensional image analysis packages have provided many opportunities for IVUS to continue to play an expanding set of roles.

In the field of vascular tissue characterization, and in particular with respect to the identification of vulnerable plaques, no single diagnostic technology has clearly proved itself to provide markedly superior performance over the others. IVUS is subject to the low signal-to-noise ratio which is inherent to all ultrasound images. It also suffers from signal attenuation and geometric effects that cause similar tissues to produce different backscattered signal properties as a result of differences in their position and orientation relative to the imaging transducer. These factors all affect the ease with which tissue classification algorithms can be developed and applied, yet in many cases, they are obstacles which are surmountable. As a core technology, IVUS also has several advantages that distinguish it from other imaging modalities. IVUS has excellent blood penetration. In the absence of calcium, it is able to penetrate deeply enough into the vascular tissue to visualize the entire vessel area, which provides important clues as to the presence and extent of disease by allowing measurement of plaque areas or volumes and eccentricity. The ability to produce real-time images is of use to investigators and clinicians alike. With foreseeable improvements in affordable computational power, many of the algorithms used to generate IVUS-RF based images also have the potential to be generated in real-time.

Several adaptations and improvements to IVUS technology may enable fundamental improvements in enabling the sought after ability to detect vulnerable lesions. Geometric compensation mechanisms may make it possible to substantially minimize the effects of angle of incidence and attenuation by interposed tissues,[32] thus improving the accuracy of classification algorithms. Alternatively, modifications to the IVUS catheter system that allow for imaging at several positions within a single cross-section would allow investigators to exploit the angle and position dependencies of ultrasound imaging for the purposes of tissue identification. As described above, ultrasonic imaging is not position dependent, but also frequency dependent. Enabling the acoustic interrogation of tissues with a wider bandwidth of frequencies, would allow for the identification of more features from the backscattered ultrasonic signal. This could be accomplished by either using single transducers with wider bandwidths or incorporating several transducers with different center frequencies on the same catheter. Ultra-high frequency components could be used to generate high resolution images to better image subluminal structures, such as fibrous caps, while lower frequency components could be used to provide depth of penetration and to further discriminate between plaque components. Another general possibility is to combine IVUS with other complementary technologies, such as thermography. This would allow for the generation of composite images that would demonstrate both the arterial wall morphology, as well as the surface

232

temperature of the vessel, thus combining structural and inflammatory indicators of disease to identify pathologic processes such as the vulnerable plaque. The introduction of guidewire-sized 0.025″ IVUS catheters[33] will allow for imaging of a greater longitudinal extent of the coronary arteries, while potentially being more easily delivered through smaller introducers and guide catheters.

While a majority of tissue characterization studies to date have been performed in vitro, we can expect to see an increasing amount of research in the near future demonstrating the use and advantages of IVUS and IVUS-RF analyses in the in vivo settings for tissue characterization purposes. Studies similar to that of Schärtl, wherein the effects of statins on the structural and acoustic properties plaques have been in progress using both IVUS[34] and IVUS-RF. Several studies combining different imaging modalities, such as IVUS-RF, optical coherence tomography and thermography, where the different technologies provide complementary information, will enable cross-validation of the different techniques. Ultimately, we anticipate and look forward to long term, in vivo, outcome-based studies using IVUS-RF and other technologies, so that an appropriately specific and sensitive definition of vulnerable plaques can be made, based on features extracted from the backscattered signals. Such a definition would have significant consequences on the ability to study and dispatch appropriate interventional measures that might substantially alter the clinical outcomes of patients with cardiovascular disease.

References

1. Nissen SE, P Yock. Intravascular ultrasound: novel pathophysiological insights and current clinical applications. *Circulation* 2001; **103**:604–16.

2. Stone GW, St Goar FG, Hodgson JM et al. Analysis of the relation between stent implantation pressure and expansion. Optimal Stent Implantation (OSTI) Investigators. *Am J Cardiol* 1999; **83**:1397–400, A8.

3. Nakamura M, Yock PG, Kataoka T et al. Impact of deep vessel wall injury on acute response and remodeling of coronary artery segments after cutting balloon angioplasty. *Am J Cardiol* 2003; **91**:6–11.

4. Mehran R, Dangas G, Mintz GS et al. Treatment of in-stent restenosis with excimer laser coronary angioplasty versus rotational atherectomy: comparative mechanisms and results. *Circulation* 2000; **101**:2484–9.

5. Mintz GS, Weissman NJ, Fitzgerald PJ. Intravascular ultrasound assessment of the mechanisms and results of brachytherapy. *Circulation* 2001; **104**:1320–5.

6. Kataoka T, Grube E, Honda Y et al. 7-Hexanoyltaxol-eluting stent for prevention of neointimal growth: an intravascular ultrasound analysis from the Study to COmpare REstenosis rate between QueST and QuaDS-QP2 (SCORE). *Circulation* 2002; **106**:1788–93.

7. Schiele F, Meneveau N, Gilard M et al. Intravascular ultrasound-guided balloon angioplasty compared with stent: immediate and 6-month results of the multicenter, randomized Balloon Equivalent to Stent Study (BEST). *Circulation* 2003; **107**:545–51.

8. Prati F, Pawlowski T, Gil R et al. Stenting of culprit lesions in unstable angina leads to a marked reduction in plaque burden: a major role of plaque embolization? A serial intravascular ultrasound study. *Circulation* 2003; **107**:2320–5.

9. Bom N, Lancee CT, Honkoop J et al. Ultrasonic viewer for cross-sectional analyses of moving cardiac structures. *Biomed Engl* 1971; **6**:500–3.

10. Yock PG, Linker DT, Angelsen BA. Two-dimensional intravascular ultrasound: technical development and initial clinical experience. *J Am Soc Echocardiogr* 1989; **2**:296–304.

11. Foster FS, Pavlin CJ, Harasiewicz KA, Christopher DA, Turnbull DH. Advances in ultrasound biomicroscopy. *Ultrasound Med Biol* 2000; **26**:1–27.

12. Klingensmith JD, Schoenhagen P, Tajaddini A et al. Automated three-dimensional assessment of coronary artery anatomy with intravascular ultrasound scanning. *Am Heart J* 2003; **145**:795–805.

13. Cothren RM, Shekhar R, Tuzcu EM et al. Three-dimensional reconstruction of the coronary artery wall by image fusion of intravascular ultrasound and bi-plane angiography. *Int J Card Imaging* 2000; **16**:69–85.

14. Stahr PM, Hofflinghaus T, Voigtlander T et al. Discrimination of early/intermediate and advanced/complicated coronary plaque types by radiofrequency intravascular ultrasound analysis. *Am J Cardiol* 2002; **90**:19–23.

15. Wilson LS, Neale ML, Talhami HE, Appleberg M. Preliminary results from attenuation-slope mapping of plaque using intravascular ultrasound. *Ultrasound Med Biol* 1994; **20**:529–42.

16. Nair A, Kuban BD, Obuchowski N, Vince DG. Assessing spectral algorithms to predict atherosclerotic plaque composition with normalized and raw intravascular ultrasound data. *Ultrasound Med Biol* 2001; **27**:1319–31.

17. Kolodgie FD, Burke AP, Farb A et al. The thin-cap fibroatheroma: a type of vulnerable plaque: the major precursor lesion to acute coronary syndromes. *Curr Opin Cardiol* 2001; **16**:285–92.

18. Mintz GS, Nissen SE, Anderson WD et al. American College of Cardiology Clinical Expert Consensus Document on Standards for Acquisition, Measurement and Reporting of Intravascular Ultrasound Studies (IVUS). A report of the American College of Cardiology Task Force on Clinical Expert Consensus Documents. *J Am Coll Cardiol* 2001; **37**:1478–92.

19. Yamagishi M, Terashima M, Awano K et al. Morphology of vulnerable coronary plaque: insights from follow-up of patients examined by intravascular ultrasound before an acute coronary syndrome. *J Am Coll Cardiol* 2000; **35**:106–11.

20. Picano E, Landini L, Distante A et al. Angle dependence of ultrasonic backscatter in arterial tissues: a study in vitro. *Circulation* 1985; **72**:572–6.

21. Di Mario C, Madretsma S, Linker D et al. The angle of incidence of the ultrasonic beam: a critical factor for the image quality in intravascular ultrasonography. *Am Heart J* 1993; **125(2 Pt 1)**:442–8.

22. Hiro T, Fujii T, Yasumoto K et al. Detection of fibrous cap in atherosclerotic plaque by intravascular ultrasound by use of color mapping of angle-dependent echo-intensity variation. *Circulation* 2001; **103**:1206–11.

23. Schartl M, Bocksch W, Koschyk DH et al. Use of intravascular ultrasound to compare effects of different strategies of lipid-lowering therapy on plaque volume and composition in patients with coronary artery disease. *Circulation* 2001; **104**:387–92.

24. de Korte CL, Pasterkamp G, van der Steen AF, Woutman HA, Bom N. Characterization of plaque components with intravascular ultrasound elastography in human femoral and coronary arteries in vitro. *Circulation* 2000; **102**:617–23.

25. Komiyama N, Berry GJ, Kolz ML et al. Tissue characterization of atherosclerotic plaques by intravascular ultrasound radiofrequency signal analysis: an in vitro study of human coronary arteries. *Am Heart J* 2000; **140**:565–74.

26. Jeremias A, Kolz ML, Ikonen TS et al. Feasibility of in vivo intravascular ultrasound tissue characterization in the detection of early vascular transplant rejection. *Circulation* 1999; **100**:2127–30.

27. Linker DT, Yock PG, Gronningsaether A, Johansen E, Angelsen BA. Analysis of backscattered ultrasound from normal and diseased arterial wall. *Int J Card Imaging* 1989; **4**:177–85.

28. Moore MP, Spencer T, Salter DM et al. Characterisation of coronary atherosclerotic morphology by spectral analysis of radiofrequency signal: in vitro intravascular ultrasound study with histological and radiological validation. *Heart* 1998; **79**:459–67.

29. Kawasaki M, Takatsu H, Noda T et al. In vivo quantitative tissue characterization of human coronary arterial plaques by use of integrated backscatter intravascular ultrasound and comparison with angioscopic findings. *Circulation* 2002; **105**:2487–92.

30. Stary HC, Chandler AB, Dinsmore RE et al. A definition of advanced types of atherosclerotic lesions and a histological classification of atherosclerosis. A report from the Committee on Vascular Lesions of the Council on Arteriosclerosis, American Heart Association. *Circulation* 1995; **92**:1355–74.

31. Nair A, Kuban BD, Tuzcu EM et al. Coronary plaque classification with intravascular ultrasound radiofrequency data analysis. *Circulation* 2002; **106**:2200–6.

32. Courtney BK, Robertson AL, Maehara A et al. Effects of transducer position on backscattered intensity in coronary arteries. *Ultrasound Med Biol* 2002; **28**:81–91.

33. Degawa T, Yagami H, Takahashi K, Yamaguchi T. Validation of a novel wire-type intravascular ultrasound imaging catheter. *Catheter Cardiovasc Interv* 2001; **52**:127–33.

34. Hagenaars T, Gussenhoven EJ, Poldermans D, van Urk H, van der Lugt A. Rationale and design for the SARIS trial; effect of statin on atherosclerosis and vascular remodeling assessed with intravascular sonography. Effect of Statin on Atherosclerosis and vascular Remodeling assessed with Intravascular Sonography. *Cardiovasc Drugs Ther* 2001; **15**:339–43.

13. Non-Invasive Visualization of Coronary Atherosclerosis with Multislice Computed Tomography

Pim J de Feyter, Nico Mollet, Karen Nieman,
Fhilippo Cademartiri, Peter Pattynama and
Patrick W Serruys

Electron beam computed tomography (EBCT) has been used for many years for detection and quantification of coronary calcium[1] but only recently to establish the presence of coronary obstructive lesions (Figure 13.1).[2,3] More recently the introduction of multidetector spiral CT has also allowed visualization of the coronary arteries and coronary plaques including obstructive and non-obstructive plaques[4,5] which can be classified as calcific and non-calcific plaques.[4] In addition CT has the potential to distinguish between low and high-risk plaques, and currently much research is evolving to establish the role of CT to identify non-invasively high-risk coronary plaque.

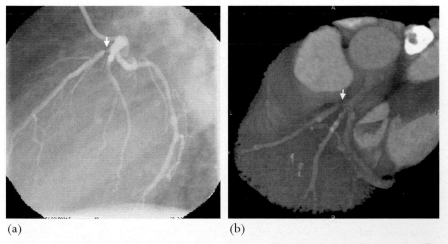

(a)   (b)

Figure 13.1 *Patient with stable angina pectoris and severe proximal obstruction of the left anterior descending coronary artery and calcification of the intermediate branch (bright spots) as assessed by (a) coronary angiography and (b) electron beam computed tomography.*

Coronary calcium as prognostic indicator of adverse coronary events

Coronary calcium is an indicator of the presence of coronary atherosclerosis.[6,7] The only exception is Mönckeberg's calcific medial sclerosis, which is associated with calcium deposition in the media and occurs particularly among patients with diabetes mellitus. The amount of coronary calcium is directly related to the extent of the underlying atherosclerotic plaque burden. However, the amount of calcium underestimates the total atherosclerotic plaque burden and the amount of coronary calcium detected is about one-fifth of the measured total atherosclerotic plaque burden.[6,7]

Higher amounts of calcium are associated with a higher likelihood of adverse coronary events, but the direct relation of higher calcium scores with increased likelihood of adverse events should be regarded as a reflection of the higher extent of underlying coronary atherosclerosis rather than the instability of a calcified plaque.[8-11] The absence of calcium does not exclude the presence of coronary atherosclerosis but is associated with a low likelihood of advanced coronary atherosclerosis and very low likelihood of an adverse coronary event.[8-11] Thus calcium is neither a marker for plaque vulnerability nor for plaque stability. The prevalence and amount of coronary calcium increases with age in both men and women, although in women there appears to be a lag time of 10 years compared to men. Men generally have higher calcium scores than women (Table 13.1).[12] Men and women with diabetes or markers of insulin resistance have an increased amount of coronary calcification (Table 13.2).[13]

The prognostic value of coronary calcium in asymptomatic subjects has been established in three studies (Table 13.3).[14-16] Although all three studies indicate that calcium is a risk factor, it remains difficult to draw definitive conclusions from these studies because there appears to be a selection bias (many individuals were self-referrals or responders to advertisements), the follow-up period is relatively short and the number of hard adverse events (cardiac death or myocardial infarction (MI)) is low. It has been shown that individuals with an above average coronary calcium score, adjusted for age and sex have a substantial higher risk of adverse coronary events (Figure 13.2).[17] The data about the independent prognostic value of calcium, in addition to the traditional risk factors, are inconsistent and remain to be determined in general populations of various ages and backgrounds.

The American College of Cardiology and American Heart Association consensus conference does not recommend screening of the general population,[8] but suggests that in individuals at intermediate risk a calcium score may be of benefit to adjust classification of an individual to a lower risk (no calcium present) or to a higher risk group (calcium present) which does have consequences for risk factor modification.[18]

Table 13.1 EBCT calcium score percentiles for 25 251 men and 9995 women within age strata.

Calcium score percentiles	Age (years)								
	<40	40–44	45–49	50–54	55–59	60–64	65–69	70–74	>74
Men (n)	3504	4238	4940	4825	3472	2288	1209	540	235
25th percentile	0	0	0	1	4	13	32	64	166
50th percentile	1	1	3	15	48	113	180	310	473
75th percentile	3	9	36	103	215	410	566	892	1071
90th percentile	14	59	154	332	554	994	1299	1774	1982
Women (n)	641	1024	1634	2184	1835	1334	731	438	174
25th percentile	0	0	0	0	0	0	1	3	9
50th percentile	0	1	0	0	1	3	24	52	75
75th percentile	1	1	2	5	23	57	145	210	241
90th percentile	3	4	22	55	121	193	410	631	709

(Reprinted with permission from JA Hoff et al. *J Am Coll Cardiol* 2003; **41**:1008–12.[12])

EBCT, electron beam computed tomography.

Table 13.2 Median CAC scores of men and women with and without diabetes

Men Age group in years	n	Diabetes Median CAC score	No Diabetes n	Median CAC score	P Value
<40	46	4	3.005	1	<0.001
40–44	63	13	3.653	1	<0.001
45–49	100	9.5	4.322	3	0.001
50–54	144	42	4.142	14	<0.001
55–59	160	111	2.192	43	<0.001
60–64	117	192	1.860	105	<0.001
65–69	72	378	955	152	<0.001
≥70	45	343	592	301	0.77
Total	747	63	21.441	6	<0.001
Women Age group in years	**n**	**Diabetes Median CAC score**	**No Diabetes n**	**Median CAC score**	**P Value**
<40	21	1	514	0	<0.001
40–44	32	0	846	0	0.14
45–49	32	1	1.398	0	0.01
50–54	74	8.5	1.826	0	<0.001
55–59	52	7.5	1.522	1	<0.001
60–64	47	21	1.105	2	0.003
65–69	34	104	712	5	0.006
≥70	36	114	465	52	0.54
Total	328	5	8.388	1	<0.001

The Mann–Whitney U-test was used to compare CAC scores between diabetic and non-diabetic subjects within each 5-year age group. The analysis was performed separately for men and women.

CAC, coronary artery calcium.

Table 13.3 Relative risks of coronary calcification for coronary heart disease in prospective electron beam computed tomography studies

	Subjects (n)	Mean age (years)	Follow-up (months)	Events (n)	Cutoff calcium score	Relative risk
Arad et al (2000)[14]	1173	53	43	39	160	22.2
Raggi et al (2001)[15]	676	52	32	30	≥0	0.12 vs 3.0*
Detrano et al (1999)[16]	1196	66	41	46	44	2.3

*Relative risk was 4.9 for subjects with low C-reactive protein level, and 6.0 for subjects with a high C-reactive protein level.

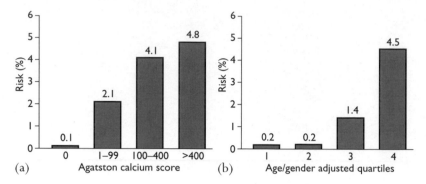

Figure 13.2 *Agatston score in patients with (a) non-significant and (b) significant coronary obstructions.*

Coronary calcium to predict significant coronary obstructive disease

The greater the amount of calcium, the greater the likelihood of a significant coronary obstruction which, however, is not site specific. The prevalence of calcium and the absolute amount of calcium, adjusted for age and presented by the Agatston score is higher in patients with coronary angiographic significant obstructions (Figure 13.3).[1]

The prediction of calcium for the presence of a significant coronary obstruction was established in 4.394 patients (67% males), mean age 55.3, who all underwent coronary angiography with a prevalence of significant coronary

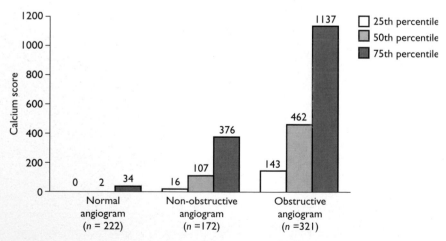

Figure 13.3 *Calcium score, adjusted for age and sex, and risk of adverse coronary events.*

Table 13.4 Predictive value of calcium after diagnostic coronary angiography

	Detrano et al[19] n=442	Keelan et al[20] n=288
Age (years)	55±12	56±11
Follow-up (months)	30±13	71
Death/MI (n)	13/8	22
CCS (Agatston)	≥ 75	≥10
Risk	6 : 1*	3.2*

CCS, coronary calcium score; MI, myocardial infarction.
*Compared to patients with lower calcium threshold.

artery disease of 52%.[8] The presence of calcium to predict a significant obstruction was high with a sensitivity of 93%, but with a low specificity of 45% and a predictive accuracy of 70%.

The value of calcium to predict adverse coronary events in patients who have undergone coronary angiography is significant with an increase in risk of death and MI between three to six times as high compared to patients with no or less calcium (Table 13.4)[19,20]

CT – coronary angiography

The diagnostic value of non-invasive coronary angiography with EBCT or four-slice MSCT (multislice computed tomography) to assess the luminal coronary integrity is tabulated in Tables 13.5 and 13.6.[1–5,21–26] The main limitation of both techniques is the insufficient robustness which is exemplified by the approximately 30% exclusion of non-assessable vessel segments predominantly caused by the limited spatial and temporal resolutions.

The newest generation spiral MSCT scanners applying 16-row detectors and if needed β-blockade to reduce heart rate are now being used to visualize the coronary arteries. These 16 MSCT scanners acquire data continuously at a rotation time of 420 ms. The data acquisition is synchronized to the patient's heart cycle and the data are retrospectively reconstructed according to the ECG from data acquired in mid diastolic cardiac phase when coronary displacement is minimal. To optimize the image quality, image acquisition (temporal resolution) is improved by reduction of the heart rate (longer motion free diastolic phase) by use of β-blockers prior to the investigation. To reduce respiratory motion artifacts the CT data are acquired during a single breath hold of approximately 20 seconds. For assessment of the coronary lumen, an iodine contrast medium, 120–150 ml, is intravenously injected and the data are acquired during the first-pass contrast

Table 13.5 Diagnostic accuracy of electron beam computed tomography for detection of a significant (>50% luminal diameter coronary stenosis

	Patients (n)	Sensitivity (%)	Specificity (%)
Schmermund et al (1998)[21]	28	82	88
Nakasnishi et al (1997)[22]	37	74	94
Reddy et al (1998)[23]	23	88	79
Budoff et al (1999)[24]	52	78	71
Achenbach et al (1998)[2]	125	92	94
Rensing et al (1998)[3]	37	77	94

Table 13.6 Diagnostic accuracy of four-slice multislice computed tomography for detection of a significant (>50% diameter luminal reduction) coronary stenosis

	Patients (n)	Assessable (%)	Sensitivity (%)	Specificity (%)
Nieman et al (2001)[4]	31	73	81	97
Achenbach et al (1998)[5]	64	68	91[*]	84[*]
Knez et al (2001)[25]	44	94	78	98
Vogl et al (2002)[26]	64	NR	75	91
Overall[†]	203	–	80	89

NR, not reported; assessable: image quality adequate for classification.
[*]High grade (>75% diameter reduction) stenoses.
[†]Corrected for patient number.

Table 13.7 16 multislice computed tomography coronary angiography: accuracy to detect significant (>50% diameter reduction) stenoses

	Patients (n)	Assessable (%)	Sensitivity (%)	Specificity (%)
Nieman et al (2002)[27]	54	100	96	84
Ropers et al (2003)[28]	77	88	92	93

plateau. These 16 MSCT scanners produce high-quality images with an in-plane resolution of 0.6 mm and a through-plane resolution of 0.8 mm. To date two studies have been published comparing 16-slice MSCT and diagnostic coronary angiography (Table 13.7).[27,28] Both studies used β-blockers to reduce the heart rate. Nieman et al evaluated the entire coronary tree including branches with a minimal luminal diameter of 2 mm. They found a sensitivity and specificity of 96%

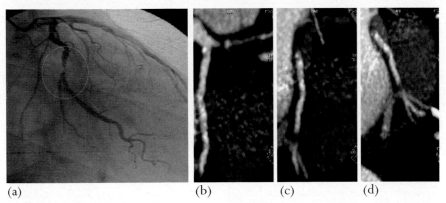

(a)   (b)   (c)   (d)

Figure 13.4 *(a–d) Multislice computed tomography: significant obstructive coronary stenosis.*

and 84%, respectively, to detect significant (>50% luminal diameter reduction) coronary obstructions (Figure 13.4). The positive and negative predictive values were 80% and 97%, respectively. Ropers et al excluded 12% of vessel segments for assessment and found a sensitivity and specificity of 92% and 93%, respectively to detect significant obstructions. However, if they had included all vessel segments (including insufficient quality images) the sensitivity would have decreased to 73%.

Sixteen-slice MSCT coronary angiography in combination with β-blockade appears to be a robust, fairly reliable technique to adequately assess the coronary lumen integrity. Remaining limitations of the technique are severe coronary calcifications, which obscure the underlying coronary lumen, and patients with irregular heart rhythm causing mis-reconstruction of slices, which precludes proper assessment.

CT – coronary plaque imaging

Visualization of coronary atherosclerotic plaques is even more challenging than visualization of the coronary lumen, due to the smaller size of the plaques. Based on the tissue-specific x-ray attenuation characteristics, CT is able to distinguish fat tissue, fibrous tissue, contrast medium and calcium and thus in theory should be able to differentiate plaques that are calcified, predominantly fibrous or plaques that contain a large lipid pool (Figure 13.5).

Schroeder et al compared contrast-enhanced MSCT images of coronary plaques with intracoronary ultrasound.[29] The echogenicity of the plaques was compared to the CT-attenuation values (Hounsfield units, HU) of the same plaque. Intracoronary ultrasound classified plaques as 'soft', 'intermediate' and calcific. The CT density of these soft, intermediate and calcific plaques was

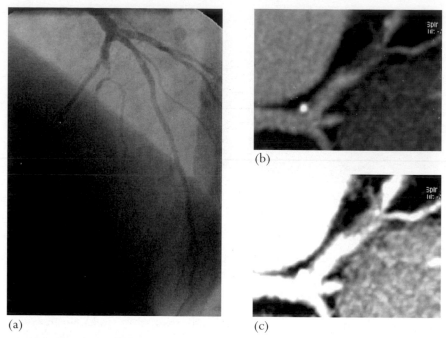

(a) (b) (c)

Figure 13.5 *(a–c) Multislice computed tomography: soft plaque in the left anterior descending coronary artery.*

14±26 HU (range −42 to +47 HU), 91±21 HU (61–112 HU) and 419±194 HU (126–736 HU), respectively.

Leber et al compared the composition of coronary atherosclerotic plaques with four-slice MSCT in patients with acute MI and stable angina.[30] A coronary plaque was defined as a structure >1 mm^2 within the coronary artery whose density differed from the contrast-enhanced vessel lumen. Plaques were classified as calcific (>130 HU) and non-calcific (<130 HU). In the stable angina group 230 coronary plaques were detected in 19 patients: 14 (7%) non-calcified, 183 (79%) calcified and 30 (13%) mixed. In the acute MI group 217 plaques were detected in 21 patients: 53 (24%) non-calcified, 125 (56%) calcified and 39 (18%) mixed. They demonstrated that non-calcified plaques contributed more to the total plaque burden in patients with acute MI compared to stable angina patients. Although these initial results are promising there are limitations. Both studies used a four-slice spiral CT scanner which has a relatively limited resolution: an effective acquisition time of 250 sec, slice thickness of 1.25 mm and an in-plane resolution of 0.6 mm. These limitations can largely be overcome by the significantly better diagnostic performance of the newest 16-slice MSCT scanner and confirmation by studies using this technique are eagerly awaited.

Progression of coronary atherosclerosis

The amount of coronary calcium is a measure of the total amount of coronary atherosclerosis and thus serial assessment of coronary calcification may give an indirect assessment of progression of coronary atherosclerosis.

Current CT scanners allow accurate repeat measurements of coronary calcification which can be obtained with a less than 10% variability. The rate of progression is related to the baseline calcium quantity and may be different in various populations. The annual increase of calcium varies between 20 and 50% in low-risk and statin-treated patients at the lower end and untreated persons at the high end of the spectrum (Table 13.8).[31–37] It is to be noted that progression of calcium may be difficult to assess in patients with low scores because interscan variability may be greater than the rate of progression.[38,39] The use of coronary calcification as a surrogate endpoint of progression or regression of coronary atherosclerosis is an interesting non-invasive alternative to quantitative intracoronary angiography or quantitative coronary ultrasound to serially monitor the effectiveness of new pharmacologic compounds to reduce or prevent progression of coronary atherosclerosis. Whether progression or regression of

Table 13.8 Annual progression of coronary calcification in generally asymptomatic subjects in observational studies

	Subjects (n)	Follow-up (months)	Progression without therapy (%)	Progression with statins (%)
Maher et al (1999)[31]	82	42	24	
Pohle et al (2001)[32]	104	15	27	
Yoon et al (2002)[33]	217	25	38	
Janowitz et al (1991)[34]	20	13		
Asymptomatic CAD			20	48
Callister et al (1998)[35]	149* (105 treated)	14	52**	5**
Budoff et al (2000)[36]	131* (60 treated)	26	39	15
Achenbach et al (2002)[37]	66	14/21†	25	9

*Study among hypercholesterolemic patients.
**Progression rate for whole follow-up period.
†14 months without treatment, then 12 months with treatment.
CAD, coronary artery disease.

calcium is representative of true plaque progression or regression is largely unknown, and even more uncertain is the fact whether calcium changes can be translated into plaque stability or instability.

In case of regression of a plaque it remains unclear which components of the plaque regress – for instance, lipid or calcium. In atherosclerotic monkeys fed an antiatherosclerotic diet the plaque size decreased but the volume of calcium remained unchanged leading to an increase in the proportion of calcium in the plaque from 20% at baseline to 50% in the regressed lesion.[40] More studies are needed to ascertain the role of calcium in progression/regression studies.

MSCT and high-risk plaque

The identification of high-risk plaques is currently the subject of much debate and research. Non-invasive detection of a high-risk plaque would be highly desirable and it has been shown that MSCT can identify characteristics of coronary plaques which may be useful to identify a high-risk plaque (Box 13.1). A potential problem using computed tomography is the radiation exposure to patients and high-risk individuals, which is, in some protocols, substantial and precludes unlimited re-investigations (Table 13.9).

Intriguing is the possibility that MSCT can be used as an initial non-invasive technique to establish the presence and localization of coronary lesion, and possibly identify a high-risk lesion in a high-risk individual (Figure 13.6). Subsequently, invasive techniques, such as intracoronary ultrasound and its derivatives: palpography, virtual histology and thermography or optical coherence tomography may then establish the 'vulnerability' of the plaque. We have devised an algorithm which includes the non-invasive role of spiral CT-scanning (Figure 13.7). However, the viability of this approach requires clinical testing to confirm these high expectations.

Box 13.1 Computed tomography coronary plaque imaging: plaque characteristics

Obstructive plaque (>50% luminal diameter reduction)
Non-obstructive plaque
Calcific plaque (quantification)
Non-calcific 'soft' plaque
Remodeling vessel wall
Total coronary plaque burden

Table 13.9 Radiation dose in computed tomography scanning of the coronary arteries in men and women

	Effective dose (mSv)	
	Coronary calcium	Coronary angiography
EBCT	0.7–1.3	1.1–2.0 (triggered)
4 MSCT	1.0	9.3–11.3
	1.5–6.2	6.7–13
Catheter angiography	–	2.1– 2.5

Annual environmental dose: 2.4 mSv

EBCT, electron beam computed tomography; MSCT, multislice computed tomography. (Adapted from Morin et al. *Circulation* 2003; **107**:917–22[41] and Hunold et al. *Radiology* 2003; **226**:145–152.[42] (MS-CT with retrospective gating))

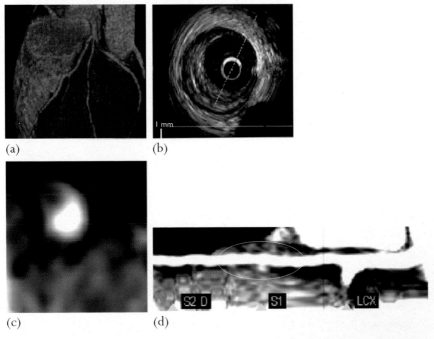

(a) (b) (c) (d)

Figure 13.6 *Multislice computed tomography (MSCT) of soft plaque detected in a high-risk individual, confirmed with intra-coronary ultrasound. (a) Volume rendered three-dimensional MSCT coronary angiogram. (b) Ultrasound cross-section with eccentric plaque. (c) MSCT cross-section at plaque site in the left anterior descending coronary artery. Bright is coronary lumen, gray zone is eccentric plaque. (d) Longitudinal MSCT view of the left anterior descending coronary artery. LCX, left coronary circumflex; S1, first septal branch; S2, second septal branch, D, diagonal branch.*

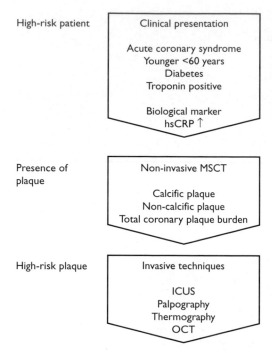

Figure 13.7. *Algorithm to detect high-risk plaque in a high-risk patient. MSCT, multislice computed tomography; ICUS, intracoronary ultrasound; OCT, optical coherence tomography; hsCRP, high sensitivity C-reactive protein.*

References

1. Agatston AS, Janowitz WR, Hildner FJ et al. Quantification of coronary artery calcium using ultrafast computed tomography. *J Am Coll Cardiol* 1990; **15**:827–32.

2. Achenbach S, Moshage W, Ropers D, Nossen J, Daniel WG. Value of electron-beam computed tomography for the noninvasive detection of high-grade coronary-artery stenoses and occlusions. *N Engl J Med* 1998; **339**:1964–71.

3. Rensing BJ, Bongaerts A, van Geuns RJ et al. Intravenous coronary angiography by electron beam computed tomography: a clinical evaluation. *Circulation* 1998; **98**:2509–12.

4. Nieman K, Oudkerk M, Rensing BJ. Coronary angiography with multi-slice computed tomography. *Lancet* 2001; **357**:599–603.

5. Achenbach S, Giesler T, Ropers D et al. Detection of coronary artery stenoses by contrast-enhanced, retrospectively electrocardiographically-gated, multislice spiral computed tomography. *Circulation* 2001; **103**:2535–8.

6. Rumberger JA, Simons DB, Fitzpatrick LA et al. Coronary artery calcium area by electron-beam computed tomography and coronary atherosclerotic plaque area. A histopathologic correlative study. *Circulation* 1995; **92**:2157–62.

7. Sangiorgi G, Rumberger JA, Severson A et al. Arterial calcification and not lumen stenosis is highly correlated with atherosclerotic plaque burden in humans: a

histologic study of 723 coronary artery segments using nondecalcifying methodology. *J Am Coll Cardiol* 1998; **89**:36–44.

8. O'Rourke RA, Brundage BH, Froelicher VF et al. American College of Cardiology/American Heart Association Expert Consensus document on electron-beam computed tomography for the diagnosis and prognosis of coronary artery disease. *Circulation* 2000; **102**:126–140.

9. Schmermund A, Erbel R. Unstable coronary plaque and its relation to coronary calcium. *Circulation* 2001; **104**:1682–7.

10. Schmermund A, Baumgart D, Gorge G et al. Coronary artery calcium in acute coronary syndromes: a comparative study of electron-beam computed tomography, coronary angiography, and intracoronary ultrasound in survivors of acute myocardial infarction and unstable angina. *Circulation* 1997; **96**:1461–9.

11. Schmermund A, Schwartz RS, Adamzik M et al. Coronary atherosclerosis in unheralded sudden coronary death under age 50: histo-pathologic comparison with 'healthy' subjects dying out of hospital. *Atherosclerosis* 2001; **155**:499–508.

12. Hoff JA, Chomka EV, Krainik AJ et al. Age and gender distributions of coronary artery calcium detected by electron beam tomography in 35 246 adults. *Am J Cardiol* 2001; **87**:1335–9.

13. Hoff JA, Quinn L, Sevrukov A et al. The prevalence of coronary artery calcium among diabetic individuals without known coronary artery disease. *J Am Coll Cardiol* 2003; **41**:1008–12.

14. Arad Y, Spadaro LA, Goodman K, Newstein D, Guerci AD. Prediction of coronary events with electron beam computed tomography. *J Am Coll Cardiol* 2000; **36**:1253–60.

15. Raggi P, Cooil B, Callister TQ. Use of electron beam tomography data to develop models for prediction of hard coronary events. *Am Heart J* 2001; **141**:375–82.

16. Detrano RC, Doherty R, Wong ND et al. Coronary calcium does not accurately predict near-term future coronary events in high-risk adults. *Circulation* 1999; **99**:2633–8.

17. Raggi P, Callister RQ, Cooil B. Identification of patients at increased risk of first unheralded acute myocardial infarction by electron-beam computed tomography. *Circulation* 2000; **101**:850–5.

18. Greenland P, Abrams J, Aurigemma, GP et al. Prevention Conference V: Beyond secondary prevention: identifying the high-risk patient for primary prevention: noninvasive tests of atherosclerotic burden: Writing Group III. *Circulation* 2000; **101**:e16–e22.

19. Detrano R, Hsiai T, Wang S et al. Prognostic value of coronary calcification and angiographic stenoses in patients undergoing coronary angiography. *J Am Coll Cardiol* 1996; **27**:285–90.

251

20. Keelan PC, Bielak LF, Ashai K et al. Long-term prognostic value of coronary calcification detected by electron-beam computed tomography in patients undergoing coronary angiography. *Circulation* 2001; **104**:412–17.

21. Schmermund A, Rensing BJ, Sheedy PF et al. Intravenous electron-beam computed tomographic coronary angiography for segmental analysis of coronary artery stenoses. *J Am Coll Cardiol* 1998; **31**:1547–54.

22. Nakanishi T, Ito K, Imazu M et al. Evaluation of coronary artery stenoses using electron-beam CT and multiplanar reformation. *J Comput Assist Tomogr* 1997; **21**:121–7.

23. Reddy G, Chernoff DM, Adams JR et al. Coronary artery stenoses: assessment with contrast-enhanced electron-beam CT and axial reconstructions. *Radiology* 1998; **208**:167–172.

24. Budoff MJ, Oudiz RJ, Zalace CP et al. Intravenous three-dimensional coronary angiography using contrast enhanced electron beam computed tomography. *Am J Cardiol* 1999; **83**:840–5.

25. Knez A, Becker CR, Leber A et al. Usefulness of multislice spiral computed tomography angiography for determination of coronary artery stenoses. *Am J Cardiol* 2001; **88**:1191–4.

26. Vogl TJ, Abolmaali ND, Diebold T et al. Techniques for the detection of coronary atherosclerosis: multi-detector row CT coronary angiography. *Radiology* **223**:212–20.

27. Nieman K, Cademartiri F, Lemos PA et al. Reliable noninvasive coronary angiography with fast submillimeter multislice spiral computed tomography. *Circulation* 2002; **106**:2051–4.

28. Ropers D, Baum U, Pohle K et al. Detection of coronary artery stenoses with thin-slice multi-detector row spiral computed tomography and multiplanar reconstruction. *Circulation* 2003; **107**:664–6.

29. Schroeder S, Kopp AF, Baumbach A et al. Noninvasive detection and evaluation of atherosclerotic coronary plaques with multislice computed tomography. *J Am Coll Cardiol* 2001; **37**:1430–5.

30. Leber AW, Knez A, Mukherjee R et al. Usefulness of calcium scoring using electron beam computed tomography and noninvasive coronary angiography in patients with suspected coronary artery disease. *Am J Cardiol* 2003; **91**:714–18.

31. Maher JE, Bielak LF, Raz JA et al. Progression of coronary artery calcification: a pilot study. *Mayo Clin Proc* 1999; **74**:347–55.

32. Pohle K, Maffert R, Ropers D et al. Progression of aortic valve calcification: association with coronary atherosclerosis and cardiovascular risk factors. *Circulation* 2001; **104**:1927–32.

33. Yoon HC, Emerick AM, Hill JA, Gjertson DW, Goldin JG. Calcium begets calcium: progression of coronary artery calcification in asymptomatic subjects. *Radiology* 2002; **224**:236–41.

34. Janowitz WR, Agatston AS, Viamonte M Jr. Comparison of serial quantitative evaluation of calcified coronary artery plaque by ultrafast computed tomography in persons with and without obstructive coronary artery disease. *Am J Cardiol* 1991; **68**:1–6.

35. Callister TQ, Raggi P, Cooil B, Lippolis NJ, Russo DJ. Effect of HMG-CoA reductase inhibitors on coronary artery disease as assessed by electron-beam computed tomography. *N Engl J Med* 1998; **208**:807–14.

36. Budoff MJ, Gillespie R, Georgiou D et al. Comparison of exercise electron beam computed tomography and sestamibi in the evaluation of coronary artery disease. *Am J Cardiol* 2000; **86**:8–11.

37. Achenbach S, Ropers D, Pohle K et al. Influence of lipid-lowering therapy on the progression of coronary artery calcification: a prospective evaluation. *Circulation* 2002; **106**:1077–82.

38. Möhlenkamp S, Behrenbeck TR, Pump H et al. Reproducibility of two coronary calcium quantification algorithms in patients with different degrees of calcifications. *Int J Card Imag* 2001; **17**:133–42.

39. Bielak LF, Sheedy PF, Peyser PA. Coronary artery calcification measured at electron-beam CT: agreement in dual scan runs and change over time. *Radiology* 2001; **218**:224–9.

40. Stary HC. Natural history of calcium deposits in atherosclerosis progression and regression. *Z Kardiol* 2000; **89 (suppl 2)**:28–35.

41. Morin RL, Gerber TC, McCollough H. Radiation dose in computed tomography of the heart. *Circulation* 2003; **107**:917–22.

42. Hunold P, Vogt FM, Schmermund A et al. Radiation exposure during cardiac CT: effective doses at multi-detector row CT and electron-beam CT. *Radiology* 2003; **226**:146–152.

14. DRUG THERAPY FOR THE VULNERABLE PLAQUE

John A Ambrose and David J D'Agate

The concept of plaque stabilization was proposed to explain how lipid-lowering therapy could decrease acute adverse coronary events without a substantial regression in atherosclerosis.[1] In the published angiographic lipid-lowering trials, there was an approximate 22–34% reduction by pooled analysis in major acute cardiac events, which was similar to the percent reduction in many of the large primary and secondary prevention trials utilizing lipid-lowering therapy.[2] Furthermore, in some of these angiographic studies the reduction in events exceeded 50%. It was postulated that regression of atherosclerosis as determined by angiography was unlikely to completely explain this large reduction in clinical events. Several factors were hypothesized to contribute to this reduction and these became known as the 'pleiotropic effects' of lipid-lowering therapy.[3,4] Several lines of evidence indicated that lipid-lowering therapy and in particular the statins possessed anti-inflammatory and anti-thrombotic effects as well as effects on normalizing endothelial function. In addition, lipid lowering in experimental animals had been shown to reduce plaque lipid, which in itself promoted plaque stabilization.[5]

The vulnerable atherosclerotic plaque

A major challenge in medicine today is to prevent future acute cardiac events including myocardial infarction (MI) and sudden cardiac death. It is now universally accepted that nearly all cases of ST-elevation MI and a significant percentage of sudden coronary deaths are caused by acute intracoronary thrombus formation on a disrupted or eroded atherosclerotic plaque.

The term, vulnerable atherosclerotic plaque, was first utilized by Muller et al to describe any plaque prone to disruption or thrombus resulting in an acute coronary event.[6] However, subsequently in the literature, the term vulnerable was usually limited to the presence of a lipid-rich atherosclerotic plaque with a thin fibrous cap infiltrated by inflammatory cells.[7] While this lipid-rich plaque was the substrate for a majority of acute coronary events, over one-third of major acute thrombi originated from superficial erosion of non-lipid-rich lesions.[8] Thus, the original definition of a vulnerable plaque (i.e. the Muller definition) appears preferable as it does not exclude plaques that might be a substrate for thrombus

---

Box 14.1 Plaque stabilizing therapeutic agents

Drugs/therapies that possess or likely possess plaque stabilizing effects due to a reduction in cardiovascular events
HMG-CoA-reductase inhibitors (statins)
Angiotensin-converting enzyme (ACE) inhibitors
Antihypertensive agents
β-blocking agents
ω-3 fatty acids
Antiplatelet agents (aspirin/clopidogrel)

Drugs/therapies that may possess plaque stabilizing effects although existing data on reducing cardiovascular events is inconclusive or negative
Peroxisome proliferative-activated receptor (PPAR) agonists
Anti-inflammatory agents
Antibiotics
Antioxidants

Drugs/therapies in the future that may possess plaque stabilizing effects
Gene therapy
Metalloproteinase inhibitors
CD-40 pathway inhibitors

---

formation. Furthermore, when considering medical management to promote plaque stabilization, we believe it is appropriate to consider all agents that reduce future acute coronary events in vulnerable lesions as being potentially plaque stabilizing.[9] This would include several different classes of drug in addition to lipid-lowering agents (Box 14.1).

Drugs/therapies that have been demonstrated to reduce subsequent acute events and possess or likely possess plaque stabilizing effects

HMG-CoA-reductase inhibitors (statins)
The first class of medications with the most proven benefit for plaque stabilization consists of the 3-hydroxy-3-methylglutaryl coenzyme A reductase inhibitors (statins). Statins may contribute to plaque stabilization via several different

mechanisms (pleiotropic effects) including a change in plaque composition, reduction in inflammation, decreased thrombosis risk, and improvement in endothelial dysfunction (Figure 14.1).

The first mechanism involves an alteration in plaque composition through the depletion of plaque lipid particularly cholesterol ester. Animal studies have demonstrated a decrease in the lipid content of atheromatous plaques after normalization of cholesterol levels.[21] Lipid depletion and removal of plaque-softening cholesteryl ester, with a relative increase in cholesterol monohydrate crystals may increase the mechanical strength of a plaque. Furthermore, it has been shown in model atherosclerotic lesion lipid pools that the stiffness of the plaque is directly related to the concentration of cholesterol monohydrate crystals.[19] Statins have been observed to decrease the number of microvessels in the intima, which may serve as a point of entry for leukocytes and various other inflammatory cells. It has been hypothesized that these microvessels are fragile and may lead to leakage or hemorrhage. Subsequent thrombosis in situ may cause the release of substances such as thrombin which contribute to plaque growth via smooth muscle proliferation.[22] Thus, a reduction in neovascularization during lipid lowering may help promote plaque stabilization.

Second, statins have been demonstrated to reduce inflammatory mediators and inflammatory cell activity, including the number of macrophage-rich foam cells.[23] Recently, C-reactive protein (CRP) has emerged as an important and reliable predictor and potential contributor of future cardiovascular events.[24] Statins have been demonstrated to reduce levels of high sensitivity CRP (hsCRP)[16]

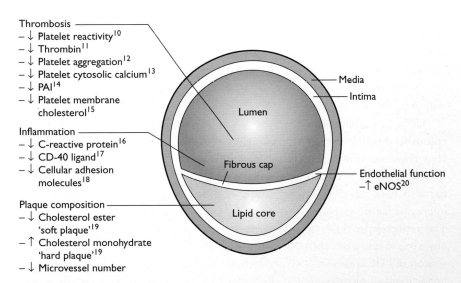

Thrombosis
 – ↓ Platelet reactivity[10]
 – ↓ Thrombin[11]
 – ↓ Platelet aggregation[12]
 – ↓ Platelet cytosolic calcium[13]
 – ↓ PAI[14]
 – ↓ Platelet membrane cholesterol[15]

Inflammation
 – ↓ C-reactive protein[16]
 – ↓ CD-40 ligand[17]
 – ↓ Cellular adhesion molecules[18]

Plaque composition
 – ↓ Cholesterol ester 'soft plaque'[19]
 – ↑ Cholesterol monohydrate 'hard plaque'[19]
 – ↓ Microvessel number

Media
Intima
Lumen
Fibrous cap
Endothelial function –↑ eNOS[20]
Lipid core

Figure 14.1 *Pleiotropic effects of statins. PAI, plasminogen activator inhibitor; eNOS, endothelial nitric oxide synthase.*

257

and other inflammatory markers including soluble CD-40 ligand.[17] In the Cholesterol and Recurrent Events (CARE) trial,[25] Sacks et al. reported a direct relationship between the degree of risk reduction and baseline values of CRP. Furthermore, pravastatin resulted in a 54% relative risk reduction of coronary artery disease (CAD) in patients with active inflammation (defined as elevated serum amyloid-A and CRP) compared to a 25% reduction in those without inflammation despite similar baseline lipid profiles in both groups. Statins have been shown to prevent the oxidation of low-density lipoprotein (LDL) and thus reduce the avidity with which macrophages ingest oxidized LDL possibly through the preservation of the endogenous antioxidant, superoxide dismutase.[26] Statins have also been shown to decrease the vascular expression of adhesion molecules,[18] monocyte expression of CD11b expression, and monocyte adhesion in hypercholesterolemic patients.[27] These anti-inflammatory responses may be a consequence of statins improving endothelial function.

Statins also appear to reduce thrombosis risk. Hypercholesterolemia has been associated with both hypercoagulability and enhanced platelet activation. Patients with elevated LDL have platelets that are also more sensitive to aggregation than patients who have normal LDL or triglyceride (TG) levels.[28,29] These changes have been demonstrated to decrease both platelet reactivity,[10] platelet-dependent thrombin production,[11] adenosine diphosphate-induced platelet aggregation,[12] and cytosolic calcium in platelets.[13] Statins can reverse blood hypercoagulability by reducing oxidized LDL and improving fibrinolysis,[30] decreasing thrombus formation,[31] maintaining a favorable balance between prothrombotic and fibrolytic mechanisms,[32] and increasing the expression of plasminogen activator (PA) and decrease the expression of its inhibitor, PAI-1.[14] The membrane cholesterol content of platelets is reduced by pravastatin, which alters platelet membrane fluidity, thus making platelets less likely to provoke thrombosis.[15] Since statins have the ability to reduce both the thrombotic tendency of blood and the thrombogenicity of plaques they may help promote vulnerable plaque stabilization.

These agents have also been shown to improve endothelial function in both the epicardial coronary arteries[33] and in the coronary microvascular circulation.[34] Hypercholesterolemia is a known cause of endothelial dysfunction and abnormal vasoreactivity in epicardial coronary arteries.[35] Likewise, hypercholesterolemia has also been observed to decrease coronary flow reserve thus affecting the microvasculature in patients without overt epicardial coronary artery disease.[36] The reduction of LDL and improvement in endothelial dysfunction has been observed in one study showing improvement in forearm blood flow after a single session of LDL apheresis.[37] Hypercholesterolemia has also been implicated in the impairment of nitric oxide (NO) synthesis.[38] Hypercholesterolemia may reduce endothelial nitric oxide synthase (eNOS) activity through several mechanisms including increased cytokine activity and by increasing dimethylarginine, an inhibitor of eNOS.[39] By treating hypercholesterolemia it is hypothesized that the above processes may be prevented. Furthermore, statins have been reported to directly upregulate the production of eNOS.[20] These findings may help explain the improvement in coronary vasospasm observed with statin use. The above mechanisms may translate into clinically anti-ischemic effects as observed by a decrease in the incidence of myocardial ischemia on quantitative ST-segment monitoring during 24-hour ambulatory electrocardiography.[40]

The pleiotropic effects of statins have also been attributed in part to their ability to effect Rho signaling. By blocking mevalonate the statins also inhibit isoprenoid synthesis which is necessary for post-translational modification of Rho.[41] Activation of Rho leads to several potentially detrimental effects including increased expression of pro-endothelin-1 in vascular endothelial cells,[42] increased endothelial tissue factor induction by thrombin,[43] activation of nuclear factor (NF)-κB by cytokines[44] and upregulation of NAD(P)H oxidase leading to increased oxidase stress.[45]

All of the above actions of statins likely contribute in varying degrees to the reduction in clinical events with lipid lowering. Most or nearly all of these favorable effects appear to be class specific. The time course of these favorable changes in the pathobiology of the vessel wall have varied. Changes in endothelial function could be demonstrated within 1 month of lipid lowering with use of statins and may be immediate in cases of LDL apheresis in patients with elevated cholesterol. Reductions in thrombosis risk have been demonstrated at 3 and 6 months after initiation of lipid-lowering therapy. Changes in the lipid and macrophage content of the plaque probably require at least 6 months to occur based on animal data.[23] In most randomized clinical trials of lipid lowering, adverse events began to diverge between placebo and treatment arms only after 6–18 months, suggesting a long latency between the initiation of lipid lowering and the reduction in MI and cardiac death. While it is presumed that some of these effects are independent of LDL reduction it is presently unknown in humans how much of the above experimental and clinical data are truly independent of LDL lowering. Finally, while most data presented on plaque stabilization utilized statins, any measure that reduces LDL cholesterol or increases HDL will conceivably possess plaque stabilizing effects.

Angiotensin-converting enzyme inhibitors

Clinical trials have documented the beneficial effects of angiotensin-converting enzyme (ACE) inhibitors with notable reductions in vascular events despite only moderate effects on blood pressure. For example, in the recent Heart Outcomes Prevention Evaluation (HOPE) trial, ACE inhibitor therapy produced little reduction in blood pressure but markedly diminished cardiovascular events.[46] In this same study of patients at risk of vascular disease, the benefit of the ACE inhibitor, ramipril, was roughly three-fold greater than would be expected from blood pressure reduction alone.[47] Furthermore, ACE inhibitors have been shown to have a beneficial effect on vascular biology partly due to the inhibition of angiotensin II and thus possibly inflammation. Within the vascular wall, angiotensin II contributes to the instability of the plaque by stimulating growth factors, adhesion molecules, chemotactic proteins, cytokines, macrophage uptake of oxidized LDL and matrix metalloproteinases (MMPs).[48,49] Angiotensin II has been shown to have a proinflammatory effect by increasing levels of NF-κB, vascular cell adhesion molecule (VCAM), interleukin (IL)-6, and tumor necrosis factor (TNF)-α.[50] Angiotensin II alters fibrinolytic balance by augmenting PAI-1 expression.[51] Finally, activation of the renin–angiotensin system increases the production of reactive oxygen species from vascular cells, contributing to the process of atherogenesis.[52]

Inhibition of ACE leads to increased formation of bradykinin and an increase in vasodilator substances such as NO, endothelium-derived hyperpolarizing factor, and prostacyclin.[53] The ability of ACE inhibitors to increase endothelial NO and prostacyclin production may, in part, explain the vasodilator, antithrombotic and antiproliferative effects of ACE inhibitors. It has recently been proposed ACE inhibitors may have important implications for vascular oxidative stress.[54] ACE inhibition limits the stimulation of vascular NAD(P)H oxidase, thereby reducing superoxide and its downstream effects. Thus, ACE inhibition increases NO bioactivity.[55] Direct evidence for plaque stabilization of ACE inhibition has been suggested in various animal studies. In these studies ACE inhibitors have been shown to decrease plaque area.[55,56] Furthermore, ACE inhibitors have been shown to decrease macrophage content,[57] while increasing the extracellular matrix of plaques.[58] Therefore, suppression of the increased ACE activity within the plaque may promote stabilization of the vulnerable plaque by reducing plaque size and inflammation in the vascular wall, and reducing the risk of rupture and thrombosis (Figure 14.2).[59]

Other antihypertensive agents

Antihypertensive agents (not necessarily only ACE inhibitors) have been shown to modify and thus potentially stabilize atherosclerotic plaques.[60] Oscillating shear stress may alter endothelial function and promote atherogenesis below intact endothelium.[61] High blood velocity within stenotic lesions may shear the endothelium away.[62] Furthermore, turbulent pressure fluctuations distal to severe asymmetric stenoses could promote plaque fatigue, thus promoting disruption.[63] Through computer modeling in simulated plaques, it has been shown that circumferential stress in a plaque with an eccentric lipid pool is concentrated near the shoulder of the plaque, the most common site of plaque rupture at autopsy.[64] A reduction in blood pressure and pulse rate at rest or with exercise with antihypertensive agents may reduce the propensity for plaque disruption by reducing circumferential stress on the fibrous caps of lipid-rich plaques. Although

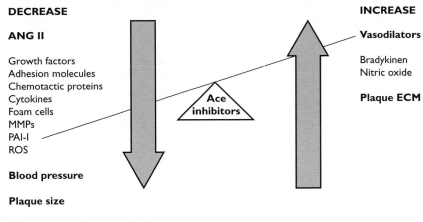

DECREASE

ANG II

Growth factors
Adhesion molecules
Chemotactic proteins
Cytokines
Foam cells
MMPs
PAI-I
ROS

Blood pressure

Plaque size

Plaque macrophage content

INCREASE

Vasodilators

Bradykinen
Nitric oxide

Plaque ECM

Ace inhibitors

Figure 14.2 Potential plaque stabilizing properties of ACE inhibitors.
*ANG, angiotensin; MMP, matrix metalloproteinases; PAI-1, plasminogen activator
inhibitor-1; ROS, reactive oxygen species; ECM, extracellular matrix;
ACE, angiotensin-converting enzyme.*

different antihypertensives may have antihypertensive independent properties
that may contribute to plaque stabilization it may be hypothesized that any agent
that lowers blood pressure may subsequently decrease circumferential stress and
promote plaque stabilization. Recently, the Antihypertensive and Lipid Lowering
treatment to prevent Heart Attack Trial (ALLHAT) reported their findings in
33 000 patients with hypertension and at least one other heart disease risk factor
who were assigned to one of three therapies including a diuretic (chlorthalidone),
calcium-channel blocker (amlodipine) or ACE inhibitor (lisinopril).[65] In patients
with hypertension, amlodipine, lisinopril and chlorthalidone all had similar effects
on CAD death and non-fatal MI. The diuretic was as efficacious as the calcium-
channel blocker and more efficacious than the ACE inhibitor ($P < 0.001$) in
reducing subsequent combined cardiovascular disease events. The results suggest
that blood pressure reduction may be the main determinant of the reduction in
future acute coronary events.

β-blocking agents

The clinical benefit of β-blockade in the secondary prevention of MI supports the
theory that hemodynamic forces may trigger plaque disruption. β-Blocker therapy
has been shown to reduce reinfarction by 25%[66,67] without antiatherogenic,
antithrombotic, profibrinolytic or antispasmodic benefits in humans. Interestingly,
β-blockers appear to have proatherogenic effects including dyslipoproteinemia,
increased platelet aggregation and vasoconstriction.[68]

Thus, the beneficial effect of β-blockers on reinfarction may be partly related to the reduction in heart rate,[69] as has been obtained by the heart rate reducing calcium antagonists verapamil and diltiazem,[70] but not with the heart rate increasing calcium antagonist, nifedipine.[71]

ω-3 Fatty acids

Epidemiologic and randomized clinical trial data suggest that ingestion of ω-3 fatty acids possess plaque stabilizing effects related to their ability to reduce the risk of future fatal or non-fatal MIs. N-3 polyunsaturated fatty acids are either plant-derived (α-linolenic acid) or derived from marine animals (eicosapentaenoic acid (EPA) and docosahexaenoic acid (DHA)). Prospective epidemiologic studies indicated that men who ingested fish on a weekly basis had a lower incidence of coronary heart disease mortality compared to men who ate none.[72,73] While other epidemiologic data were controversial showing no beneficial effect of fish ingestion, fish consumption has also been shown in some studies to reduce the incidence of sudden cardiac death.[74] Other recent epidemiologic data have shown that the plant-derived α-linolenic acid was also associated with a lower risk of fatal ischemic heart disease and MI in both men and women.[75,76] Randomized clinical trial data also support the role of ω-3 fatty acids in the secondary prevention of CAD. Several studies have indicated that the intake of oily fish or other sources of ω-3 fatty acids will reduce the risk of fatal and non-fatal MI.[77–79] Although not all of the data support this conclusion, a meta analysis of 11 randomized trials indicated significant reductions of non-fatal and fatal MI as well as reductions in sudden coronary death in patients ingesting dietary and/or supplemental ω-3 fatty acids.[80]

There are several potential mechanisms by which these N-3 polyunsaturated fatty acids may reduce cardiovascular risk. These mechanisms include an anti-arrhythmic effect based on stabilization of the myocardium, leading to a reduced susceptibility to ventricular arrhythmias,[81,82] antithrombotic[83,84] and anti-inflammatory effects[85,86] as well as improved endothelial function.[87] ω-3 Fatty acids reduce platelet aggregation and can prolong bleeding times. An antiatherogenic role has also been proposed and both EPA and DHA will reduce levels and expression of VCAM-1, intercellular adhesion molecule (ICAM)-1 and other cytokines. High dose ω-3 fatty acids will also significantly reduce triglyceride levels.

The American Heart Association (AHA) has recently summarized their recommendations for ω-3 fatty acid intake.[88] In patients without documented CAD, it has suggested to eat a variety of fish, preferably oily fish at least twice a week. Vegetable oils are the usual source of α-linolenic acid and these are additional sources of ω-3 fatty acids. In patients with documented CAD, the AHA recommends consuming approximately 1 g of EPA and DHA per day preferably from oily fish or from ω-3 fatty acid supplements. To significantly reduce triglyceride levels, at least 2–4 g of DHA and EPA per day are required.

Antiplatelet agents

Aspirin

Aspirin reduces platelet aggregability by irreversible inhibition of cyclo-oxygenase (COX).[89] Aspirin may also improve endothelium-dependent vasodilation.[90] In animal studies aspirin has been shown to increase the number of smooth muscle cells and the content of collagen, while reducing the number of foam cells within aortic atherosclerotic lesions.[91] These findings suggest that aspirin treatment results in the development of a more stable plaque phenotype. Aspirin has also been demonstrated to reduce various inflammatory cytokines.[91] The anti inflammatory effects have been clinically recognized in a large randomized study of aspirin for the primary prevention of cardiovascular events among men; the magnitude of benefit of aspirin in preventing MI was directly related to baseline levels of CRP. Specifically, the risk reduction for aspirin was 56% ($P = 0.02$) among those with baseline levels of CRP in the highest quartile, while there was a small, non-significant reduction (14%; $P = 0.8$) among those with CRP levels in the lowest quartile.[89] Aspirin may help to decrease the progression of atherosclerosis by protecting LDL from oxidative modification[92] and also improves endothelial dysfunction in atherosclerotic vessels.[93] Recently, the antioxidant properties of aspirin on vascular tissues has been described in both normotensive and hypertensive animals.[94]

Clopidogrel

Clopidogrel, another commonly used antithrombotic agent, reduces platelet aggregation by irreversibly blocking the ADP receptor. In the Clopidogrel versus Aspirin in Patients at Risk of Ischaemic Events (CAPRIE) trial, the benefit of clopidogrel over aspirin for preventing the endpoint of MI was substantial, a statistically significant 19.2% relative risk reduction.[95] There is a synergistic effect of aspirin and clopidogrel on platelet function. The long-term use of both aspirin and clopidogrel for patients with an acute coronary syndrome was analyzed in the Clopidogrel in Unstable angina to prevent Recurrent Events (CURE) study.[96] The results of the trial after a mean follow-up of 9 months revealed an approximately 20% relative reduction in the risk of vascular death, MI and stroke. It is unclear from this study if the effect of clopidogrel on reducing subsequent infarction and vascular death is related to the original destabilized culprit lesion or to stabilizing the potentially vulnerable plaques.

Drugs/therapies that may possess or likely possess plaque stabilizing effects although data are presently inconclusive or negative

Peroxisome proliferative-activated receptor agonists

Activators of the ligand-activated nuclear transcription factor, peroxisome proliferator-activated receptor γ (PPARγ), have emerged as a promising target to modify vascular inflammation. PPARγ activators inhibit the release of proinflammatory cytokines and matrix-degrading enzymes in monocytes and macrophages; they modulate the expression of chemokines and endothelin in endothelial cells; and PPARγ ligands have been shown to reduce the secretion of interferon (IFN)-γ in T cells.[97] In vascular smooth muscle cells, PPARγ activators decrease the release of MMPs. Because PPARγ can be activated by the novel group of clinically used antidiabetic thiazolidinediones (TZDs, glitazones),[98] like troglitazone, rosiglitazone and pioglitazone, clinical data revealed a reduction of inflammatory serum markers of arteriosclerosis[99] as well as a reduction of intima–media thickness upon TZD treatment in diabetic patients. PPARs also regulate chemoattraction and cellular adhesion to endothelial cells reducing cytokine-induced expression of VCAM-1 and ICAM-1.[100,101] Incubation of human monocytes with natural prostaglandin (J_2) and synthetic PPARγ ligands inhibits the production of inflammatory cytokines, such as TNF-α, IL-1β, IL-6, IL-8 and IL-10.[102–104] In vivo studies have demonstrated that troglitazone significantly reduced monocyte/macrophage recruitment to atherosclerotic lesions in apoE-null mice.[105] The atheroprotective role of PPARγ has been further documented in animal models of atherosclerosis.[106] Similarly, rosiglitazone treatment of patients with type 2 diabetes significantly reduces plasma levels of IL-6 and CRP PPARγ activators inhibit the expression of MMP-9, a secreted MMP. PPAR agonists may also possess antithrombotic effects through several mechanisms including reduced platelet activation, tissue factor expression in lymphocytes and PAI-1[107–114] which may prevent subsequent thrombosis (Box 14.2). Long-term clinical trials appear warranted.

Anti-inflammatory agents

Selective COX-2 inhibitors were developed to improve the treatment of arthritis with less gastrointestinal effects associated with aspirin and other non-steroidal anti-inflammatory drugs (NSAIDs), which effect both COX-1 and COX-2 activity. Theoretically, prostacyclin (PGI-2) inhibition with relatively unopposed platelet thromboxane (TX)A_2 generation, as seen with selective COX-2 inhibition, may lead to increased thrombosis.[115] These concerns were sustained by the Vioxx Gastrointestinal Outcomes Research (VIGOR) trial during which a five-fold increase in atherothrombotic cardiovascular events associated with

---

Box 14.2 Potential plaque stabilizing effects of PPAR agonists

Anti-inflammatory
↓TNF-α, IL-1β, IL-6, IL-8, IL-10
↓Monocyte/macrophage recruitment
↓C-reactive protein

Antithrombotic
↓Platelet activation
↓Tissue factor
↓PAI-1

Fibrous cap protection
↓Metalloproteinase

TNF, tumor necrosis factor; IL, interleukin; PAI, plasminogen activator inhibitor; PPAR, peroxisome proliferative-activated receptor.

---

rofecoxib was observed.[116] However, the Celecoxib Long-Term Arthritis Safety Study (CLASS)[117] did not support this finding of increased risk with COX-2 inhibition.

It has also been suggested that selective COX-2 inhibition could have a beneficial effect on cardiovascular events in atherosclerosis since COX-2 expression is upregulated in atherosclerotic plaques which may promote inflammation.[118,119] COX-2 inhibition may decrease vascular inflammation and enhance plaque stability, possibly resulting in a net decrease in atherothrombotic events. In the Non-steroidal Anti-Inflammatory Drugs in Unstable Angina Treatment-2 (NUT-2) pilot study, the COX-2 inhibitor meloxicam was administered intravenously and continued orally for 30 days.[120] Patients assigned meloxicam had a significant reduction in the primary composite outcome consisting of recurrent angina, MI, or death (15% vs 38%, $P = 0.007$) and a secondary composite outcome consisting of coronary revascularization procedures, MI, and death (10% vs 26.7%, $P = 0.034$) at 30 days. These results suggest a possible favorable effect for meloxicam. However, this pilot study was open-labeled and single blind and should, therefore, be confirmed by larger randomized double-blind trials.

Antibiotics

There is considerable evidence supporting inflammation, immune activation and infectious agents as potentially important components in the pathogenesis of

265

atherosclerosis.[121,122] Multiple organisms have been implicated including cytomegalovirus (CMV), herpes simplex virus (HSV-1), hepatitis virus, *Chlamydia pneumoniae*, and *Helicobacter pylori*.[123,124] *Chlamydia pneumoniae* remains the most studied infectious agent with regard to its association to atherosclerosis and acute coronary events.[125] Epidemiologic studies have demonstrated an association between elevated *Chlamydia pneumoniae* antibody titers and atherosclerosis.[126] However, prospective and well controlled seroepidemiologic studies have failed to support retrospective observations of a consistent causative link between infectious agents, atherosclerosis and coronary events.[127] Studies have also been conflicting with respect to identification of the most important pathogens.[128] Two antibiotic trials utilizing macrolide antibiotics have been recently presented and these are WIZARD (Weekly Intervention with Zithromax for Atherosclerosis and its Related Disorders) and AZACS (AZithromycin in Acute Coronary Syndromes).[129] The negative results of these trials have decreased the enthusiasm for the causative role of infectious agents in atherosclerosis. Additional randomized trials will add to our understanding of this relationship including Azithromycin and Coronary Events Study (ACES) and Pravastatin or Atorvastatin Evaluation and Infection Therapy (PROVE-IT) trial. The results will be reported in the next few years.

Macrolide antibiotics are also known to have anti-inflammatory properties.[130] Previous investigations have shown that roxithromycin is able to penetrate into atherosclerotic plaques and eradicate microorganisms in the plaques.[131] Macrolide antibiotics have also been shown to decrease clinical progression of lower limb atherosclerosis,[132] favorably effect endothelial function,[133] and decrease markers of inflammation.[134] Due to limited sample sizes, however, most of the above data should be cautiously interpreted.[135] Currently, the use of antibiotics, although mechanistically attractive, cannot be recommended for treatment or prevention of MI or other acute coronary events.

Antioxidants

Antioxidants theoretically may promote plaque stabilization via decreased oxidation of LDL and reduced matrix degradation of the vulnerable plaque. Oxidized LDL, as discussed above, has the ability to contribute to progression and destabilization of the vulnerable plaque via several mechanisms including increased macrophage population and endothelium binding,[136,137] increased macrophage transformation to foam cells and activation,[138] increased tissue factor expression by monocytes,[139] endothelial cell damage,[140,141] decreased NO synthesis[142] and recruitment of leukocytes via monocyte chemoattractant protein-1 (MCP-1).[143] A decrease in matrix degradation may also be a method by which antioxidants promote plaque stabilization. Reactive oxygen species (ROS) can promote the activation of MMP precursors.[144] Furthermore, a decrease in the expression and activation of MMP-9 in hypercholesterolemic rabbits has been demonstrated with the ROS scavenger, *N*-acetylcysteine.[145]

Despite a theoretical benefit of antioxidants in plaque stabilization this has not conclusively translated into a clinical benefit. At the time of writing of this chapter, several large, double-blind, placebo-controlled trials have shown that neither β-carotene,[146] nor vitamin E,[147] alone or in combination with other antioxidant vitamins,[148] reduces the risk of fatal or non-fatal MI in an unselected population of people with established coronary heart disease or at high risk of coronary heart disease.

Drugs / therapies in the future that may possess plaque stabilizing effects

Gene therapy

Genetic therapy has seen advances in lowering the LDL, increasing HDL, increasing eNOS, decreasing VCAM and promoting MMP inhibition.[149] LDL-targeted gene therapy has been used particularly in the field of familial hypercholesterolemia.[149] Several studies have focused on increasing the number of LDL receptors in animals and humans.[150–151] The animal model for familial hypercholesterolemia using the Watanabe heritable hyperlipidemia (WHHL) rabbit transduced ex vivo the LDL receptor gene which resulted in stable expression of the gene and a decrease in serum cholesterol levels.[152] In a pilot study of five patients with homozygous familial hypercholesterolemia, the LDL receptor gene was transferred. However, a sustained reduction in serum LDL only occurred in two patients.[153]

It has been shown that an increase in HDL correlates with a reduction in the incidence of acute coronary syndromes and plaque regression.[154–155] HDL may reduce the cholesterol content entering the plaque.[156] One study showed that intravenous administration of HDL both inhibited progression and promoted regression of aortic lipid deposits and fatty streaks.[157,158] This strategy of HDL infusion may become, in the future, a novel method for plaque stabilization.[159] Apo-1, a major protein component of HDL, was overexpressed via a transgenic mouse gene and subsequently demonstrated a decrease in the development of early atherosclerotic lesions.[160] Thus, an elevation in HDL may promote plaque stabilization and may be another possible target for gene therapy. In the future, it is likely that several new targets for gene therapy will be identified in this area.

Metalloproteinase inhibitors

The importance of MMPs in the pathogenesis of vascular disorders is increasingly being recognized, particularly with respect to atherosclerotic lesions. Degradation of the extracellular matrix scaffold of the thin fibrous cap appears to be an important step in the destabilization of the lipid-rich vulnerable plaque. The fibrous cap components usually consist of collagen which make them stable and do not break down. However, MMPs are capable of degrading the fibrous cap of the vulnerable plaques. MMPs are generally localized in atherosclerotic lesions around the lipid core.[161] The MMP family of enzymes includes collagenases, gelatinases, stromelysins, matrilysins, and metalloelastases.[162] In normal vascular tissues the main sources of MMPs are endothelial cells, medial smooth muscle cells and adventitial connective tissue cells most of which are present in inactive form. During inflammatory conditions, macrophages and T lymphocytes along with other types of infiltrating cells become important sources of MMPs.[163] Cells of atherosclerotic plaques have been observed to express increased MMP levels in regions of increased circumferential tensile stress in the fibrous cap.[164] Increased MMP activity has also been observed with inflammatory cytokines and oxidized LDL.[165] Currently there is no direct evidence of an association between an individual's MMP activity and plaque destabilization, but this concept has been supported by the finding of an increase in intracellular gelatinase B production in atherectomy specimens from patients with unstable angina compared with specimens from patients with stable angina.[166] Furthermore, gelatinase B has been identified from homogenates of the luminal aspect of atherosclerotic aortas but not normal aortas.[167]

Despite being an attractive target from a therapeutic standpoint, the increasing number and complexity of this family makes it challenging to determine precisely which enzyme(s) should be targeted. However, current therapy may have beneficial effects on MMPs. New data suggest that statins diminish accumulation of macrophages in aortic atheroma and macrophage expression of MMP-1, MMP-3 and MMP-9.[168] PPAR agonists at least in vitro will inhibit macrophage activation and MMP expressions.[169] Finally, tissue inhibitors of metalloproteinases (TIMPs), are specific endogenous inhibitors that bind to MMPs and control their activity. In the future they might also serve as an attractive target.[170]

CD-40 pathway inhibitors

The CD-40 immune mediator pathway appears to have an important role in the increased expression of matrix degrading enzymes by smooth muscle cells, macrophages, and activated T lymphocytes that may promote rupture of the vulnerable plaque. Recent work has demonstrated overexpression of the potent immune mediator CD-40 and its counterpart CD-40 ligand (CD-40L) in experimental and human atherosclerotic lesions.[171,172] An example of this has been the administration of anti-CD-40L antibody to hyperlipidemic mice which resulted in a 79% reduction in lipid content and a 59% reduction in atherosclerotic lesion size.[173] CD-40 receptor binding induces production of inflammatory cytokines, chemokines, MMPs and atheroma tissue factor, while inhibiting endothelial cell migration, which can lead to the weakening of the collagen frame of the plaque rendering it prone to rupture and thrombosis.[174]

Patients with unstable angina have enhanced plasma concentrations of soluble CD-40L (sCD-40L).[175] Recently it has been shown that even apparently healthy women with high plasma concentrations of sCD-40L may have an increased vascular risk.[176]

CD-40 signaling and CD-40/CD-40L interactions expressed on vascular endothelial cells, smooth muscle cells, mononuclear phagocytes and platelets become an attractive therapeutic target for plaque stabilization by favorably altering the expression of cytokines, chemokines, growth factors, MMPs, and procoagulants. Common cardiovascular therapies appear to alter the CD-40 pathway. Statins decrease the expression of the CD-40 receptor/ligand dyad both directly as well as through diminished lipoprotein levels.[177] Glycoprotein (GP) IIb/IIIa blockade, in addition to inhibiting platelet aggregation at the vulnerable plaque and thereby preventing physical vessel occlusion, may also prevent platelet–CD-40L-mediated inflammatory cascades.[178] Large randomized clinical trials will be needed to further elucidate the clinical role of interrupting the CD-40 signaling system on atherosclerosis and ultimately plaque stabilization.

References

1. Brown ZG, Zhao XQ, Sacco DE et al. Lipid lowering and plaque regression. New insights into prevention of plaque disruption and clinical events in coronary disease. *Circulation* 1993; **87**:1781–91.

2. Vos J, Roygrok PN, de Feyter PJ. Progression and regression of coronary atherosclerosis: a review of trials by quantitative angioplasty. In: Fuster V, ed. *Syndromes of Atherosclerosis. Correlations of Clinical Imaging and Pathology*. Armonk NY: Futura Publishing, 1996:437–53.

3. Libby P, Schoenbeck U, Mach F et al. Current concepts in cardiovascular pathology: the role of LDL cholesterol in plaque rupture and stabilization. *Am J Med* 1998; **104(2A)**: 14S–18S.

4. Shepherd J, Cobbe SM, Ford I et al. Prevention of coronary heart disease with pravastatin in men with hypercholesterolemia. West of Scotland Coronary Prevention Study Group. *N Engl J Med* 1995; **333**:1301–7.

5. Wissler RW, Vesselinovitch D. Can atherosclerotic plaques regress? Anatomic and biochemical evidence from non-human animal models. *Am J Cardiol* 1990; **65**:33–40.

6. Fuster V, Lewis A. Conner Memorial Lecture. Mechanisms leading to myocardial infarction: insights from studies of vascular biology. *Circulation* 1994; **90**:2126–46.

7. Ambrose JA, Weinrauch M. Thrombosis in ischemic heart disease. *Arch Int Med* 1996; **156**:1382–94.

8. Ambrose JA, Dangas G. Unstable angina: current concepts of pathogenesis and treatment. *Arch Int Med* 2000; **160**:25–37.

9. Ambrose JA, Martinez EE. A new paradigm for plaque stabilization. *Circulation* 2002; **105**:2000–4.

10. Yokoyama I, Ohtake T, Momomura S et al. Reduced coronary flow reserve in hypercholesterolemic patients without overt coronary stenosis. *Circulation* 1996; **94**:3232–8.

11. Lacoste L, Lam JY, Hung J et al. Hyperlipidemia and coronary disease. Correction of the increased thrombogenic potential with cholesterol reduction. *Circulation* 1995; **92**:3172–7.

12. Mayer J, Eller T, Brauer P et al. Effects of long-term treatment with lovastatin on the clotting system and blood platelets. *Ann Hematol* 1992; **64**:196–201.

13. Le Quan Sang KH, Levenson J, Megnien JL, Simon A, Devynck MA. Platelet cytosolic Ca^{2+} and membrane dynamics in patients with primary hypercholesterolemia. Effects of pravastatin. *Arterioscler Thromb Vasc Biol* 1995; **15**:759–64.

14. Bourcier T, Libby P. HMG CoA reductase inhibitors reduce plasminogen activator inhibitor-1 expression by human vascular smooth muscle and endothelial cells. *Arterioscler Thromb Vasc Biol* 2000; **20**: 556–62.

15. Lijnen P, Celis H, Fagard R et al. Influence of cholesterol lowering on plasma membrane lipids and cationic transport systems. *J Hypertens* 1994; **12**:59–64.

16. Ross R. Atherosclerosis – an inflammatory disease. *N Engl J Med* 1999; **340**: 115–26.

17. Cipollone F, Mezzetti A, Porreca E et al. Association between enhanced soluble CD40L and prothrombotic state in hypercholesterolemia: effects of statin therapy. *Circulation* 2002; **106**:399–402.

18. Kimura M, Kurose I, Russell J, Granger DN. Effects of fluvastatin on leukocyte-endothelial cell adhesion in hypercholesterolemic rats. *Arterioscler Thromb Vasc Biol* 1997; **17**:1521–6.

19. Loree HM, Tobias BJ, Gibson LJ et al. Mechanical properties of model atherosclerotic lesion lipid pools. *Arterioscler Thromb* 1994; **14**:230–4.

20. Laufs U, La Fata V, Plutzky J et al. Upregulation of endothelial nitric oxide synthase by HMG CoA reductase inhibitors. *Circulation* 1998; **97**:1129–35.

21. Armstrong ML, Megan MB. Lipid depletion in atheromatous coronary arteries in Rhesus monkeys after regression diets. *Circ Res* 1972; **30**:675–80.

22. Moulton KS, Heller E, Konerding MA et al. Angiogenesis inhibitors endostatin or TNP-470 reduce intimal neovascularization and plaque growth in apolipoprotein E-deficient mice. *Circulation* 1999; **99**:1726–32.

23. Aviram M., Dankner G Cogan U et al. Lovastatin inhibits LDL oxidation and alters its fluidity and uptake by macrophages: in vitro and in vivo studies. *Metabolism* 1992; **41**:229–35.

24. Ridker PM. Evaluating novel cardiovascular risk factors: can we better predict heart attacks? *Ann Intern Med* 1999; **130**:933–7.

25. Sacks FM, Pfeffer MA, Moye LA et al. The effect of pravastatin on coronary events after myocardial infarction in patients with average cholesterol levels. Cholesterol and Recurrent Events Trial investigators. *N Engl J Med* 1996; **335**:1001–9.

26. Chen L, Haught WH, Yang B et al. Preservation of endogenous antioxidant activity and inhibition of lipid peroxidation as common mechanisms of antiatherosclerotic effects of vitamin E, lovastatin and amlodipine. *J Am Coll Cardiol* 1997; **30**:569–75.

27. Weber C, Erl W, Weber KS, Weber PC. HMG-CoA reductase inhibitors decrease CD11b expression and CD11b-dependent adhesion of monocytes to endothelium and reduce increased adhesiveness of monocytes isolated from patients with hypercholesterolemia. *J Am Coll Cardiol* 1997; **30**:1212–17.

28. Aikawa M, Rabkin E, Okada Y et al. Lipid lowering by diet reduces matrix metalloproteinase activity and increases collagen content of rabbit atheroma: a potential mechanism of lesion stabilization. *Circulation* 1998; **97**:2433–44.

29. Notarbartolo A, Davi G, Averna M et al. Inhibition of thromboxane biosynthesis and platelet function by simvastatin in type IIa hypercholesterolemia. *Arterioscler Thromb Vasc Biol* 1995; **15**:247–51.

30. Wada H, Mori Y, Kaneko T et al. Elevated plasma levels of vascular endothelial cell markers in patients with hypercholesterolemia. *Am J Hematol* 1993; **44**:112–16.

31. Lacoste L, Lam JY, Hung J et al. Hyperlipidemia and coronary disease. Correction of the increased thrombogenic potential with cholesterol reduction. *Circulation* 1995; **92**:3172–7.

32. Waters D, Higginson L, Gladstone P et al. Effects of monotherapy with an HMG-CoA reductase inhibitor on the progression of coronary atherosclerosis as assessed by serial quantitative arteriography. The Canadian Coronary Atherosclerosis Intervention Trial. *Circulation* 1994; **89**:959–68.

33. Treasure CB, Klein JL, Weintraub WS et al. Beneficial effects of cholesterol-lowering therapy on the coronary endothelium in patients with coronary artery disease. *N Engl J Med* 1995; **332**:481–7.

34. Eichstadt HW, Eskotter H, Hoffman I, Amthauer HW, Weidinger G. Improvement of myocardial perfusion by short-term fluvastatin therapy in coronary artery disease. *Am J Cardiol* 1995; **76**:122A–125A.

35. Seiler C, Hess OM, Buechi M, Suter TM, Krayenbuehl HP. Influence of serum cholesterol and other coronary risk factors on vasomotion of angiographically normal coronary arteries. *Circulation* 1993; **88(5 Pt 1)**:2139–48.

36. Yokoyama I, Ohtake T, Momomura S et al. Reduced coronary flow reserve in hypercholesterolemic patients without overt coronary stenosis. *Circulation* 1996; **94**:3232–8.

37. Tamai O, Matsouka JP, Itabe H et al. Single LDL apheresis improves endothelium-dependent vasodilation in hypercholesterolemic humans. *Circulation* 1997; **95**:76–82.

38. Liao JK, Shin WS, Lee WY, Clark SL. Oxidized low-density lipoprotein decreases the expression of endothelial nitric oxide synthase. *J Biol Chem* 1995; **270**:319–24.

39. Cooke JP, Tsao PS. Arginine: a new therapy for atherosclerosis? *Circulation* 1997; **95**:311–12.

40. Andrews TC, Raby K, Barry J et al. Effect of cholesterol reduction on myocardial ischemia in patients with coronary disease. *Circulation* 1997; **95**:324–8.

41. Koh KK. Effects of statins on vascular wall: vasomotor function, inflammation, and plaque stability. *Cardiovasc Res* 2000; **47**:648–57.

42. Hernandez-Perera O, Perez-Sala D, Soria E, Lamas S. Involvement of Rho GTPases in the transcriptional inhibition of preproendothelin-1 gene expression by simvastatin in vascular endothelial cells. *Circ Res* 2000; **87**:616–22.

43. Eto M, Kozai T, Cosentino F, Joch H, Luscher TF. Statin prevents tissue factor expression in human endothelial cells: role of Rho/Rho-kinase and Akt pathways. *Circulation* 2002; **105**:1756–9.

44. Pruefer D, Scalia R, Lefer AM. Simvastatin inhibits leukocyte-endothelial cell interactions and protects against inflammatory processes in normocholesterolemic rats. *Arterioscler Thromb Vasc Biol* 1999; **19**:2894–900.

45. Wagner AH, Kohler T, Ruckschloss U, Just I, Hecker M. Improvement of nitric oxide-dependent vasodilatation by HMG-CoA reductase inhibitors through attenuation of endothelial superoxide anion formation. *Arterioscler Thromb Vasc Biol* 2000; **20**:61–9.

46. Yusuf S, Sleight P, Pogue J et al. Effects of an angiotensin-converting-enzyme inhibitor, ramipril, on cardiovascular events in high-risk patients: the Heart Outcomes Prevention Evaluation Study Investigators. *N Engl J Med* 2000; **342**:145–53.

47. Sleight P, Yusuf S, Pogue J et al. Blood-pressure reduction and cardiovascular risk in HOPE study. *Lancet* 2001; **358**:2130–1.

48. Brasier AR, Recinos A III, Eledrisi MS et al. Vascular inflammation and the renin-angiotensin system. *Arterioscler Thromb Vasc Biol* 2002; **22**:1257–66.

49. Schieffer B, Schieffer E, Hilfiker-Kleiner D et al. Expression of angiotensin II and interleukin 6 in human coronary atherosclerotic plaques: potential implications for inflammation and plaque instability. *Circulation* 2000; **101**:1372–8.

50. Han Y, Runge MS, Brasier AR et al. Angiotensin II induces interleuken-6 transcription in vascular smooth muscle cells through pleiotropic activation of nuclear factor-kappa B transcription factors. *Circ Res* 1999; **84**:695–703.

51. Brown NJ, Vaughan DE. Prothrombotic effects of angiotensin. *Adv Intern Med* 2000; **45**:419–29.

52. Fukai T, Siegfried MR, Ushio-Fukai M et al. Modulation of extracellular superoxide dismutase expression by angiotensin II and hypertension. *Circ Res* 1999; **85**:23–8.

53. Vanhoutte PM, Boulanger CM, Illiano SC et al. Endothelium-dependent effects of converting-enzyme inhibitors. *J Cardiovasc Pharmacol* 1993; **22 (suppl 5)**:S10–S16.

54. Thomas M, Keaney JF Jr. Are ACE inhibitors a 'magic bullet' against oxidative stress? *Circulation* 2001; **104**:1571–4.

55. Mancini GB, Henry GC, Macaya C et al. Angiotensin-converting enzyme inhibition with quinapril improves endothelial vasomotor dysfunction in patients with coronary artery disease: the TREND (Trial on Reversing Endothelial Dysfunction) Study. *Circulation* 1996; **94**:258–65.

56. Chobanian AV. The effects of ACE inhibitors and other antihypertensive drugs on cardiovascular risk factors and atherogenesis. *Clin Cardiol* 1990; **13(6 Suppl 7)**:VII43–8.

57. Chobanian AV, Haudenschild CC, Nickerson C, Drago R. Antiatherogenic effect of captopril in the Watanabe heritable hyperlipidemic rabbit. *Hypertension* 1990; **15**:327–31.

58. Aberg G, Ferrer P. Effects of captopril on atherosclerosis in cynomolgus monkeys. *J Cardiovasc Pharmacol* 1990; **15 (Suppl 5)**:S65–S72.

59. Rolland PH, Charpiot P, Friggi A et al. Effects of angiotensin-converting enzyme inhibition with perindopril on hemodynamics, arterial structure, and wall rheology in the hindquarters of atherosclerotic mini-pigs. *Am J Cardiol* 1993; **71**:22E–27E.

60. Chobanian AV, Brecher PI, Haudenschild CC et al. Effects of hypertension and of antihypertensive therapy on atherosclerosis. *Hypertension* 1986; **8(suppl I)**:I-15–I-21.

61. Glagov S, Zarins C, Giddens DP, Ku DN. Hemodynamics and atherosclerosis: insights and perspectives gained from studies of human arteries. *Arch Pathol Lab Med* 1988; **112**:1018–31.

62. Gertz SD, Uretzky G, Wajnberg RS, Navot N, Gotsman MS. Endothelial cell damage and thrombus formation after partial arterial constriction: relevance to the role of coronary artery spasm in the pathogenesis of myocardial infarction. *Circulation* 1981; **63**:476–86.

63. Loree HM, Kamm RD, Atkinson CM, Lee RT. Turbulent pressure fluctuations on surface of model vascular stenoses. *Am J Physiol* 1991; **261(3 Pt 2)**:H644–50.

64. Richardson PD, Davies MJ, Born GV. Influence of plaque configuration and stress distribution on fissuring of coronary atherosclerotic plaques. *Lancet* 1989; **2**:941–4.

65. Major outcomes in high-risk hypertensive patients randomized to angiotensin-converting enzyme inhibitor or calcium channel blocker vs diuretic: The Antihypertensive and Lipid-Lowering Treatment to Prevent Heart Attack Trial (ALLHAT). *JAMA* 2002; **288**:2981–97.

66. Yusuf S, Peto J, Lewis J, Collins R, Sleight P. Beta blockade during and after myocardial infarction: an overview of the randomized trials. *Prog Cardiovasc Dis* 1985; **27**:335–71.

67. Held PH, Yusuf S. Effects of beta-blockers and calcium channel blockers in acute myocardial infarction. *Eur Heart J* 1993; **14(Suppl F)**:18–25.

68. Leren P. Ischaemic heart disease: how well are the risk profiles modulated by current beta blockers? *Cardiology* 1993; **82(Suppl 3)**:8–12.

69. Kjekshus JK. Importance of heart rate in determining beta-blocker efficacy in acute and long-term acute myocardial infarction intervention trials. *Am J Cardiol* 1986; **57(Suppl F)**:43F–49F.

70. The Danish Study Group on Verapamil in Myocardial Infarction. The effect of verapamil on mortality and major events after myocardial infarction: the Danish Verapamil Infarction Trial II (DAVIT II). *Am J Cardiol* 1990; **66**:779–85.

71. Held PH, Yusuf S. Calcium antagonists in the treatment of ischemic heart disease: myocardial infarction. *Coron Artery Dis* 1994; **5**:21–6.

72. Stone NJ. Fish consumption, fish oil, lipids, and coronary heart disease. *Circulation* 1996; **94**:2337–40.

73. Krauss RM, Eckel RH, Howard B et al. AHA dietary guidelines: revision 2000: a statement for healthcare professionals from the Nutrition Committee of the American Heart Association. *Circulation* 2000; **102**:2284–99.

74. Siscovick DS, Raghunathan TE, King I et al. Dietary intake and cell membrane levels of long-chain n-3 polyunsaturated fatty acids and the risk of primary cardiac arrest. *JAMA* 1995; **274**:1363–7.

75. Hu FB, Stampfer MJ, Manson JE et al. Dietary intake of alpha-linolenic acid and risk of fatal ischemic heart disease among women. *Am J Clin Nutr* 1999; **69**:890–7.

76. Djousse L, Pankow JS, Eckfeldt JH et al. Relation between dietary linolenic acid and coronary artery disease in the National Heart, Lung, and Blood Institute Family Heart Study. *Am J Clin Nutr* 2001; **74**:612–19.

77. Dolecek TA, Granditis G. Dietary polyunsaturated fatty acids and mortality in the Multiple Risk Factor Intervention Trial (MRFIT). *World Rev Nutr Diet* 1991; **66**:205–16.

78. Daviglus ML, Stamler J, Orencia AJ et al. Fish consumption and the 30-year risk of fatal myocardial infarction. *N Engl J Med* 1997; **336**:1046–53.

79. Zhang J, Sasaki S, Amano K et al. Fish consumption and mortality from all causes, ischemic heart disease, and stroke: an ecological study. *Prev Med* 1999; **28**:520–9.

80. Bucher HC, Hengstler P, Schindler C et al. N-3 polyunsaturated fatty acids in coronary heart disease: a meta-analysis of randomized controlled trials. *Am J Med* 2002; **112**:298–304.

81. de Lorgeril M, Salen P, Martin JL et al. Mediterranean diet, traditional risk factors, and the rate of cardiovascular complications after myocardial infarction: final report of the Lyon Diet Heart Study. *Circulation* 1999; **99**:779–85.

82. Dietary supplementation with n-3 polyunsaturated fatty acids and vitamin E after myocardial infarction: results of the GISSI-Prevenzione trial. Gruppo Italiano per lo Studio della Sopravvivenza nell'Infarto miocardico. *Lancet* 1999; **354**:447–55.

83. Mori TA, Beilin LJ, Burke V et al. Interactions between dietary fat, fish, and fish oils and their effects on platelet function in men at risk of cardiovascular disease. *Arterioscler Thromb Vasc Biol* 1997; **17**:279–86.

84. Knapp HR. Dietary fatty acids in human thrombosis and hemostasis. *Am J Clin Nutr* 1997; **65 (Suppl 5)**:1687S–98S.

85. Endres S, von Schacky C. n-3 polyunsaturated fatty acids and human cytokine synthesis. *Curr Opin Lipidol* 1996; **7**:48–52.

86. Lee RT, Libby P. The unstable atheroma. *Arterioscler Thromb Vasc Biol* 1997; **17**:1859–67.

87. McVeigh GE, Brennan GM, Cohn JN et al. Fish oil improves arterial compliance in non-insulin-dependent diabetes mellitus. *Arterioscler Thromb* 1994; **14**:1425–9.

88. Sheard NF. Fish consumption and risk of sudden cardiac death. *Nutr Rev* 1998; **56**:177–9.

89. Ridker PM, Cushman M, Stampfer MJ et al. Inflammation, aspirin, and the risk of cardiovascular disease in apparently healthy men. *N Engl J Med* 1997; **336**:973–9.

90. Husain S, Andrews NP, Mulcahy D, Panza JA et al. Aspirin improves endothelial dysfunction in atherosclerosis circulation 1998; **97**:716–20.

91. Cyrus T, Sung S, Zhao L et al. Effect of low-dose aspirin on vascular inflammation, plaque stability, and atherogenesis in low-density lipoprotein receptor-deficient mice. *Circulation* 2002; **106**:1282–7.

92. Steer KA, Wallace TM, Bolton CH, Hartog M. Aspirin protects low density lipoprotein from oxidative modification. *Heart* 1997; **77**:333–7.

93. Husain S, Andrews NP, Mulcahy D, Panza JA, Quyyumi AA. Aspirin improves endothelial dysfunction in atherosclerosis. *Circulation* 1998; **97**:716–20.

94. Wu R, Lamontagne D, de Champlain J et al. Antioxidative properties of acetylsalicylic acid on vascular tissues from normotensive and spontaneously hypertensive rats. *Circulation* 2002; **105**:387–92.

95. CAPRIE Steering Committee. A randomised, blinded, trial of clopidogrel versus aspirin in patients at risk of ischaemic events (CAPRIE). *Lancet* 1996; **348**:1329–39.

96. The Clopidogrel in Unstable Angina to Prevent Recurrent Events Trial Investigators. Effects of clopidogrel in addition to aspirin in patients with acute coronary syndromes without ST-segment elevation. *N Engl J Med* 2001; **345**:494–502.

97. Marx N, Kehrle B, Kohlhammer K et al. PPAR activators as antiinflammatory mediators in human T lymphocytes: implications for atherosclerosis and transplantation-associated arteriosclerosis. *Circ Res* 2002; **90**:703–10.

98. Lehmann JM, Moore LB, Smith-Oliver TA et al. An antidiabetic thiazolidinedione is a high affinity ligand for peroxisome proliferator-activated receptor gamma (PPARγ). *J Biol Chem* 1995; **270**:12953–6.

99. Cominacini L, Garbin U, Pasini A et al. Troglitazone reduces LDL oxidation and lowers plasma E-selectin concentration in NIDDM patients. *Diabetes* 1998; **47**:130–3.

100. Marx N, Sukhova GK, Collins T, Libby P, Plutzky J. PPARalpha activators inhibit cytokine-induced vascular cell adhesion molecule-1 expression in human endothelial cells. *Circulation* 1999; **99**:3125–31.

101. Jackson SM, Parhami F, Xi XP et al. Peroxisome proliferator-activated receptor activators target human endothelial cells to inhibit leukocyte-endothelial cell interaction. *Arterioscler Thromb Vasc Biol* 1999; **19**:2094–104.

102. Ricote M, Huang JT, Welch JS, Glass CK. The peroxisome proliferator-activated receptor (PPARgamma) as a regulator of monocyte/macrophage function. *J Leukoc Biol* 1999; **66**:733–9.

103. Azuma Y, Shinohara M, Wang PL, Ohura K. 15-Deoxy-delta(12,14)-prostaglandin J(2) inhibits IL-10 and IL-12 production by macrophages. *Biochem Biophys Res Commun* 2001; **283**:344–6.

104. Staels B, Koenig W, Habib A et al. Activation of human aortic smooth-muscle cells is inhibited by PPARalpha but not by PPARgamma activators. *Nature* 1998; **393**:790–3.

105. Pasceri V, Wu HD, Willerson JT, Yeh ET. Modulation of vascular inflammation in vitro and in vivo by peroxisome proliferator-activated receptor-gamma activators. *Circulation* 2000; **101**:235–8.

106. Li AC, Brown KK, Silvestre MJ et al. Peroxisome proliferator-activated receptor gamma ligands inhibit development of atherosclerosis in LDL receptor-deficient mice. *J Clin Invest* 2000; **106**:523–31.

107. Ikeda Y, Sugawara A, Taniyama Y et al. Suppression of rat thromboxane synthase gene transcription by peroxisome proliferator-activated receptor gamma in macrophages via an interaction with NRF2. *J Biol Chem* 2000; **275**:33142–50.

108. Sugawara A, Takeuchi K, Uruno A et al. Differential effects among thiazolidinediones on the transcription of thromboxane receptor and angiotensin II type 1 receptor genes. *Hypertens Res* 2001; **24**:229–33.

109. Neve BP, Corseaux D, Chinetti G et al. PPARalpha agonists inhibit tissue factor expression in human monocytes and macrophages. *Circulation* 2001; **103**:207–12.

110. Marx N, Mackman N, Schonbeck U et al. PPARalpha activators inhibit tissue factor expression and activity in human monocytes. *Circulation* 2001; **103**:213–19.

111. Durrington PN, Mackness MI, Bhatnagar D et al. Effects of two different fibric acid derivatives on lipoproteins, cholesteryl ester transfer, fibrinogen, plasminogen activator inhibitor and paraoxonase activity in type IIb hyperlipoproteinaemia. *Atherosclerosis* 1998; **138**:217–25.

112. Kato K, Yamada D, Midorikawa S, Sato W, Watanabe T. Improvement by the insulin-sensitizing agent, troglitazone, of abnormal fibrinolysis in type 2 diabetes mellitus. *Metabolism* 2000; **49**:662–5.

113. Pasceri V, Chang J, Willerson JT, Yeh ET. Modulation of C-reactive protein-mediated monocyte chemoattractant protein-1 induction in human endothelial cells by anti-atherosclerosis drugs. *Circulation* 2001; **103**:2531–4.

114. Staels B, Koenig W, Habib A et al. Activation of human aortic smooth-muscle cells is inhibited by PPARalpha but not by PPARgamma activators. *Nature* 1998; **393**:790–3.

115. Pitt B, Pepine C, Willerson JT. Cyclooxygenase-2 inhibition and cardiovascular events. *Circulation* 2002; **106**:167–9.

116. Bombardier C, Laine L, Reicin A et al. Comparison of upper gastrointestinal toxicity of rofecoxib and naproxen in patients with rheumatoid arthritis: VIGOR study group. *N Engl J Med* 2000; **343**:1520–8.

117. Silverstein FE, Faich G, Goldstein JL et al. Gastrointestinal toxicity with celecoxib vs nonsteroidal anti-inflammatory drugs for osteoarthritis and rheumatoid arthritis: the Celecoxib Long-Term Arthritis Safety Study (CLASS): a randomized controlled trial. *JAMA* 2000; **284**:1247–55.

118. Baker CS, Hall RJ, Evans TJ et al. Cyclooxygenase-2 is widely expressed in atherosclerotic lesions affecting native and transplanted human coronary arteries and colocalizes with inducible nitric oxide synthase and nitrotyrosine particularly in macrophages. *Arterioscler Thromb Vasc Biol* 1999; **19**:646–55.

119. Schonbeck U, Sukhova GK, Graber P et al. Augmented expression of cyclooxygenase-2 in human atherosclerotic lesions. *Am J Pathol* 1999; **155**:1281–91.

120. Altman R, Luciardi HL, Muntaner J et al. Efficacy of assessment of meloxicam, a preferential COX-2 inhibitor in acute coronary syndromes without ST-segment elevation: the NUT-2 pilot study. *Circulation* 2002; **106**:191–5.

121. Ross R. Atherosclerosis: an inflammatory disease. *N Engl J Med* 1999; **340**:115–26.

122. Libby P, Egan D, Skarlatos S. Roles of infectious agents in atherosclerosis and restenosis: an assessment of the evidence and need for future research. *Circulation* 1997; **96**:4095–103.

123. Nicholson AC, Hajjar DP. Herpes virus in atherosclerosis and thrombosis: etiologic agents or ubiquitous bystanders. *Arterioscler Thromb Vasc Biol* 1998; **18**:339–48.

124. Kuvin JT, Kimmelstiel CD. Infectious causes of atherosclerosis. *Am Heart J* 1999; **137**:216–26.

125. Zebrack JS, Anderson JL. The role of inflammation and infection in the pathogenesis and evolution of coronary artery disease. *Curr Cardiol Rep* 2002; **4**:278–88.

126. Leinonen M, Saikku P. Evidence for infectious agents in cardiovascular disease and atherosclerosis. *Lancet Infect Dis* 2002; **2**:11–17.

127. Danesh J, Whincup P, Walker M et al. *Chlamydia pneumoniae* IgG titres and coronary heart disease: prospective study and meta-analysis. *BMJ* 2000; **321**:208–13.

128. Kuvin JT, Kimmelstiel CD. Infectious causes of atherosclerosis. *Am Heart J* 1999; **137**:216–26.

129. Dunne MW. Weekly Intervention with Zithromax for Atherosclerosis and its Related Disorders (WIZARD) trial. American College of Cardiology 51st Annual Scientific Session, Atlanta, 17–20 March 2002.

130. Ianaro A, Ialenti A, Maffia P et al. Anti-inflammatory activity of macrolide antibiotics. *J Pharmacol Exp Ther* 2000; **292**:156–63.

131. Melissano G, Blasi F, Esposito G et al. *Chlamydia pneumoniae* eradication from carotid plaques: results of an open, randomised treatment study. *Eur J Vasc Endovasc Surg* 1999; **18**:355–9.

132. Wiesli P, Czerwenka W, Meniconi A et al. Roxithromycin treatment prevents progression of peripheral arterial occlusive disease in *Chlamydia pneumoniae* seropositive men: a randomized, double-blind, placebo-controlled trial. *Circulation* 2002; **105**:2646–52.

133. Parchure N, Zouridakis EG et al. Effect of azithromycin treatment on endothelial function in patients with coronary artery disease and evidence of *Chlamydia pneumoniae* infection. *Circulation* 2002; **105**:1298–303.

134. Stone A, Mendall MA, Northfield J et al. Effect of treatment for *Chlamydia pneumoniae* and *Helicobacter pylori* on markers of inflammation and cardiac events in patients with acute coronary syndromes: South Thames Trial of Antibiotics in Myocardial Infarction and Unstable Angina (STAMINA). *Circulation* 2002; **106**:1219–23.

135. Gupta S, Leatham EW, Carrington D et al. Elevated *Chlamydia pneumoniae* antibodies, cardiovascular events, and azithromycin in male survivors of myocardial infarction. *Circulation* 1997; **96**:404–7.

136. Quinn MT, Parthasarathy S, Steinberg D et al. Lysophosphatidylcholine: a chemotactic factor for human monocytes and its potential role in atherogenesis. *Proc Natl Acad Sci USA* 1988; **85**:2805–9.

137. Vora DK, Fang ZT, Liva SM et al. Induction of P-selectin by oxidized lipoproteins. Separate effects on synthesis and surface expression. *Circ Res* 1997; **80**:810–18.

138. Libby P. Molecular bases of the acute coronary syndromes. *Circulation* 1995; **91**:2844–50.

139. Rosenson RS, Tangney CC. Antiatherothrombotic properties of statins: implications for cardiovascular event reduction. *JAMA* 1998; **279**:1643–50.

140. Hessler JR, Morel DW, Lewis LJ et al. Lipoprotein oxidation and lipoprotein-induced cytotoxicity. *Arteriosclerosis* 1983; **3**:215–22.

141. Yagi K. Increased serum lipid peroxides initiate atherogenesis. *Bioessays* 1984; **1**:58–60.

142. Drexler H, Hornig B. Endothelial dysfunction in human disease. *J Mol Cell Cardiol* 1999; **31**:51–60.

143. Parhami F, Fang ZT, Fogelman AM et al. Minimally modified low density lipoprotein-induced inflammatory responses in endothelial cells are mediated by cyclic adenosine monophosphate. *J Clin Invest* 1993; **92**:471–8.

144. Rajagopalan S, Meng XP, Ramasamy S et al. Reactive oxygen species produced by macrophage-derived foam cells regulate the activity of vascular matrix metalloproteinases in vitro. Implications for atherosclerotic plaque stability. *J Clin Invest* 1996; **98**:2572–9.

145. Galis ZS, Asanuma K, Godin D et al. N-acetyl-cysteine decreases the matrix-degrading capacity of macrophage-derived foam cells: new target for antioxidant therapy? *Circulation* 1998; **97**:2445–53.

146. Omenn GS, Goodman GE, Thornquist MD et al. Effects of a combination of beta carotene and vitamin A on lung cancer and cardiovascular disease. *N Engl J Med* 1996; **334**:1150–5.

147. Yusuf S, Dagenais G, Pogue J et al. Vitamin E supplementation and cardiovascular events in high-risk patients: the Heart Outcomes Prevention Evaluation Study Investigators. *N Engl J Med* 2000; **342**:154–60.

148. Brown BG, Xue-Qiao Z, Chait A et al. Simvastatin and niacin, antioxidant vitamins, or the combination for the prevention of coronary disease. *N Engl J Med* 2001; **345**:1583–92.

149. Grossman M, Raper SE, Kozarsky K et al. Successful ex vivo gene therapy directed to liver in a patient with familial hypercholesterolaemia. *Nat Genet* 1994: **6**:335–41.

150. Schneider MD, French BA. The advent of adenovirus. Gene therapy for cardiovascular disease. *Circulation* 1993; **88(4 Pt 1)**:1937–42.

151. Wilson JM, Chowdhury NR, Grossman M et al. Temporary amelioration of hyperlipidemia in low density lipoprotein receptor-deficient rabbits transplanted with genetically modified hepatocytes. *Proc Natl Acad Sci USA* 1990; **87**:8437–41.

152. Isner Chowdhury JR, Grossman M, Gupta S. Long-term improvement of hypercholesterolemia after ex vivo gene therapy in LDLR-deficient rabbits. *Science* 1991; **254**:1802–5.

153. Grossman M, Rader DJ, Muller DW et al. A pilot study of ex vivo gene therapy for homozygous familial hypercholesterolaemia. *Nat Med* 1995; **1**:1148–54.

154. Brown G, Albers JJ, Fisher LD et al. Regression of coronary artery disease as a result of intensive lipid-lowering therapy in men with high levels of apolipoprotein B. *N Engl J Med* 1990; **323**:1289–98.

155. Buchwald H, Varco RL, Matts JP et al. Effect of partial ileal bypass surgery on mortality and morbidity from coronary heart disease in patients with hypercholesterolemia. Report of the Program on the Surgical Control of the Hyperlipidemias (POSCH). *N Engl J Med* 1990; **323**:946–55.

156. Reichl D, Miller NE. Pathophysiology of reverse cholesterol transport. Insights from inherited disorders of lipoprotein metabolism. *Arteriosclerosis* 1989; **9**:785–97.

157. Badimon JJ, Badimon L, Galvez A et al. High density lipoprotein plasma fractions inhibit aortic fatty streaks in cholesterol-fed rabbits. *Lab Invest* 1989; **60**:455–61.

158. Badimon JJ, Badimon L, Fuster V. Regression of atherosclerotic lesions by high density lipoprotein plasma fraction in the cholesterol-fed rabbit. *J Clin Invest* 1990; **85**:1234–41.

159. Newton RS, Krause BR. HDL therapy for the acute treatment of atherosclerosis. *Atheroscler Suppl* 2002; **3**:31–8.

160. Paszty C, Maeda N, Verstuyft J et al. Apolipoprotein AI transgene corrects apolipoprotein E deficiency-induced atherosclerosis in mice. *J Clin Invest* 1994; **94**:899–903.

161. Henney AM, Wakeley PR, Davies MJ et al. Localization of stromelysin gene expression in atherosclerotic plaques by in situ hybridization. *Proc Natl Acad Sci USA* 1991; **88**:8154–8.

162. Ye S, Humphries S, Henney A. Matrix metalloproteinases: implication in vascular matrix remodelling during atherogenesis. *Clin Sci (Lond)* 1998; **94**:103–10.

163. Sukhova GK, Schonbeck U, Rabkin E et al. Evidence for increased collagenolysis by interstitial collagenases-1 and -3 in vulnerable human atheromatous plaques. *Circulation* 1999; **99**:2503–9.

164. Lee RT, Schoen FJ, Loree HM et al. Circumferential stress and matrix metalloproteinase 1 in human coronary atherosclerosis: implications for plaque rupture. *Arterioscler Thromb Vasc Biol* 1996; **16**:1070–3.

165. Xu XP, Meisel SR, Ong JM et al. Oxidized low-density lipoprotein regulates matrix metalloproteinase-9 and its tissue inhibitor in human monocyte-derived macrophages. *Circulation* 1999; **99**:993–8.

166. Brown DL, Hibbs MS, Kearney M, Loushin C, Isner JM. Identification of 92 kD gelatinase in human coronary atherosclerotic lesions. *Circulation* 1995; **91**:2125–31.

167. Vine N, Powell J. Metalloproteinases in degenerative aortic disease. *Clin Sci* 1991; **81**:233–9.

168. Aikawa M, Rabkin E, Sugiyama S et al. An HMG-CoA reductase inhibitor, cerivastatin, suppresses growth of macrophages expressing matrix metalloproteinases and tissue factor in vivo and in vitro. *Circulation* 2001; **103**:276–83.

169. Ricote M, Li AC, Willson TM, Kelly CJ, Glass CK. The peroxisome proliferator-activated receptor-gamma is a negative regulator of macrophage activation. *Nature* 1998; **391**:79–82.

170. Dollery CM, McEwan JR, Henney AM. Matrix metalloproteinases and cardiovascular disease. *Circ Res* 1995; **77**:863–8.

171. Schonbeck U, Sukhova GK, Shimizu K et al. Inhibition of CD40 signaling limits evolution of established atherosclerosis in mice. *Proc Natl Acad Sci USA* 2000; **97**:7458–63.

172. Lutgens E, Cleutjens KB, Heeneman S et al. Both early and delayed anti-CD40L antibody treatment induces a stable plaque phenotype. *Proc Natl Acad Sci USA* 2000; **97**:7464–9.

173. Mach F, Shonbeck U, Sukhova GK et al. Reduction of atherosclerosis in mice by inhibition of CD40 signaling. *Nature* 1998; **394**:200–3.

174. Mach F, Schonbeck U, Libby P. CD40 signaling in vascular cells: a key role in atherosclerosis? *Atherosclerosis* 1998; **137**:S89–S95.

175. Aukrust P, Muller F, Ueland T et al. Enhanced levels of soluble and membrane-bound CD40 ligand in patients with unstable angina: possible reflection of T lymphocyte and platelet involvement in the pathogenesis of acute coronary syndromes. *Circulation* 1999; **100**:614–20.

176. Schönbeck U, Varo N, Libby P, Buring J, Ridker PM. Soluble CD40L and cardiovascular risk in women. *Circulation* 2001; **104**:2266–8.

177. Schönbeck U, Gerdes N, Varo N et al. Oxidized low-density lipoprotein augments and 3-hydroxy-3-methylglutaryl coenzyme A reductase inhibitors limit CD40 and CD40L expression in human vascular cells. *Circulation* 2002; **106**:2888–93.

178. May AE, Kalsch T, Massberg S et al. Engagement of glycoprotein IIb/IIIa (alpha(IIb)beta3) on platelets upregulates CD40L and triggers CD40L-dependent matrix degradation by endothelial cells. *Circulation* 2002; **106**:2111–17.

15. PHOTODYNAMIC THERAPY

Ron Waksman

Photodynamic therapy (PDT) involves photosensitizing (light-sensitive) drugs, light and tissue oxygen to treat a wide range of medical conditions primarily in the field of oncology. Photosensitizing agents, many of which are porphyrins or chemicals of similar structure, are administered locally or parenterally and selectively absorbed or retained within the tissues targeted for therapy. This differential selectivity or retention promotes selective damage when the target tissue is exposed to light of an appropriate wavelength; the surrounding normal tissue, containing little or no drug, absorbs little light and is thus spared injury.[1,2] PDT clinical research has historically focused primarily and successfully on cancer treatment,[3–6] however, it has shown promise as a breakthrough treatment in ophthalmic, urologic, autoimmune and cardiovascular diseases. Any disease associated with rapidly growing tissue, including the formation of abnormal blood vessels, can potentially be treated with this technology. For the cardiovascular system, selectivity renders PDT particularly appealing in the treatment of restenosis and atherosclerotic illnesses such as coronary artery disease (CAD), in which other catheter-based approaches are relatively non-selective and carry a substantial risk of damage to the normal arterial wall.[7] Recently there have been preclinical and clinical studies targeted to examine the utility of PDT for vascular applications. This chapter will summarize the mechanisms of action, PDT systems, and the results of these preclinical and clinical studies.

Mechanisms of action

PDT is a non-thermal, photochemical process that involves the administration of a photosensitizer followed by light activation, which corresponds to the sensitizer's profile. Based on the differential accumulation of a photosensitizer in the target tissue, PDT uses light absorption to produce photochemical reactions through the production of free radical moieties without the generation of heat. These free radical moieties are produced either by the photosensitizer itself or by energy transfer to ambient molecular oxygen causing cytotoxic effects on tissue and cells. The tissue is subsequently photo-illuminated at the wavelength that favors maximal absorption by the photosensitized drug. Light is usually in the form of red light derived from a laser, however it can originate from collimated or diffuse illuminators as well (e.g. high-power lamps and light-emitting diode panels).[8] For intravascular application, light is delivered to the treatment site directly with either balloon catheter-based illumination systems[9,10] or optical fibers with cylindrically emitting diffusing fibers.

The photobiologic response (direct, rapid cell apoptosis and delayed necrosis from neovascular damage) becomes maximal within several days.[1,11–13] Throughout this process, the drug serves as a catalyst for energy transfer, whereas light absorption leads to the formation of cytotoxic-reactive oxygen species such as singlet oxygen, a highly reactive, oxidizing agent with very short diffusion distances (≤ 0.1 µm). Cell death is thus confined to those illuminated areas in which there is an adequate presence of the sensitized drug.[14] PDT demonstrated in numerous trials and in different animal (rat and rabbit) models the potential of eradication of medial smooth muscle proliferation following endothelial denudation. A strong correlation exists between depletion of potential neointimal precursor cells at acute time points and inhibition of intimal hyperplasia over the long term after PDT.[15,16] This observation suggests that the main mechanisms are by apoptosis and DNA fragmentation.

Photosensitizers and PDT systems

While laser balloon systems have been purported to have therapeutic vascular effects,[17,18] the goal of illumination for PDT is to have no intrinsic biologic activity due to thermal effects from the light source. Early PDT agents were activated at wavelengths between 630 and 670 nm. At those wavelengths, blood and tissue substantially attenuated the delivery of light to target cells.[19] Tissue optics suggested that higher wavelengths were desired for penetration and photosensitizer activation, with a maximal absorption in the range of 700–800 or 950–1100 nm.[20] Hematoporphyrin derivative (HpD) was the first of a number of photosensitizers with demonstratable, selective accumulation within atherosclerotic plaque,[21] which displays in vitro preferential uptake by human plaque. Administration of the photosensitizing agent 5-aminolevulinic acid (ALA) has been accomplished by topical, systemic and local internal routes in a variety of malignant and dysplastic conditions.[14,22] However, its administration can elicit hemodynamic changes (depression of systemic and pulmonary pressures and pulmonary resistance) that could limit its ultimate utility in cardiovascular applications.[23]

Biotechnology has developed a new generation of selective photosensitizers and catheter-based technological advances in light delivery, which have allowed the introduction of PDT into the vasculature. Two of these systems include Antrin® phototherapy (Pharmacyclics, Inc., Sunnyvale, CA) and PhotoPoint™ PDT (Miravant Medical Technologies, Santa Barbara, CA).

Antrin® phototherapy is a combination of endovascular illumination and motexafin lutetium (MLu, Antrin), an expanded porphyrin (texaphyrin) that accumulates in plaque (Figure 15.1). Texaphyrins can disrupt the intracellular oxidation–reduction balance and alter bioenergetic processes within target cells. When activated by various energy forms (e.g., ionizing radiation, chemotherapy or light), they may also be able to reduce or eliminate diseased tissue targets. Interest in the texaphyrin family of molecules as therapeutic agents for cardiovascular disease is based on tissue selectivity, cellular localization and light activation properties. This phototherapy has been shown to reduce plaque in animal models and generates cytotoxic singlet oxygen that has been shown to induce apoptosis in macrophages and smooth muscle cells.[8] Antrin® is excited by red light that penetrates tissue and blood, is synthetic and water soluble, localizes in atheroma and has a short plasma half-life.[24]

A specialized diode laser (Figure 15.2) has been developed for use with MLu in the catheterization laboratory, which produces a consistent 730 nm red light. This approximates the size of a standard desk top PC with a touch screen control system that allows easy testing of the light fiber and calibration before endovascular illumination. The optical fiber is 0.018″ in diameter (Figure 15.3), can be delivered through angioplasty balloon catheters and standard transfer catheters, and has been delivered to allow illumination at sites where standard interventional technologies can be delivered.[8]

PhotoPoint™ PDT is a newly developed proprietary catheter-based system involving photoselective delivery of a non-ionizing, non-thermal energy source of visible light to activate a photosensitizer localized in the artery wall (Figure 15.4). MV0611, gallium chloride mesoporphyrin dimethyl ester (Miravant Pharmaceuticals Inc., Santa Barbara, CA), was discovered through rational drug screening for use in cardiovascular applications. The interaction between MV0611 and intravascular light generates reactive oxygen species, causing targeted medial

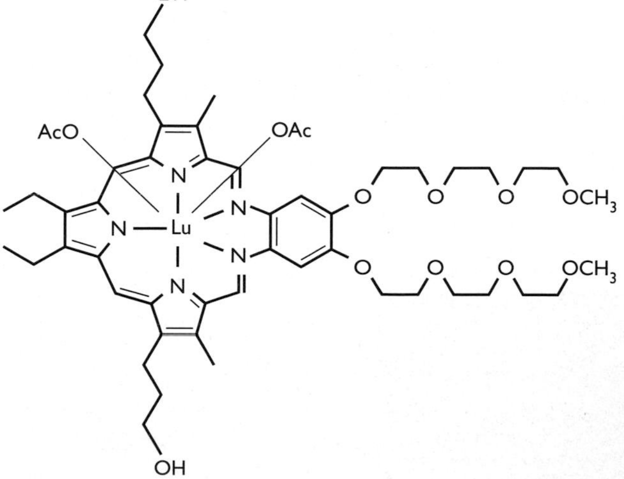

Figure 15.1
Motexafin lutetium (MLu) photosensitizer.

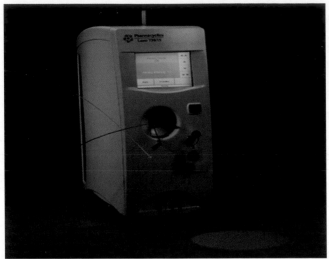

Figure 15.2
Antrin®
phototherapy diode
laser.

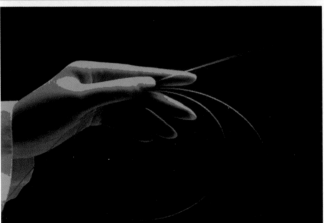

Figure 15.3
Antrin®
phototherapy optical
0.018″ fiber.

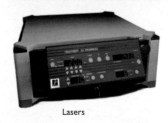

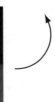

Figure 15.4
PhotoPoint™ – an
integrated system.

Lasers

Light-activated
compounds

Light-delivery devices

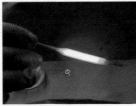

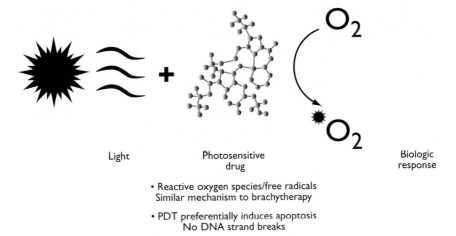

Light   Photosensitive drug   Biologic response

- Reactive oxygen species/free radicals
  Similar mechanism to brachytherapy

- PDT preferentially induces apoptosis
  No DNA strand breaks

Figure 15.5 *PhotoPoint*[TM] *mechanism.*

smooth muscle cell apoptosis and depletion of neointimal precursor cells (Figure 15.5) in rat carotid and porcine coronary arteries.[7,25,26]

PDT for restenosis prevention

Smooth muscle cell migration and proliferation are the main mechanisms for restenosis following intervention. PDT has shown its ability to eradicate smooth muscle cells following injury in animal models. Also PDT is known to increase collagen cross linkage in the extracellular matrix, creating a barrier to smooth muscle cell attachment, proliferation and migration.[27] Restenosis, the major limitation of the long-term success of percutaneous coronary interventions, is probably best treated with brachytherapy, which uses ionizing radiation. PDT, however, which in contrast to brachytherapy uses non-ionizing radiation, has emerged as another possible strategy.[28]

Using the novel photosensitizer molecule, MV0611, Waksman et al examined the effects of intracoronary PhotoPoint[TM] PDT in a porcine stented model of restenosis (Figure 15.6).[29] The photosensitive drug, MV0611, was given systemically followed by intravascular laser light, which was selectively delivered to porcine coronary arteries using a light diffuser centered with a balloon catheter. Bare metal stents were then implanted at the treatment site in the PDT ($n = 5$) or control ($n = 4$) arteries (Figure 15.7). Thirty days later, vessels were analyzed by histopathology and histomorphometry and showed that PDT reduced percent area stenosis compared to controls ($39\pm3\%$ vs $55\pm4\%$, $P<0.01$). Luminal area was increased with PDT and a maximal re-endothelialization score was observed by gross histology in all PDT and control stents. No cases of aneurysm formation or thrombosis presented. Here, intracoronary PDT inhibited

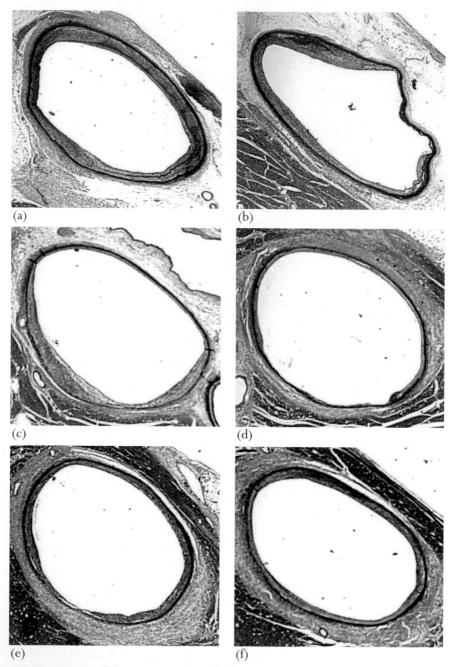

Figure 15.6 (a–f) Porcine stented model of restenosis – sections through single artery 14 days post treatment.

vascular neointima formation without impairing endothelial regeneration in the 30-day porcine model of in-stent restenosis.[29]

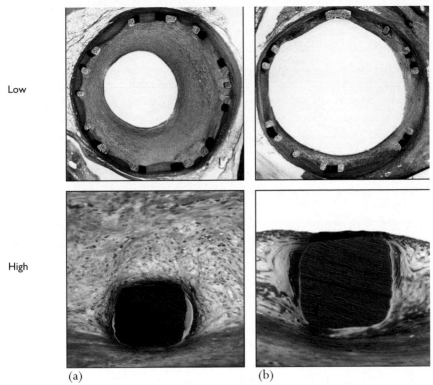

Low

High

(a)   (b)

Figure 15.7 *Bare metal stents implanted (a) in control and (b) at treatment site in photodynamic therapy treated arteries.*

Further studies with the use of the same system on porcine balloon overstretch injury model demonstrated significant inhibition of neointima formation, with vascular remodeling and absence of fibrin deposition or thrombus formation. Other studies on the use of PDT on arteriovenous grafts demonstrated depletion of neointimal precursor cells in the vessel wall. These observations support that PDT can be selectively targeted to smooth muscle cells and fibroblasts and attenuates the restenosis process following intervention.

Photodynamic therapy and atherosclerotic plaque

Atherosclerosis, a vascular inflammatory disease, involves the pathologic development of fatty plaques in a heterogeneous cell matrix.[30] The atherosclerotic plaque target requires radial light delivery, with penetration to a specific target depth, to gain the desired vascular effect. Interest in PDT for treating atherosclerosis has increased in recent years because of the advent of new drugs with fewer side effects and more powerful, less expensive devices. PDT has the potential to provide safe attenuation of macrophages and lipid content, and reduce the atheroma mass through selective effect on macrophages (Figure 15.8) and perhaps cytokines promoting the atherosclerosis process. PDT application can be integrated into traditional vascular procedures with or without stent implantation.[8]

Chen et al explored the effect of altering the intracellular redox state on PDT-induced cell death by depleting intracellular glutathione stores with the use of butathionine sulfoximine (BSO), a specific inhibitor of γ-glutamyl cysteine synthetase.[31] Alone, BSO had no effect on macrophage viability, however treatment of the cells with the antioxidant N-acetylcysteine (NAC) significantly reduced cell death induced by PDT. In contrast to PDT, macrophage apoptosis induced by exogenous C2-ceramide was largely unaffected by treatment with BSO or NAC. The investigators concluded that taken together, these observations suggested that apoptosis initiated by PDT is redox sensitive and that distinct signaling cascades may be operative in PDT compared with certain non-PDT pathways.[31]

Chen et al also examined the mechanism of cell death induced by PDT with MLu by using annexin V staining of macrophages and smooth muscle cells.[31] Here, PDT increased the number of apoptotic macrophages 4.2 ± 1.2-fold (mean$\pm$SD, $n = 4$) and the number of apoptotic smooth muscle cells 4.0 ± 1.9-fold ($n = 3$). The percentage of necrotic cells did not increase from baseline after PDT.

In a vein-graft model, Yamaguchi et al found that PDT could effectively reduce intimal hyperplasia.[32] Inferior vena cava grafted rats were injected with MLu (10 mg/kg) 4 or 12 weeks after grafting. Light therapy was performed 24 hours

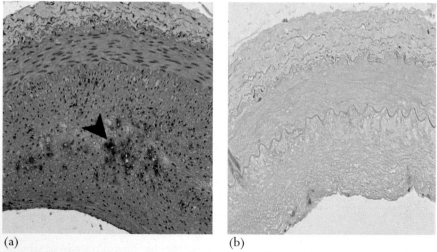

(a)   (b)

Figure 15.8 Photodynamic therapy-induced loss of 'foam cell' macrophages (arrowhead). (a) Control and (b) 7 days post-PDT treatment.

after MLu injection. PDT at 4 weeks after surgery significantly reduced the intima/media ratio, whereas treatment at 12 weeks did not. Activated macrophages were observed 4 weeks after grafting; however, a significant reduction occurred in these cells by 12 weeks. Thus, it appeared that the mechanism by which PDT works may be related to the targeting of activated macrophages in these models of vascular disease.[8]

Targeting entire plaque cell populations, in their study, Waksman et al also examined the effects of the photosensitizing drug MV0611.[30] New Zealand White rabbits received MV0611 (intravenous 2 mg/kg) followed by light delivery using a Miravant catheter-based diode laser (15 J/cm^2) 4 hours post-injection. PDT induced a significant reduction (92±6%) in the population of nuclei of all cell types in plaques relative to controls (P<0.01). Results indicated that PDT with MV0611 induces significant depletion of plaque cell populations.[30]

Clinical trials

In a phase 1 trial of PDT with Antrin®, Rockson et al demonstrated that photoangioplasty with Antrin® is well tolerated and safe in the endovascular treatment of atherosclerosis. This was an open-label, single-dose, escalating drug and light-dose study that was originally not designed to examine clinical efficacy, however, several secondary endpoints suggested a favorable therapeutic effect. Clinical evaluation, serial quantitative angiography, and intravascular ultrasonography were performed on a study population, which consisted of patients with symptomatic claudication and objectively documented peripheral arterial insufficiency (n = 47; 51 procedures). The standardized classification of clinical outcomes of the 47 patients at follow-up showed improvement in 29 (62%), no change in 17 (36%), and moderate worsening in one (2%).[33]

Bisaccia et al used photopheresis for the first time to prevent restenosis.[34] A total of 78 patients with single-vessel coronary artery disease were enrolled, 41 in the control group and 37 in the photopheresis group. Clinical restenosis occurred in significantly less photopheresis patients than in the control patients (8% vs 27%; P = 0.04), with a relative risk of 0.30 (95% confidence interval 0.09–1.00). A multicenter clinical trial following a US Food and Drug Administration recommended protocol is currently underway to better determine what, if any, impact photopheresis has in preventing restenosis.[34]

In an original study including seven patients with symptomatic restenosis of the superficial femoral artery within 6 months of angioplasty (one with two lesions in the same artery), Mansfield et al determined that at 48 (mean) months after PDT, no patients developed critical limb ischemia or ulceration and there were no arterial complications.[35] Only one of eight lesions treated by angioplasty with adjuvant PDT developed symptomatic restenosis at the treated site over a 4-year interval. Although the study was uncontrolled and had a small number of patients, the authors reported that adjunctive PDT seems to hold considerable promise as a new strategy to prevent restenosis after angioplasty.[35]

Kereiakes et al, in an open-label, phase I, drug and light dose-escalation clinical trial of MLu phototherapy, enrolled 80 patients undergoing de novo coronary stent deployment. MLu was administered to 79 patients by intravenous infusion 18 to 24 hours before procedure, and photoactivation was performed after balloon predilatation and before stent deployment. Clinical evaluation, serial quantitative angiography, and intravascular ultrasound were performed periprocedurally and at 6 months follow-up. Beyond 30 days (range, 71 to 189 days), 15 (19%) patients experienced adverse outcomes, including non-Q-wave myocardial infarction ($n = 6$) and symptomatic target lesion revascularization ($n = 11$), with 2 patients experiencing both infarction and revascularization. MLu phototherapy was well tolerated without serious dose-limiting toxicities, and side

Table 15.1 QCA at follow-up by study stage and segment analyzed

	Stent	Injury	Illumination	Entire analysis
Stage 1				
Late loss, mm				
Median	1.1	0.8	0.6	0.6
Mean (SD)	1.1 (0.59)	0.9 (0.64)	0.6 (0.48)	0.6 (0.55)
95% CI	(0.9, 1.3)	(0.7, 1.1)	(0.5, 0.8)	(0.4, 0.8)
Binary restenosis (>50%), %	39.5	42.1	42.1	44.7
Stage 2				
Late loss, mm				
Median	1.0	0.9	0.6	0.4
Mean (SD)	0.9 (0.62)	0.9 (0.64)	0.6 (0.58)	0.6 (0.59)
95% CI	0.7 to 1.2	0.7 to 1.2	0.4 to 0.8	0.4 to 0.8
Binary restenosis (>50%), %	27.3	30.3	30.3	30.3

(Adapted with permission from Kereiakes et al, 2003.[24])

There were no clinically significant differences between the stent, balloon injury, illumination and analysis segments.

MLD, minimal lumen diameter.

Stage 1: MLu dose escalation was performed in 7 sequential cohorts of 5 patients, each beginning at 0.05 mg/kg and ending with 4.0 mg/kg MLu. The far red laser light dose was held constant at 100 J/cm-fiber in this stage.

Stage 2: MLu was administered sequentially in doses of 2 and 3 mg/kg, and light dose escalation was performed (200, 400, and 600 J/cm-fiber) in cohorts of 5 patients at both MLu dose levels administered. Each patient cohort was individually assessed by the steering committee of the trial for safety and tolerability before enrolling subsequent patient cohorts.

effects (paresthesia and rash) were minor. No adverse angiographic outcomes were attributed to phototherapy.[25] QCA at follow-up by study stage and segment analyzed is depicted in Table 1.

Conclusion

Photodynamic technology for vascular applications holds promise and is expected to play a role in the prevention of restenosis, as a modality to attenuate atherosclerotic plaques, and perhaps to pacify vulnerable plaques. Nevertheless, the challenge lies in finding the optimal dose for both the drug (photosensitizer) and the light energy source to achieve these targets safely without affecting the integrity of the vessel or exposing the patients to additional risk. If this technology is proved in clinical trials, catheter-based photodynamic therapy will play a pivotal role in interventional cardiology.

Acknowledgments

The author would like to acknowledge Pauline McEwan, Ian Leitch and Robert Scott of Miravant Medical Technologies.

References

1. Henderson B, Dougherty T. How does photodynamic therapy work? *Photochem Photobiol* 1992; **55**:145–57.

2. Dougherty T. Photosensitizers: therapy and detection of malignant tumors. *Photochem Photobiol* 1987; **45**:879–89.

3. Dougherty TJ, Gomer CJ, Henderson BW et al. Photodynamic therapy. *J Natl Cancer Inst* 1998; **90**:889–905.

4. Pass HI. Photodynamic therapy in oncology: mechanisms and clinical use. *J Natl Cancer Inst* 1993; **85**:443–56.

5. Prewitt TW, Pass HI. Photodynamic therapy for thoracic cancer: biology and applications. *Semin Thorac Cardiovasc Surg* 1993; **5**:229–37.

6. Woodburn KW, Fan Q, Kessel D et al. Phototherapy of cancer and atheromatous plaque with texaphyrins. *J Clin Laser Med Surg* 1996; **14**:343–8.

7. Rockson SG, Lorenz DP, Cheong W-F et al. Photoangioplasty: an emerging clinical cardiovascular role for photodynamic therapy. *Circulation* 2000; **102**:591–6.

8. Chou TM, Woodburn KW, Cheong W-F et al. Photodynamic therapy: applications in atherosclerotic vascular disease with motexafin lutetium. *Catheter Cardiovasc Interv* 2002; **57**:387–94.

9. Spears JR. Percutaneous laser treatment of atherosclerosis: an overview of emerging techniques. *Cardiovasc Interv Radiol* 1986; **9**:303–12.

10. Jenkins MP, Buonaccorsi GA, Mansfield R et al. Reduction in the response to coronary and iliac artery injury with photodynamic therapy using 5-aminolaevulinic acid. *Cardiovasc Res* 2000; **45**:478–85.

11. Kessel D, Luo Y, Deng Y et al. The role of subcellular localization in initiation of apoptosis by photodynamic therapy. *Photochem Photobiol* 1997; **65**:422–6.

12. Sluiter W, de Vree W, Pietersma A et al. Prevention of late lumen loss after coronary angioplasty by photodynamic therapy: role of activated neutrophils. *Mol Cell Biochem* 1996; **157**:233–8.

13. Reed M, Miller F, Wieman T et al. The effect of photodynamic therapy on the microcirculation. *J Surg Res* 1988; **45**:452–9.

14. Nyamekye I, Anglin S, McEwan J et al. Photodynamic therapy of normal and balloon-injured rat carotid arteries using 5-amino-levulinic acid. *Circulation* 1995; **91**:417–25.

15. Grove RI, Leitch I, Rychnovsky S et al. Current status of photodynamic therapy for the prevention of restenosis. In: Waksman R, ed. *Vascular Brachytherapy*. 3rd edn. New York: Futura Publishing Co, 2002:339–45.

16. Barton JM, Nielsen HV, Rychnovsky S et al. PhotoPoint™ PDT inhibits intimal hyperplasia in arteriovenous grafts. Presented at CRT 2003, January 26–29. Washington, DC.

17. Spears JR, James LM, Leonard BM et al. Plaque-media rewelding with reversible tissue optical property changes during receptive cw Nd:YAG laser exposure. *Lasers Surg Med* 1988; **8**:477–85.

18. Cheong WF, Spears JR, Welch AJ. Laser balloon angioplasty. *Crit Rev Biomed Engineer* 1991; **19**:113–46.

19. Vincent GM, Fox J, Charlton G et al. Presence of blood significantly decreases transmission of 630 nm laser light. *Lasers Surg Med* 1991; **11**:399–403.

20. Doiron DR, Keller GS. Porphyrin photodynamic therapy: principles and clinical applications. *Curr Prob Dermatol* 1986; **15**:85–93.

21. Spears J, Serur J, Shropshire D et al. Fluorescence of experimental atheromatous plaques with hematoporphyrin derivative. *J Clin Invest* 1983; **71**:395–9.

22. Kennedy J, Marcus S, Pottier R. Photodynamic therapy (PDT) and photodiagnosis (PD) using endogenous photosensitization induced by 5-aminolevulinic acid (ALA): mechanisms and clinical results. *J Clin Laser Med Surg* 1996; **14**:289 304.

23. Herman M, Webber J, Fromm D et al. Hemodynamic effects of 5-aminolevulinic acid in humans. *J Photochem Photobiol B* 1998; **43**:61–5.

24. Kereiakes DJ, Szyniszewski AM, Wahr D, et al. Phase 1 drug and light dose-escalation trial of motexafin lutetium and far red light activation (phototherapy) in subjects with coronary artery disease undergoing percutaneous coronary intervention and stent deployment: procedural and long-term results. *Circulation* 2003; **108**:1310–15.

25. Wilson A, Leitch IM, Diaz E et al. Endovascular photodynamic therapy with the new photosensitizer MV0611 reduces neo-intimal cell content in a rodent arterial injury model [abstract 3133]. *Circulation* 2001; **104(suppl II)**:II–663.

26. Yazdi H, Kim H-S, Seabron R et al. Cellular effects of intracoronary photodynamic therapy with the new photosensitizer MV0611 in normal and balloon-injured porcine coronary arteries. Acute and long term effects [abstract 1849]. *Circulation* 2001; **104(suppl II)**:II–388.

27. Overhaus M, Heckenkamp J, Kossodo S et al. Photodynamic therapy generates a matrix barrier to invasive vascular cell migration. *Circ Res* 2000; **86**:334–40.

28. Mansfield R, Bown S, McEwan J. Photodynamic therapy: shedding light on restenosis. *Heart* 2001; **86**:612–18.

29. Waksman R, Leitch I, Roessler J et al. Intracoronary PhotoPoint photodynamic therapy reduces neointimal growth without suppressing re-endothelialization in a porcine model of restenosis. Submitted for publication, October 2003.

30. Waksman R, Leborgne L, Seabron R et al. Novel PhotoPoint photodynamic therapy for the treatment of atherosclerotic plaques. *JACC* (Suppl. A)2003; **41**:259A.

31. Chen Z, Woodburn KW, Shi C et al. Photodynamic therapy with motexafin lutetium induces redox-sensitive apoptosis of vascular cells. *Arterioscler Thromb Vasc Biol* 2001; **21**:759–64.

32. Yamaguchi A, Woodburn KW, Hayase M et al. Reduction of vein graft disease using photodynamic therapy with monotexafin lutetium in a rodent isograft model. *Circulation* 2000; **102**:III275–III280.

33. Rockson SG, Kramer P, Razavi M et al. Photoangioplasty for human peripheral atherosclerosis: results of a phase I trial of photodynamic therapy with motexafin lutetium (Antrin). *Circulation* 2000; **102**:2322–4.

34. Bisaccia E, Palangio M, Gonzalez J et al. Photopheresis: therapeutic potential in preventing restenosis after percutaneous transluminal coronary angioplasty. *Am J Cardiovasc Drugs* 2003; **3**:43–51.

35. Mansfield RJR, Jenkins MP, Pai ML et al. Long-term safety and efficacy of superficial femoral artery angioplasty with adjuvant photodynamic therapy to prevent restenosis. *BJ Surg* 2002; **89**:1538–9.

16. SHOULD WE TREAT THE VULNERABLE PLAQUE WITH DRUG ELUTING STENTS?

Willibald Maier and Bernard Meier

The principal manifestations of coronary atherosclerosis derive from two mechanisms. Significant degrees of coronary artery stenosis result in flow limitation at least during conditions of increased demand such as physical exercise.[1] Symptomatic coronary artery disease (angina and angina equivalents) ensues. Surgical[2] and percutaneous[3] treatment modalities have been developed in the past three decades for its treatment. The more ominous manifestation of coronary atherosclerosis is plaque rupture resulting in thrombotic partial or complete vessel obstruction.[4] This complication is associated with grave consequences such as myocardial infarction (MI), heart failure, life threatening arrhythmias and death. Although high-grade coronary artery stenoses have a higher potential for vessel occlusion than mild stenoses, they are responsible only for the minority of the acute coronary syndromes (ACS). The majority of ruptured plaques have been observed in non-flow limiting stenoses because they outnumber the flow limiting lesions by a factor of 10 or more.

Stenting has largely resolved the problem of acute vessel closure during PCI (percutaneous coronary intervention)[5] and reduced the incidence of restenosis. Yet, with conventional stents a considerable restenosis rate persists.[6] This argues against stenting of non-significant but conspicuous lesions to prevent a future plaque rupture. Drug eluting stents prevent restenosis to a degree that this problem no longer can be called an Achilles heel.[6,7] This invites to treat angiographically non-flow limiting, but potentially vulnerable lesions to prevent a future rupture. If it was easy to screen for and identify the vulnerable plaque with the armamentarium described in this handbook, one could argue to treat these and not the others. However, most of these methods are not routinely available. And low vulnerability today may change tomorrow. Therefore, the hypothesis to seal plaques with angioplasty deserves to be discussed. Clinical aspects will be merged with the sparse data from randomized trials on that subject to extrapolate the potential of plaque sealing with drug eluting stents.[8,9]

Clinical examples

Figures 16.1 and 16.2 illustrate the clinical dilemma with the impossibility to predict a plaque rupture of angiographically non-significant lesions, even while exhausting pharmacological plaque passivation. Figure 16.1 shows the angiograms of a 60-year-old male with multiple risk factors (cigarette smoking, hypertension, hypercholesterolemia and positive family history). He first came to our catheterization laboratory after a non-ST-elevation MI. The first diagonal branch was recanalized and stented. The LAD (left anterior descending artery) showed

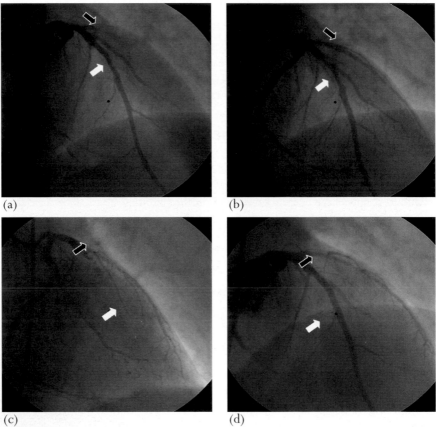

(a)　　　　　　　　　　　　　　(b)

(c)　　　　　　　　　　　　　　(d)

Figure 16.1 (a) Angiogram of the left coronary artery prior to the first intervention with an occluded first diagonal branch (black arrow) and a non-significant plaque in the mid left anterior descending (LAD) artery (white arrow). (b) Post intervention. (c) Acute reangiography five months later for an occluded LAD (white arrow) with patent diagonal branch (black arrow). (d) After successful intervention with both vessels patent.

298

only minor wall irregularities. The patient was discharged under acetylsalicylic acid, clopidogrel (for 1 month), statins and an optimally controlled risk profile. Five months later he required an acute intervention for a complete occlusion of the LAD, which again was successfully recanalized and stented. The diagonal branch showed a good long-term result.

Figure 16.2 shows the case of a 54-year-old female with a similar risk profile and unstable angina who was successfully stented on a subtotal stenosis of the mid LAD. In the proximal segment of the right coronary artery (RCA) an exulcerated, but angiographically non-significant plaque was seen and was left untreated. Again, acetylsalicylic acid, clopidogrel (for 1 month), state of the art risk factor management, and statin therapy were applied. Two months later the patient was readmitted with an acute inferior ST-elevation MI. Angiography demonstrated an occlusion of the RCA at the site of the formerly exulcerated plaque. The lesion was recanalized and stented. The LAD documented no restenosis at this time.

Definition of plaque sealing in clinical routine

In the pre-stent era, the term plaque sealing was coined for mechanical stabilization of non-significant stenoses at strategically important coronary artery sites. At that time, there was no possibility to identify a vulnerable plaque, but this was considered moot, anyhow, because of the fact that cold plaques may turn into hot plaques at any given time. The impressive innocuousness and stability of a dilated lesion had led to the hypothesis of mechanical plaque sealing by balloon angioplasty. Clinical experiences like the two cases support the plaque sealing approach.[10] Coronary angioplasty typically induces an extensive splitting of the plaque or the border zone. This splitting engenders proliferation of new tissue layers covering the former plaque area, hence plaque sealing. The smooth muscle-rich intima observed over the first few months after angioplasty transforms into a fibrous layer immune to fissures or rupture.[11] Thus once the acute effect with its inherent risk of acute occlusion has passed, the subsequent risk of plaque rupture is markedly reduced compared with that of an untreated plaque. Immediate, abrupt vessel closure represented one of the major shortcomings of balloon angioplasty that today can be successfully prevented or resolved with stenting.[5]

Restenosis is a major shortcoming of balloon angioplasty and remains a blemish of conventional stenting. Non-drug eluting stents in complex lesions still carry a risk for restenosis of about 30%,[6] and in-stent restenosis treated with balloon angioplasty yields a high re-restenosis rate.[12,13] In contrast to restenosis, acute occlusion due to the rupture of a plaque may cause irreversible myocardial damage or even death and should be in the focus of therapeutic endeavors.

There is no rationale from flow dynamics or structure–function relationships to dilate non-significant stenoses, since lesions with diameter reduction of 50% or

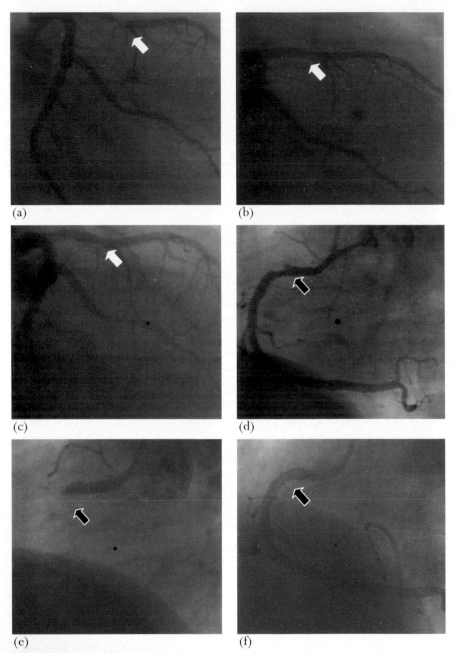

Figure 16.2 *(a) Angiogram of the left coronary artery with a high-grade stenosis of the mid left anterior descending (LAD) (white arrow), which was successfully stented (b). (c) Situation at follow-up. (d) Angiogram of the right coronary artery with an exulcerated, non-significant plaque in the proximal segment (black arrow) at the time of the LAD procedure. (e) This plaque occluded 2 months later and (f) was stented acutely.*

300

less typically have a normal coronary flow reserve.[1] The concept of measuring coronary flow reserve or fractional flow reserve[14] only relates to functional lesion severity and thus angina. The concept of plaque sealing targets prognosis and is independent of functional relevance. Dilating stenoses appearing non-significant at angiography but with a reduced coronary flow reserve or fractional flow reserve represents classic therapeutic angioplasty. Plaque sealing still is in the picture, but it is not the principal reason for the procedure. Hence, plaque sealing is a preventive action to avoid future rupture of a non-significant coronary stenosis that has been identified at the occasion of an angiography indicated by a variety of symptoms or associated disease conditions like, e.g. preoperative risk stratification, angioplasty of significant stenoses, etc. In a typical scenario, the patient's symptoms definitively are not due to flow obstruction of this stenosis – defined by any means of morphologic (angiography, intravascular ultrasound) or physiologic (coronary flow reserve, fractional flow reserve) assessment, and thus the patient does not have angina pectoris or objective signs of ischemia from this lesion. If the patient has demonstrable angina pectoris unequivocally related to this stenosis, angioplasty would be standard therapy and mechanical plaque sealing a welcome side product but not the primary intention. Plaque sealing is typically pondered at a moment when angiography has been performed on a patient for whatever reason. Vascular access and a coronary catheter are in place. A lesion of usually 40–70% diameter reduction by visual estimate or on-line quantitative coronary angiography has been identified in a proximal segment of the LAD, left circumflex, or RCA subtending a sufficiently large territory to cause a major threat in case of occlusion. About 90% of clinically relevant MI are caused by lesions in the proximal third of the major coronary arteries. An immediate decision is warranted whether to proceed with a preventive angioplasty to transform this potentially vulnerable plaque mechanically into scar tissue by intentionally cracking the fibrous cap under controlled conditions to induce a scar meant to exclude later plaque rupture. The potential risk of performing angioplasty for this lesion and for causing a significant restenosis must be taken into account.

Estimated probabilities of myocardial infarction and restenosis

The literature indicates that about 80% or more of all infarctions result from thrombosis of a lesion which by itself is not hemodynamically significant.[15–19] This does not mean that a mild stenosis is more dangerous in terms of producing an acute infarction than a severe stenosis. It rather implies that there are commonly about 10 mild stenoses to every single severe stenosis and it is the cumulative risk of all the non-significant stenoses that prevails.[20]

Figure 16.3 shows a Japanese series of 39 patients with MI in whom a coronary angiography with ergonovine provocation test had been performed a maximum of 13 years previously. More than half of infarctions resulted from stenoses, which were not significant at the initial examination.[19]

According to the CASS (Coronary Artery Surgery Study) registry, the risk of infarction over 3 years is 2% for a stenosis of less than 50%, 7% for a stenosis of 50–70%, 8% for a stenosis of 70–90%, 15% for a stenosis of 90–98%, and 7% for a functionally occlusive lesion (Figure 16.4).[21] This underscores that the tight but not subtotal stenosis is the most dangerous one. Subtotal stenoses are usually either protected by collaterals or they represent lesions that have already been occluded before. A number of other factors also influence the risk of subsequent occlusion and infarction such as an irregular surface of the lesion or a lesion in a tortuous segment,[21] a branching point stenosis[21,22] or a proximal location of the

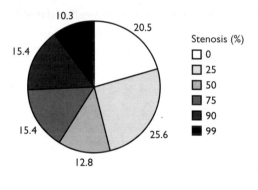

Figure 16.3 Percentages of original stenoses at the initial coronary angiogram of 39 patients who underwent reangiography for acute MI from that lesion over a period of up to 13 years.[19]

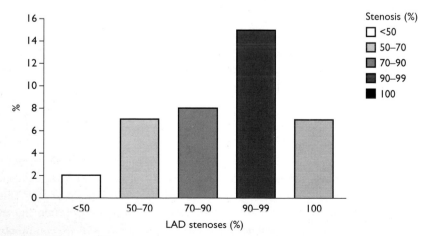

Figure 16.4 Risk of left anterior descending (LAD) artery infarction (in percent) according to the degree of coronary stenosis over 3 years according to the Coronary Artery Surgery Study registry.[21]

stenosis.[16] The latter criterion may be a misleader. The more proximal a lesion, the more likely it is that the resultant occlusion will become manifest to the clinician or the pathologist.

As to the likely outcome of the mild or moderate lesion subjected to coronary angioplasty, data have been accumulated to emphasize the fact that such lesions have a low risk of acute occlusion and restenosis after angioplasty. In the era of modern angioplasty equipment and techniques, particularly with the use of stents for suboptimal results and for impending or acute occlusions, infarctions should occur in less than 3% in the acute phase. To this we have to add roughly a 0.5% incidence of infarctions during the next year (including the risk carried by repeat angioplasty in about 10% of patients), counting only the ones being unequivocally attributable to the dilated site.[23] Beyond this period, spontaneous infarctions related to the dilated site are extremely rare. Even in case of restenosis, the highest incidence of related infarctions reported is 0.5%.[24–27]

It has also been observed that the incidence of late infarctions (related or unrelated to the dilated site) is independent of the presence of restenosis.[28] This indicates that these infarctions are not related to the dilated site itself but predominantly to other diseased segments (unsealed adjacent plaques). Although occlusions at the dilated site do occur in a few percent during long term follow-up after angioplasty of non-total lesions, these occlusions pertain typically to previously occluded or collateralized vessels and rarely cause a clinical event.[29] Though the above data largely pertain to significant stenoses, the figures for non-significant stenoses are bound to be similar, and probably even more favorable. In a study of 415 patients with angioplasty for moderately severe stenoses only one case of MI occurred subsequently.[30] Another small study addressing truly non-significant stenoses (<50% diameter stenosis assessed by quantitative coronary angiography), which had been dilated in the same session with a significant stenosis and had angiographic follow-up at 6 months, reported no major adverse cardiac events related to these stenoses during that period. There was no angiographic benefit at 6 months, i.e. the same non-significant diameter stenosis was observed,[31] but the goal of eliminating the infarct potential of the lesion was likely attained.

Retrospective and prospective evidence

There is little published evidence for the plaque sealing concept. Mercado et al have investigated the clinical and angiographic outcome of patients with mild coronary lesions treated with balloon angioplasty or coronary stenting in comparison with moderate and severe stenosis.[32] They identified 3812 patients with chronic stable angina and a single de novo lesion in a native coronary artery from 14 different studies in a core-laboratory database using identical and standardized methods of data acquisition and analysis. Quantitative coronary angiographic (QCA) analysis was performed for pre and post intervention and 6 months follow-up and clinical event rates were observed for 1 year. Stenosis severity prior to PCI was categorized into three groups: <50% diameter stenosis (DS), 50–99% DS, and >99% DS. Thirty-nine percent were successfully treated with balloon angioplasty only and 61% of the patients received stents. One year event rate (mortality, rate of non-fatal MI, and repeat revascularization) did not differ between balloon and stented angioplasty for any of the stenosis severity categories (around 20%). In other words, event rates were the same for significant and non-significant stenoses, indicating that intervention per se is associated with a certain event rate, which needs to be offset by the unknown rate of potentially prevented later plaque ruptures. However, this study was retrospective and the purpose to treat the non-significant lesion was not plaque sealing.

In the DEFER study,[8] patients with significant coronary lesions, but without documented ischemia at non-invasive stress testing were stratified according to the fractional flow reserve (FFR) into an intervention group (FFR <0.75) as reference and two study groups with FFR >0.75, indicating no significant lesion. One group was randomized to angioplasty mostly with stenting and the other was treated conservatively (deferral group). Event free survival at 24 months did not differ between the two groups, but was significantly worse in the reference group in which FFR measurements had identified a functionally significant stenosis. This study neither proved nor disproved the plaque sealing concept. The patients with an intervention did not yet show an advantage at 2 years but their lesion was sealed while the non-treated lesions continued to harbor an unchanged infarction risk.

Intravascular ultrasound measurements were suggested for discrimination of lesion significance. A low event rate for an observation period of more than 1 year was reported without an intervention with a minimal luminal area of 4.0 mm^2 at the interrogated lesion.[33] However, these observations were not targeted at plaque sealing. They were driven by the concept to optimize the detection of flow-limiting stenoses for therapeutic angioplasty.

Physiological assessment and small vessel disease

Patients with small vessel disease or syndrome X[34] need to be addressed separately in the context of plaque sealing. Microvascular dysfunction usually shows an impaired coronary flow reserve.[35] There might be symptom overlap between patients with classic syndrome X and patients with atypical angina and documentation of a coronary plaque. However, syndrome X from pure microvascular dysfunction is not linked to distinct plaques. If non-significant coronary artery lesions are treated in syndrome X, plaque sealing would be the only motive.

(Drug eluting) stents for vulnerable plaques

Initially, plaque sealing only warranted provisional stenting. First, balloon angioplasty has an excellent prognosis in mild lesions of large vessels so there is little need to improve it with stenting. Second, stents introduce a small but relevant risk of subacute thrombosis, a serious hazard virtually unheard of after balloon angioplasty. Third, the rare in-stent restenoses may be difficult to treat if they are of the long and diffuse kind. The last point is moot with the published data for drug eluting stents that are impressive. The RAVEL study showed a 0% binary restenosis rate at 6 months for the sirolimus eluting stent as compared to 27% in the standard stent group, and an overall rate of major adverse cardiac events (MACE) at 1 year of 6% versus 29%, respectively.[6] The smaller TAXUS I study demonstrated for a stent system with local delivery of paclitaxel comparable results with a 0% binary restenosis rate for the paclitaxel-eluting stent versus 10% for the bare metal control group, and MACE at 1 year of 3% versus 10%, respectively.[6a] Two-year angiographic follow-up of an observational group treated with the sirolimus eluting Bx Velocity (Cordis Johnson and Johnson, Cordis Corporation, FL) stent demonstrated no in-stent restenosis and a target *vessel* revascularization rate of 10%, indicating freedom of restenosis 'catch-up' during this period.[7] Preliminary data from the ongoing larger randomized and observational trials with the sirolimus eluting stent support the substantial improvement of restenosis without increase in other MACE rates also in complex lesion and patient subsets.

The advent of the drug eluting stents thus invites for stenting non-significant lesions to the ends of plaque sealing and preventing progression to significant obstruction, as significant restenosis induced by dilating a non-significant lesion is no longer a real issue. Plaque sealing is no option for a diffusely diseased vessel in an 80-year-old diabetic patient. It is the 50–60% plaque in the proximal LAD of a 50-year-old banker referred for diagnostic angiography with atypical chest pain and a FFR >0.75 that brings it up. Current clinical practice would mandate to send the patient home without treatment. As plain balloon angioplasty is deemed obsolete (for no good reason as it were), MACE rates around 10% with drug eluting stenting are weighed against the unknown probability of later plaque rupture at this specific site. Various methods are discussed in this handbook to assess the vulnerability of a given plaque. Some of them are not risk free and cost more than an angioplasty procedure. Moreover, a 'cold' plaque may turn 'hot' anytime. On the other hand, there is increasing evidence that in ACS multiple plaques might be involved in a generalized inflammatory disease,[36–38] relegating plaque sealing to the 'long shot in the dark' realm. Nevertheless, MACE rates of only 3–6% for 1 year open up a new dimension for preventive angioplasty in strategically important vessels with a perfusion territory carrying the risk of major disabling or lethal infarction in case of uncontrolled plaque rupture.

305

The ultimate equation

For the pre-drug eluting stent era, an ultimate equation opposed the risk of a spontaneous infarction based on a moderate (hemodynamically non-significant) lesion of 7% over 3 years to a 3% infarction rate during coronary angioplasty to which 0.5% has to be added for the next 4–5 years in the two-thirds of patients without restenosis and 2.5% in the remaining third with restenosis (factoring in a 2% infarction risk during the repeat coronary angioplasty). This yields a pessimistically calculated overall infarction risk of the hypothetical plaque sealing group of 5% which represents a relative risk reduction of about 30% over 3 years and argues in favor of angioplasty for such lesions. With a 0% restenosis using drug eluting stents, the ratio would be 3.5% versus 7% in favor of stenting. But then again, conventional treatment, particularly with statins and thienopyridines, has improved as well.

Our experience with plaque sealing

We have clinically followed 34 patients with balloon only (65%) or stented (35%) angioplasty of single de novo coronary stenoses of less than 50% diameter reduction over an average of 69±25 months. Mean reference diameter assessed by quantitative coronary angiography was 3.0±0.5 mm. Pre-intervention mean ejection fraction was 73±7%, and no wall motion abormalities were documented. The lesions were dilated from 45±4 to 16±9% diameter stenosis. No cardiac death or MI occurred. Eleven follow-up angiograms were performed for recurrence of initial symptoms and resulted in one repeat angioplasty of the dilated plaque and three angioplasties of new lesions.

Mechanically or pharmacologically targeting the vulnerable plaque

Convincing evidence is provided by large-scale lipid-lowering studies that lipid lowering reduces the incidence of coronary events[39] and may induce plaque passivation.[40,41] The effect may be even more impressive with aggressive lipid lowering[9] and sustained treatment with clopidogrel[42] and lead to the conclusion that the need for coronary intervention might be postponed or even obviated pharmacologically. However, there is no conclusive proof up to now that coronary artery disease really can be put to a halt rather than just slowed down. Interventional therapy may still only be deferred by a few years. Moreover, the reduction in events in the AVERT trial, which compared percutaneous transluminal coronary angioplasty with conservative management under aggressive lipid lowering, is mainly due to reduction in minor events (e.g. repeat hospitalization) in the medically treated group during the first 18 months of follow-up and not to reduction in hard endpoints like death or MI. For instance, mortality in the patients randomized to the invasive strategy was naught. It is obvious that once an invasive strategy is engaged, it produces consecutive medical attendance and expenditure, in part solely due to the patient's enhanced awareness of the disease, since it could not be managed medically. As long as we cannot reliably detect the vulnerable plaque in clinical practice, we appear served best with the blind plaque sealing hypothesis. And even if one day we can assess plaque vulnerability, we may not bother. The advent of the drug eluting stents has engendered several crucial advantages in favor of mechanical plaque sealing: by reduction of restenosis rate balance between the unavoidable, but nowadays fairly acceptable procedural risk plus reinterventions for restenosis versus the natural course is possibly shifted in favor of the intervention. Moreover, malignant in-stent restenosis as the sword of Damocles over conventional stenting in non-significant stenoses has been virtually eradicated. Now the time has come to prove this concept with randomized trials such as the one currently under way at our centers.

In case of multiple borderline plaques, this concept is impracticable for obvious reasons. Diffuse non-significant coronary artery disease needs aggressive medical risk factor management. Of course, the plaque sealing patient requires the same state of the art lipid lowering and antiplatelet management to fully profit from both the pharmacologic and the mechanical approach.

So, should we treat the non-significant plaque with angioplasty? If we know that it is vulnerable, most agree to go ahead. A stent appears to be a 'sine qua non' these days so it had better be a drug eluting one. Drug eluting stents may turn out to be the midwife of the plaque sealing principle, irrespective of the vulnerability of the plaque, bringing it to life at last, albeit for all the wrong reasons.

References

1. Gould KL. *Coronary Artery Stenosis*. New York, Elsevier 1991.

2. Favaloro RG. Critical analysis of coronary artery bypass graft surgery: a 30-year journey. *J Am Coll Cardiol* 1998; **31**:1B–63B.

3. Gruntzig AR, Senning A, Siegenthaler WE. Nonoperative dilatation of coronary-artery stenosis: percutaneous transluminal coronary angioplasty. *N Engl J Med* 1979; **301**:61–8.

4. Corti R, Farkouh ME, Badimon JJ. The vulnerable plaque and acute coronary syndromes. *Am J Med* 2002; **113**:668–80.

5. Bittl JA. Advances in coronary angioplasty. *N Engl J Med* 1996; **335**:1290–302.

6. Morice MC, Serruys PW, Sousa JE et al. A randomized comparison of a sirolimus-eluting stent with a standard stent for coronary revascularization. *N Engl J Med* 2002; **346**:1773–80.

6a. Grube E, Silber S, Hauptmann KE et al. TAXUS I: Six- and twelve-month results from a randomized, double-blind trial on a slow-release paclitaxel-eluting stent for de novo cornary lesions. *Circulation* 2003; **107**:38–42.

7. Sousa JE, Costa MA, Sousa AG et al. Two-year angiographic and intravascular ultrasound follow-up after implantation of sirolimus-eluting stents in human coronary arteries. *Circulation* 2003; **107**:381–3.

8. Bech GJ, De Bruyne B, Pijls NH et al. Fractional flow reserve to determine the appropriateness of angioplasty in moderate coronary stenosis: a randomized trial. *Circulation* 2001; **103**:2928–34.

9. Pitt B, Waters D, Brown WV et al. Aggressive lipid-lowering therapy compared with angioplasty in stable coronary artery disease. Atorvastatin versus Revascularization Treatment Investigators. *N Engl J Med* 1999; **341**:70–6.

10. Meier B, Ramamurthy S. Plaque sealing by coronary angioplasty. *Cathet Cardiovasc Diagn* 1995; **36**:295–7.

11. Inoue K, Nakamura N, Kakio T et al. Serial changes of coronary arteries after percutaneous transluminal coronary angioplasty: histopathological and immunohistochemical study. *J Cardiol* 1994; **24**:279–91.

12. Waksman R, Raizner AE, Yeung AC, Lansky AJ, Vandertie L. Use of localised intracoronary beta radiation in treatment of in-stent restenosis: the INHIBIT randomised controlled trial. *Lancet* 2002; **359**:551–7.

13. Leon MB, Teirstein PS, Moses JW et al. Localized intracoronary gamma-radiation therapy to inhibit the recurrence of restenosis after stenting. *N Engl J Med* 2001; **344**:250–6.

14. Pijls NH, De Bruyne B, Peels K et al. Measurement of fractional flow reserve to assess the functional severity of coronary-artery stenoses. *N Engl J Med* 1996; **334**:1703–8.

15. Hackett D, Davies G, Maseri A. Pre-existing coronary stenoses in patients with first myocardial infarction are not necessarily severe. *Eur Heart J* 1988; **9**:1317–23.

16. Ambrose JA, Tannenbaum MA, Alexopoulos D et al. Angiographic progression of coronary artery disease and the development of myocardial infarction. *J Am Coll Cardiol* 1988; **12**:56–62.

17. Little WC, Constantinescu M, Applegate RJ et al. Can coronary angiography predict the site of a subsequent myocardial infarction in patients with mild-to-moderate coronary artery disease? *Circulation* 1988; **78**:1157–66.

18. Brown BG, Gallery CA, Badger RS et al. Incomplete lysis of thrombus in the moderate underlying atherosclerotic lesion during intracoronary infusion of streptokinase for acute myocardial infarction: quantitative angiographic observations. *Circulation* 1986; **73**:653–61.

19. Nobuyoshi M, Tanaka M, Nosaka H et al. Progression of coronary atherosclerosis: is coronary spasm related to progression? *J Am Coll Cardiol* 1991; **18**:904–10.

20. Giroud D, Li JM, Urban P, Meier B, Rutishauer W. Relation of the site of acute myocardial infarction to the most severe coronary arterial stenosis at prior angiography. *Am J Cardiol* 1992; **69**:729–32.

21. Ellis S, Alderman E, Cain K et al. Prediction of risk of anterior myocardial infarction by lesion severity and measurement method of stenoses in the left anterior descending coronary distribution: a CASS Registry Study. *J Am Coll Cardiol* 1988; **11**:908–16.

22. Taeymans Y, Theroux P, Lesperance J, Waters D. Quantitative angiographic morphology of the coronary artery lesions at risk of thrombotic occlusion. *Circulation* 1992; **85**:78–85.

23. Ernst SM, van der Feltz TA, Bal ET et al. Long-term angiographic follow up, cardiac events, and survival in patients undergoing percutaneous transluminal coronary angioplasty. *Br Heart J* 1987; **57**:220–5.

24. Guiteras P, Tomas L, Varas C et al. Five years of angiographic and clinical follow-up after successful percutaneous transluminal coronary angioplasty. *Eur Heart J* 1989; **10**:42–8.

25. Kober G, Vallbracht C, Kadel C, Kaltenbach M. Results of repeat angiography up to eight years following percutaneous transluminal angioplasty. *Eur Heart J* 1989; **10**:49–53.

26. Dimas AP, Grigera F, Arora RR et al. Repeat coronary angioplasty as treatment for restenosis. *J Am Coll Cardiol* 1992; **19**:1310–14.

27. Bottner RK, Green CE, Ewels CJ et al. Recurrent ischemia more than 1 year after successful percutaneous transluminal coronary angioplasty. An analysis of the extent and anatomic pattern of coronary disease. *Circulation* 1989; **80**:1580–4.

28. Vlietstra RE, Holmes DR Jr, Rodeheffer RJ, Bailey KR. Consequences of restenosis after coronary angioplasty. *Int J Cardiol* 1991; **31**:143–7.

29. Kitazume H, Kubo I, Iwama T, Ageishi Y. Long-term angiographic follow-up of lesions patent 6 months after percutaneous coronary angioplasty. *Am Heart J* 1995; **129**:441–4.

30. Rozenman Y, Gilon D, Welber S et al. Total coronary artery occlusion late after successful coronary angioplasty of moderately severe lesions: incidence and clinical manifestations. Cardiology 1994; **85**:222–8.

31. Hamon M, Bauters C, McFadden EP, Lablanche JM, Bertrand ME. Six-month quantitative angiographic follow-up of 50% diameter stenoses dilated during multilesion percutaneous transluminal coronary angioplasty. *Am J Cardiol* 1993; **71**:1226–9.

32. Mercado N, Maier W, Boersma E et al. Clinical and angiographic outcome of patients with mild coronary lesions treated with balloon angioplasty or coronary stenting. *Eur Heart J* 2003; **24**:541–51.

33. Abizaid AS, Mintz GS, Mehran R et al. Long-term follow-up after percutaneous transluminal coronary angioplasty was not performed based on intravascular ultrasound findings: importance of lumen dimensions. *Circulation* 1999; **100**:256–61.

34. Wiedermann JG, Schwartz A, Apfelbaum M. Anatomic and physiologic heterogeneity in patients with syndrome X: an intravascular ultrasound study. *J Am Coll Cardiol* 1995; **25**:1310–17.

35. Chauhan A, Mullins PA, Petch MC, Schofield PM. Is coronary flow reserve in response to papaverine really normal in syndrome X? *Circulation* 1994; **89**:1998–2004.

36. Ross R. Atherosclerosis – an inflammatory disease. *N Engl J Med* 1999; **340**:115–26.

37. Rioufol G, Finet G, Ginon I et al. Multiple atherosclerotic plaque rupture in acute coronary syndrome: a three-vessel intravascular ultrasound study. *Circulation* 2002; **106**:804–8.

38. Goldstein JA, Demetriou D, Grines CL. Multiple complex coronary plaques in patients with acute myocardial infarction. *N Engl J Med* 2000; **343**:915–22.

39. MRC/BHF Heart Protection Study of cholesterol lowering with simvastatin in 20 536 high-risk individuals: a randomised placebo-controlled trial. *Lancet* 2002; **360**:7–22.

40. Brown BG, Zhao XQ, Sacco DE, Albers JJ. Lipid lowering and plaque regression. New insights into prevention of plaque disruption and clinical events in coronary disease. *Circulation* 1993; **87**:1781–91.

41. Effect of simvastatin on coronary atheroma: the Multicentre Anti-Atheroma Study (MAAS). *Lancet* 1994; **344**:633–8.

42. Steinhubl SR, Berger PB, Mann JT III et al. Early and sustained dual oral antiplatelet therapy following percutaneous coronary intervention: a randomized controlled trial. *JAMA* 2002; **288**:2411–20.

17. VOLCANO THERAPEUTICS

M Pauliina Margolis

Cardiovascular disease is America's number one killer. Over one million people die from cardiovascular disease each year. There are currently over 1 million people in the United States (US) each year that suffer from ischemic events (heart attacks) and over half of these people die. As recently as 5 years ago, most physicians would have described the disease process of atherosclerosis in such a way that included the understanding that the fat-laden material gradually built up on the surface of the artery walls. If the deposit or plaque grew and clogged or blocked the artery, this resulted in a heart attack. Today, scientists understand that most heart attacks may in fact stem from less obstructive plaques that rupture suddenly, triggering the emergence of a blood clot, or thrombus, that blocks the blood flow. These plaques have been classified as vulnerable plaques.

About Volcano Therapeutics, Inc.

The founding scientists of Volcano Therapeutics, Inc., the University of Texas/Texas Heart Institute-based Drs Jim Willerson and Trip Casscells, were among the first to describe the phenomenon of vulnerable plaque, to postulate a mechanism of vulnerable plaque rupture and to identify the unique signature (heat due to inflammation) for plaque vulnerable to erosion and rupture.[13] Based both on their scientific understanding of vulnerable plaque and on their clinical observations, Drs Willerson and Casscells, later joined by Dr Mort Naghavi, also a scientific founder of Volcano, conceived of, patented, and produced prototypes of a catheter to identify vulnerable plaque lesions producing heat and thus at risk of rupture.

Volcano Therapeutics, Inc. was organized in its present form in February 2001, when Domain Associates, LLC, the largest healthcare venture capital firm in the US, made the initial investment. In April 2002, an investor group including Domain, Johnson & Johnson Development Corp, Medtronic, Inc. and Mayo Medical Ventures invested $24 million in the Company. In addition to licensing the broad and encompassing intellectual property of the scientific founders, Volcano has acquired significant intellectual property in the area of thermal detection of vulnerable plaque from David Brown, MD and Farallon Medical Systems (Tom Campbell patents). The intellectual property licensed from Texas Heart Institute also includes near-infrared-based detection and thermal treatment of vulnerable plaque. In addition, Volcano has licensed from and is now co-developing with the

Cleveland Clinic Foundation unique intravascular ultrasound (IVUS)-based spectral imaging software, or IVUS Virtual Histology™, that has the potential to provide important information on plaque composition.

Volcano's mission is to develop and commercialize a full range of catheter-based diagnostic and therapeutic products for use in the areas of vulnerable plaque detection and treatment. The company's initial product, an intracoronary thermography system and catheter, is described here.

Scientific background

Inflammation has been shown to be part of or the main etiologic factor in numerous vascular disorders including atherosclerosis, vasculitis, hypertension, aneurysms and chronic venous insufficiency. The majority of ACS including unstable angina, MI and sudden death, are due to plaque rupture on a non-flow limiting, angiographically 'silent' atherosclerotic plaque.[1] In addition, even though the majority of patients with sudden coronary death have no previous history of heart disease, 61% of these patients have other healed plaque ruptures in their coronary segments with or without evidence of healed MI.[2]

Post-mortem studies on coronary arteries from patients with acute MI have demonstrated that 50–90% of plaques prone to rupture have a lipid-rich core (lipid pool) in the central portion of an eccentrically thickened intima and are bound on its luminal aspect by a thin fibrous cap with inflammatory cells.[3–6] The majority of inflammatory cells are located in the central portion of the ruptured fibrous cap and the minority are at the edge of the fibrotic cap, the so-called 'shoulder' region of the lipid pool.[7] Plaque calcification is present in approximately 70% of the cases and the fibrous cap is infiltrated by macrophages in 100% and T cells are present in 75%. Seventy-five percent of patients with acute coronary ruptures have other healed ruptures in the coronary vasculature as well (typically one to two plaque ruptures at different stage of healing). Of the acute ruptures which lead to sudden death due to coronary artery thrombosis, 33% have evidence of a single large necrotic core filled with blood at the site of the ruptured fibrous cap and 67% have evidence of two to four previous plaque ruptures at the same site.[2,8] These important post-mortem findings have clearly demonstrated that plaque rupture not only plays a major role in acute MI, but also in the development of an atherosclerotic plaque.

The presence of inflammation as a marker for plaque vulnerability has gained increasing attention during recent years due to the role of macrophages in the pathophysiology of vulnerable plaque. Macrophages are predominantly 'matrix-degrading' cells (secrete proteinases including matrix metalloproteinases (MMPs) and collagenases), that can cause thinning and possible digestion of the fibrous cap, have the ability to recruit more monocytes, stimulate further angiogenesis, promote increased modification of low-density lipoprotein (LDL) cholesterol and the arrival of T lymphocytes, and increase the apoptosis of smooth muscle cells.[9–11] Apoptosis of smooth muscle cells, the main source for collagen synthesis, increases further plaque vulnerability.[12]

Casscells and colleagues demonstrated in 1996 that 37% of plaques from human carotid atherosclerotic plaque specimens taken during endarterectomy had substantially warmer regions (0.4–2.2 °C) when compared to normal tissue.[13] Temperature measurements correlate positively with the density of inflammatory cells (mostly macrophages) and inversely with the distance of cell clusters from the luminal surface. In 1999, Stefanadis and co-authors detected thermal heterogeneity of atherosclerotic coronary arteries in vivo.[14] Temperature measurements from 90 patients showed that vessel wall temperature was constant in normal coronary arteries, but significantly higher in the majority of the atherosclerotic plaques. Temperature differences between atherosclerotic plaque and healthy coronary vessel wall increased progressively from patients with stable angina to patients with acute MI. The difference of plaque temperature from background (blood) temperature was 0.106 ± 0.110 °C in stable angina, 0.683 ± 0.347 °C in unstable angina, and 1.472 ± 0.691 °C in acute MI. In 2001, Stefanidis and co-authors showed that temperature difference was also a strong predictor of adverse cardiac events during the follow-up period (17.88 ± 7.16 months).[15] Adverse event rates in patients who had a maximum measured vessel wall temperature deviation from blood (ΔT) of 0.5 °C or greater was significantly higher when compared to patients with temperature differences of <0.5 °C (41% vs 7%, P = 0.001).

Identification of vessel wall inflammation

Over the past several years Volcano Therapeutics, Inc. has developed a thermography catheter and instrument intended as an adjunct to conventional angiographic procedures to provide thermal mapping of tissue temperature of both coronary and peripheral vasculature. The thermography catheter is designed to be used as a diagnostic tool to provide temperature information of the pathophysiology of the target tissue, which may indicate the presence or absence of tissue inflammation within the vessel wall. Thermography may be used to guide therapeutic strategy and interventional procedures. The results of the series of investigations described in Volcano preclinical and clinical studies below and conducted by several academic research institutes and hospitals were designed to study the acute procedural success, safety, feasibility and performance of the Volcano thermography system in healthy and diseased coronary arteries, and the relationship of vessel wall ΔT with the amount and location of inflammatory cells.

Description of the device

The Volcano Therapeutics thermography system consists of two primary components: the sterile, single-use thermography catheter (Catheter); and the movable instrument which houses the electronics and includes the flat panel color monitor. Additionally, the system utilizes an interface cable and power cable. A commercially available pullback device, similar to the Jomed or Endosonics Trak Back™ device may be used at the discretion of the physician. Pullback devices are commonly used during IVUS procedures.

Catheter

The thermography catheter (Catheter) consists of a handle with thumb actuator and 3.3 Fr-catheter tubing with an effective length of 135 cm (Figures 17.1 and 17.2). The Catheter is designed to accommodate a 0.014″ guidewire and a guiding catheter greater than or equal to 6 Fr. The thermography catheter is designed for the percutaneous insertion using the common over-the-wire method. The Catheter also includes the following technical characteristics:

- The Catheter tip includes a self-expanding basket made from nitinol material with five outer thermocouples, located at the apex of each of the five arms of the circular basket, for measuring vessel wall temperature and one inner

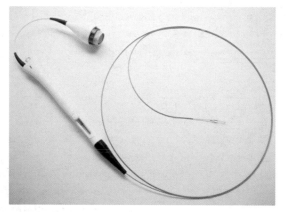

Figure 17.1 *Volcano thermography system.*

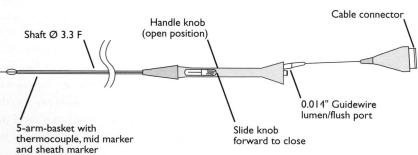

Figure 17.2 *Schematic presentation of Volcano thermography system.*

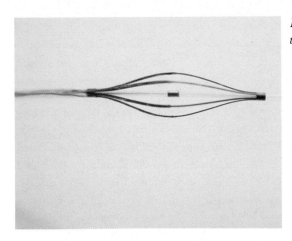

Figure 17.3 *Volcano temperature sensors.*

thermocouple for measuring the reference blood temperature (Figure 17.3). The basket when fully open has a nominal diameter of 4–5.5 mm. The basket and the device are designed for vessels 2–4 mm in size. The self-expanding basket is allowed to expand once the Catheter sheath is retracted. The sheath, which extends the length of the Catheter, is retracted by moving the thumb actuator located on the Catheter handle. The catheter sheath is positioned over the Catheter basket prior to insertion into the patient by moving the thumb actuator forward. With the sheath positioned over the basket the entire length of the Catheter has a nominal diameter of 3.3 Fr. The sheath is retracted once the Catheter is in position within the coronary vasculature. The position of the Catheter and the state of the sheath can be verified by viewing the position of radiopaque markers using fluoroscopy.

- The Catheter tubing is constructed using common biocompatible materials and has an effective length of 135 cm and has a nominal diameter of approximately 3.3 Fr. The Catheter tubing is also coated with a biocompatible material similar to the material used by the predicate devices to increase lubricity.

- Encased within the Catheter handle is a 10 000Ω (ohm) thermistor (producing resistance values consistent with −40 °C to +300 °C). It converts ambient temperature to resistance, which is then available to the data acquisition processor via the interface cable. The thermistor is essential when using thermocouples to measure temperature by providing a cold junction temperature. The cold junction temperature is sensed by a precision thermistor in good thermal contact with the input connectors of the measuring instrument. This second temperature reading, along with the readings from the thermocouples is used by the instrument to calculate the true temperature at the distal end of the catheter.

- The serial memory chip, also located within the Catheter handle retains calibration constants for the thermistor and the thermocouples. The calibration constants are determined during the manufacturing process and are referenced by the instrument when the 'calibration' sequence is actuated.

Instrument

The Volcano Therapeutics thermography system instrument is portable and can be rolled into an evaluation suite where the Volcano Therapeutics thermography system will be used (Figure 17.4). The monitor attached to the instrument provides the visual representation of temperature data acquired by the thermography Catheter (Figure 17.5). The instrument also records patient demographic information and will output information in the DICOM format using a writable CD-ROM device. The user interface devices (monitor, keyboard, and writable CD-ROM) are built into the instrument. It houses the processor

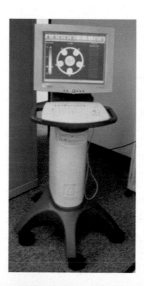
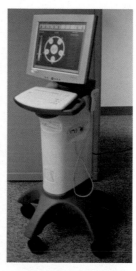

Figure 17.4 *Volcano thermography system instrument.*

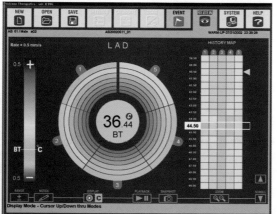

Figure 17.5 *Volcano instrument display.*

boards (user interface and data acquisition), power switching and regulating hardware, and the hard disk drive, none of which are externally accessible. It provides external connections for the interface cable and the encoder cable. The instrument can operate on either 120 VAC or 240 VAC from an external line source using a standard grounded power cord.

- The data acquisition processor acquires A/D thermal data from the thermistor, located in the Catheter handle, and the six Catheter thermocouples and position data from the encoder. The data acquisition processor displays vessel wall and blood temperature both graphically and numerically with respect to time and the position of the Catheter in the vessel. It initiates the thermal data acquisition hardware calibration.

- The user interface processor allows the user (physician) to enter patient information and then to store processed data captured during a session (for each patient) for later review. The user can also control the format in which the results are displayed.

- The Volcano Therapeutics thermography system's only user input device is a standard 101/102 keyboard, which is built into the instrument. It allows the user to perform the following functions: input patient information, calibration, control display format, save and recall session information, transfer session information to the writable CD-ROM, and review saved session information.

Principles of operation

The Volcano Therapeutics thermography system relies on the percutaneous, over-the-wire insertion of a thermography Catheter to the coronary peripheral vasculature. The position of the Catheter is verified by conventional fluoroscopy methods. Once in place a self-expanding nitinol basket moves five thermocouples into contact with the vessel wall. The Catheter is then slowly withdrawn through the vasculature by hand or by using an optional pullback device.

During the withdrawal process the thermocouples register the temperature of the vessel wall relative to blood temperature, which is measured in the same manner using a separate thermocouple. The temperature difference (ΔT) is displayed on the monitor. The instrument utilizes color scales to display the ΔT with the numeric values.

The micro processors and amplifiers within the instrument measure the DT seven times per second. This value is averaged and displayed on the instrument monitor two times per second when using a rate of 1 mm/s and displayed one time per second at 0.5 mm/s.

The withdrawal process can be done by hand by the physician or by using an automatic pullback device. When the automatic pullback device is used the temperature information is correlated to distance traveled during the pullback of the thermography Catheter.

Pre-clinical work

Bench-top

Several factors are critical in order for a thermography catheter to consistently obtain meaningful temperature data. Basket opening is defined as the ability of the catheter to fully allow the thermocouples to initially contact the vessel wall upon deployment. Wall contact is the ability of the thermocouples to maintain contact with the vessel wall as the Catheter is pulled back through the artery. The path of pullback may be straight or tortuous, and the diameter can vary from typical values of 2.0–5.0 mm. In addition to these mechanical characteristics, the signal transmission through the thermocouple is dependent upon several other factors such as thermocouple time constant, thermocouple accuracy and thermocouple precision.

An in vitro model was developed to characterize the key mechanical factors of a thermography catheter. The model consists of a molded silicone aortic arch which is attached to simulated coronary arteries of varying diameter, shape and tortuosity. The simulated vessels are clear in order to allow assessment of the catheter functionality. Clear fluid (water or normal saline) can be circulated through the model at 37 °C, so that the catheter is tested in its normal environment. Flow rate can be adjusted with the use of a roller pump. A guiding catheter is placed into the model and engaged with the simulated coronary ostium. Thermography catheters are inserted through a rotating hemostatic valve and advanced into the simulated vessel over a coronary guidewire.

Basket opening is achieved by relative axial displacement between the inner and outer catheter members. In the model, the distance between the tips of the inner and outer members is measured before and after the deployment of the thermography basket. The distance of the displacement is a determinant of the ability of the basket to open completely. In addition the contact of the basket on the inner diameter of the simulated vessel is another determinant. Studies on basket opening with Volcano thermography catheter in preclinical bench-top testing have shown good basket opening in both straight and tortuous models.

Wall contact is measured by performing a pullback of the catheter at a known rate, such as 0.5 mm/s, and recording the number of thermocouples contacting the vessel at different points along the length of the pullback. The total percentage of 'good' measurements – in which the thermocouples are contacting the wall – can be calculated from this recording. Volcano thermography catheter has shown good and consistent wall contact in both straight and tortuous models.

Animal experiments
In-vivo safety and feasibility
To assess safety and feasibility of the thermography catheter, three major coronary arteries of healthy, domestic swine were interrogated according to normal clinical

practice either once with IVUS catheter (Boston Scientific), or once, twice or three times with the thermography catheter. Animals were sacrificed either acutely, at 7 days or at 28 days. After sacrifice, coronary arteries were pressure perfusion fixed with 10% formalin and sent for histopathological evaluation. Acute vessel wall effects were assessed with light and scanning electron microscopy and arteries harvested at 7 and 28 days were studied with light microscopy.

During or after each pullback with either IVUS or temperature catheter there were no signs of vessel wall spasm, dissections or thrombus formation. However, three consecutive pullbacks of the temperature catheter induced a mild and diffuse vessel spasm in one animal that was treated with intracoronary nitroglycerin without sequelae. Light and scanning electron microscopy showed superficial endothelial denudation, but no deeper vessel wall injury after either IVUS or Volcano catheter (Figures 17.6 and 17.7). At 7 days the vessel wall was totally re-endothelialized and complete healing of the vessel wall was also confirmed at 28-day follow-up.

In-vivo performance

To assess the ability of the thermography system in measuring intracoronary temperatures copper coils were deployed by balloon in the coronary arteries of five domestic swine (35–40 kg) to induce an inflammatory response. All three major coronary arteries (left anterior descending, left circumflex, right coronary) underwent coil implant. The coronary arteries in this study were studied at 7, 10, and 28 days using the thermography catheter. After temperature recording, the swine were sacrificed and the coronary arteries pressure perfusion fixed with 10% formalin. These were then sent for histopathologic examination to correlate degree and extent of coronary artery inflammation with temperature measurements.

Seven days post copper coil implantation, no vessel wall inflammation was present, and no temperature differences measured. Inflammation developed by

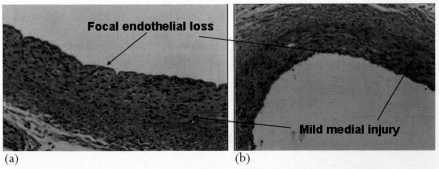

(a) (b)

Figure 17.6 *Minimal, acute vessel wall trauma after a single pullback of (a) Volcano and (b) intravenous ultrasound catheter.*

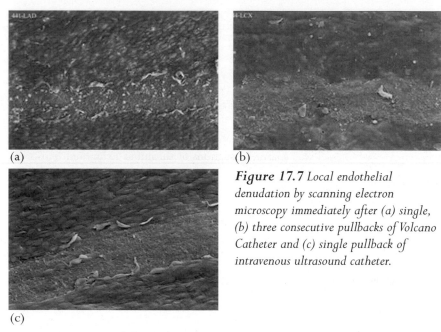

(a)

(b)

(c)

Figure 17.7 Local endothelial denudation by scanning electron microscopy immediately after (a) single, (b) three consecutive pullbacks of Volcano Catheter and (c) single pullback of intravenous ultrasound catheter.

10 days, with localized mononuclear, neutrophilic and lymphocytic cell infiltrates near the luminal surface. Maximum measured vessel wall ΔT from blood was 1.1 °C at the site of a vessel wall dissection at the distal edge of the coil (Figure 17.8). At 28 days, no significant ΔT was found in any vessel, despite marked inflammation located principally in the adventitia. Histopathology showed 300 μm or more of neointimal thickness, insulating the luminal surface from the adventitial inflammatory cell infiltrates. Control arteries showed no thermal differential and normal histopathology was found at all time points (Figure 17.9).

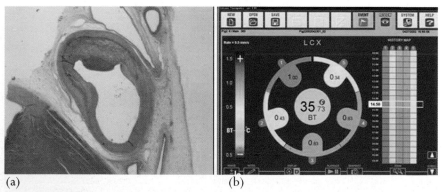

(a)   (b)

Figure 17.8 Temperature map and histopathology 10 days after copper-coil implantation and vessel wall dissection in porcine coronary artery. (a) Histopathology: chronic, superficial inflammation, mainly mononuclear cells three-quarters of the lumen circumflex. (b) Temperature map: Max ΔT 1.0 °C.

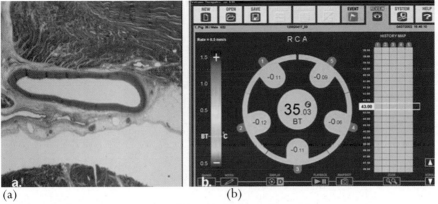

Figure 17.9 *Temperature map and histopathology of control porcine coronary artery at 10 days. (a) Histopathology: normal vessel wall. (b) Temperature map: no temperature increase.*

Clinical work

Safety and feasibility

To date, over 60 stable or unstable patients have been enrolled in the clinical safety and feasibility study conducted by Volcano Therapeutics. Patients were followed for 7 days in case of any post-procedural complications either during hospitalization or after discharge due to thermal mapping of the culprit artery.

Patients with CAD were studied with the Volcano catheter before culprit lesion intervention. Predilatation of the culprit lesion was recommended if the minimum lumen diameter of the segment of interest was by visual assessment less than 1.8 mm. Volcano catheter was advanced over the wire distal to the culprit lesion and a motorized pullback (0.5 mm/s) was used to acquire a thermal map of the artery.

No acute or short term adverse safety issues have been identified in the study. In patients with tortuous vessels or angiographic evidence of vessel calcium the performance of the catheter was moderate. The temperature profile of the first nine patients of the study have also been analyzed. Seven patients were stable and two patients were unstable. One patient had a 3-day history of angina, but during the study was symptom free and had slightly elevated Troponin-t levels. All nine patients were diagnosed with dyslipidemia, one patient had in-stent restenosis by angiography, and two patients were diagnosed with diabetes mellitus.

In these nine patients, the maximum ΔT measured was +0.23 °C (Figure 17.10). No significant ΔT was seen in two of the nine arteries (Figure 17.11). Most of the culprit lesions showed mild (<0.2 °C) eccentric ΔT (Figure 17.12), and in two arteries maximum ΔT (>0.2 °C) was identified in angiographically

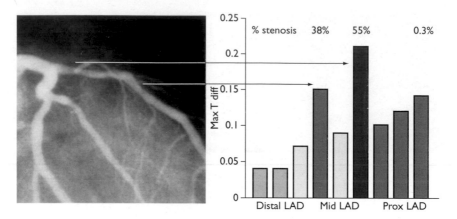

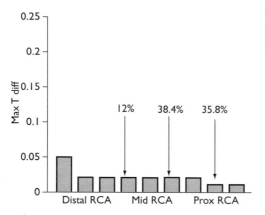

Figure 17.10 *Temperature map of the right coronary artery of a stable patient. Max ΔT (temperature difference between vessel wall temperature and blood temperature) was 0.23 °C at the site of the culprit lesion.*

Figure 17.11 *Temperature map of the right coronary artery (RCA) of a stable patient.*

normal regions (Figure 17.13). The patients with in-stent restenosis showed a moderate ΔT both within and at the edges of the stent with significant amount of neointimal regrowth (Figure 17.14).

Clinical work in progress

Volcano Therapeutics is currently conducting a clinical study called PILOT. This study aims to continue the assessment of the safety and feasibility of the catheter and system in patients with ACS. PILOT will enroll up to a 200 patients and the temperature mapping of all three major coronary arteries is encouraged. PILOT

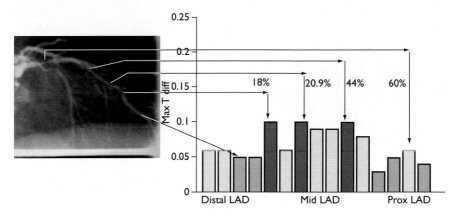

Figure 17.12 *Temperature map of the left anterior descending (LAD) artery of an unstable patient.*

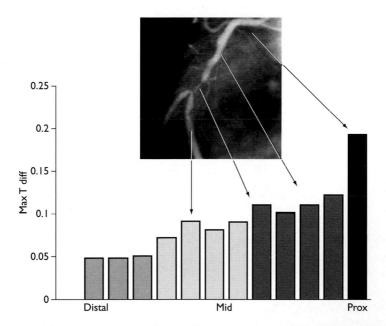

Figure 17.13 *Temperature map of the right coronary artery of a stable patient. Note max ΔT at the site of angiographically normal vessel at the ostium of the RCA.*

will also study the role of IVUS based radiofrequency-tissue characterization (IVUS Virtual Histology™) in the assessment of vulnerable plaques.

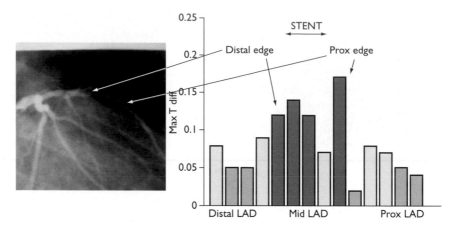

Figure 17.14. *Temperature map of the left anterior descending (LAD) artery of a stable patient with in-stent restenosis; a moderate max ΔT both within and at the edges of the stent.*

Summary

The Volcano thermography catheter and instrument have demonstrated good procedural success, safety and feasibility in both normal and diseased swine coronary arteries as well as in stable and unstable patients with diffuse or focal coronary atherosclerosis. Superficial inflammation in porcine coronary arteries has been associated with significant, focal temperature rise above blood temperature. However, inflammation-induced ΔT was found to be minimal when inflammatory cells were more than 300 μm from the lumen surface.

In patients, the maximum detected ΔT has been 0.23 °C, clearly a lower value when compared to the preclinical data and lower than previously reported by Stefanadis et al.[14] The lower temperature values seen in patients may be due to (i) the stable nature of the patients studied so far, (ii) the differences in the catheter and system design used for previous thermal mapping of coronary arteries, (iii) the effect of blood flow on the vessel wall temperature, (iv) the measurement sensitivity of the catheter, and/or (v) the heterogeneity of the vascular pathology seen in coronary atherosclerosis. Future studies are required to assess the accuracy of thermal mapping to identify lesions prone to rupture and to evaluate the role of thermal mapping in other forms of vascular inflammation and its feasibility to identify patients with high risk for coronary events.

References

1. Dalager-Pederson S, Ravn HB, Falk E. Atherosclerosis and acute coronary events. *Am J Cardiol* 1998; **82**: 37T–40T.

2. Burke AP, Kolodgie FD, Farb A, et al. Healed plaque ruptures and sudden coronary death. *Circulation* 2001; **103**:934.

3. Libby P. Molecular bases of the acute coronary syndromes. *Circulation* 1995; **91**:2844–50.

4. Davies MJ, Thomas AC. Plaque fissuring: the cause of acute myocardial infarction, sudden ischemic death, and crescendo angina. *Br Heart J* 1985; **53**:363–73.

5. Falk E. Coronary thrombosis: pathogenesis and clinical manifestations. *Am J Cardiol* 1991; **68**:28B–35B.

6. Friedman M, Van Den Bovenkamp GJ. The pathogenesis of a coronary thrombus. *Am J Pathol* 1966; **48**:19–44.

7. Farb A, Burke AP, Tang AL et al. Coronary plaque erosion without rupture into a lipid core. A frequent cause of coronary thrombosis in sudden coronary death. *Circulation* 1996; **93**: 1354–63.

8. Falk E. Plaque rupture with severe pre-existing stenosis precipitating coronary thrombosis. Characteristics of coronary atherosclerotic plaques underlying fatal occlusive thrombi. *Br Heart J* 1983; **50**:127–34.

9. Van der Wal AC, Becker AE, van der Loos CM, Das PK. Site of intimal rupture or erosion of thrombosed coronary atherosclerotic plaques is characterized by an inflammatory process irrespective of the dominant plaque morphology. *Circulation* 1994; **89**:36–44.

10. Brown DL, Hibbs MS, Kearney M et al. Expression and cellular location of 92 kDa gelatinase in coronary lesions of patients with unstable angina. *J Am Coll Cardiol (Special Issue)* 1994; 123A. [Abstract].

11. Shah PK, Falk E, Badimon JJ et al. Human monocyte-derived macrophages express collagenases and induce collagen breakdown in atherosclerotic fibrous caps: implications for plaque rupture. *Circulation* 1993; **88 (suppl I)**:I-254. [Abstract].

12. Geng Y-J, Libby P. Evidence for apoptosis in advanced human atheroma. Colocalization with interleukin-1-converting enzyme. *Am J Pathol* 1995; **147**:251–66.

13. Cassells W, Hathorn B, David M et al. Thermal detection of cellular infiltrates in living atherosclerotic plaques: possible implications for plaque rupture and thrombosis. *Lancet* 1996; **347**:1447–9.

14. Stefanadis C, Diamantopoulos L, Vlachopoulos C et al. Thermal heterogeneity within human atherosclerotic coronary arteries detected in vivo. A new method of detection by application of a special thermography catheter. *Circulation* 1999; **99**:1965–71.

15. Stefanadis C, Toutouzas K, Tsiamis E et al. Increased local temperature in human coronary atherosclerotic plaques: an independent predictor of clinical outcome in patients undergoing a percutaneous coronary intervention. *J Am Coll Cardiol* 2001; **37**:1277–83.

18. RADIOFREQUENCY-TISSUE CHARACTERIZATION AND VIRTUAL HISTOLOGY™

D Geoffrey Vince, Anuja Nair, Jon D Klingensmith,
Barry D Kuban, M Pauliina Margolis and Vince Burgess

Traditional methods for studying human coronary artery disease (CAD) have significant limitations. Angiography allows evaluation only of the geometry of the unobstructed part of the lumen; it cannot provide information on the structure of the arterial wall, which is essential to understand the processes leading to plaque rupture. Although histologic analysis directly evaluates atherosclerotic plaque composition, it cannot be used to identify plaques 'at risk' for rupture because the necessary tissue specimens can only be obtained at autopsy. Intravascular ultrasound (IVUS) can provide the necessary structural information in situ, and the development and refinement of this technique have provided a powerful in vivo method to assess plaque morphology. Until recently, IVUS has been used to guide interventional procedures. In spite of the limited accuracy of conventional IVUS images to detect plaque morphology, it has been lately used to identify ruptured atherosclerotic plaques in non-culprit arteries. Perhaps more importantly, the potential of IVUS to quantify the structure and geometry of normal and atherosclerotic coronary arteries will allow one to characterize specific lesions and to distinguish which plaques will or will not lead to coronary plaque rupture.

Intravascular ultrasound

Two approaches to transducer construction have gained popularity over the past decade: electronic arrays and mechanically rotating single-element devices. One of the prerequisites for spectral analysis of radio-frequency (RF)-data is access to the RF source. This is currently only commercially available on Boston-Scientific Corporation (Natick, MA) equipment, including the Galaxy and most Clearview consoles. These systems employ mechanically rotating transducers.

IVUS backscatter

The pulse–echo mode of ultrasound imaging is the most common method of visualizing tissues, and is also the modus operandi with IVUS. The ultrasound transducer is excited with a certain voltage, which makes it resonate and produce an ultrasound pulse. This wave propagates through the tissue and is reflected or scattered by the media back to the transducer, where it is converted back to a voltage. This voltage is known as the backscattered or RF-data. Figure 18.1 is an illustration of the IVUS catheter with the transducer at the tip. An ultrasound pulse is sent out into the tissue to be imaged in the radial direction. The backscatter is acquired by the transducer, which then rotates approximately 1.5° and sends out another ultrasound pulse, with 256 such A-scans (backscattered signals) forming one IVUS image in the clinically available consoles (Figure 18.2). It is the analysis of these A-scans that holds potential for tissue characterization.

One A-scan is thus a signal that contains information about the tissue that reflected the ultrasound energy. However, this received signal is changed slightly by catheter and console specific parameters. While the ultrasound console does not change (usually in the same clinical setting), the IVUS catheter is a single-use device, and different catheters produce a different response for each patient. It is therefore important to calibrate the A-scans to account for the aberrations introduced by the catheter. Prior to tissue characterization, these scans are calibrated for this aberration, also known as the system response or transfer function, which is the additive effect of the IVUS console and catheter and their respective electronics on these backscatter data.

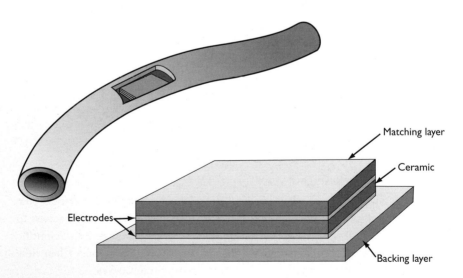

Figure 18.1 *Schematic of the transducer arrangement in a typical mechanically rotating intravenous ultrasound catheter. The transducer is mounted on a flexible drive shaft which is mounted inside a catheter. The transducer is unfocused with approximate dimensions 0.68 and 0.41 mm whilst the catheters range from 2.9 to 3.5 Fr.*

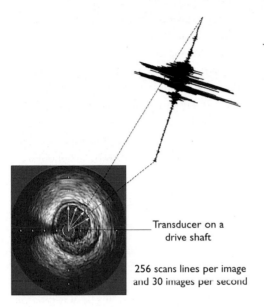

Figure 18.2 *Images obtained from Boston-Scientific Clearview and Galaxy consoles are created using 256 RF-scan lines.*

Transducer on a
drive shaft

256 scans lines per image
and 30 images per second

Plaque composition

Image analysis

Extensive research has been conducted on IVUS image analysis for determining plaque composition.[1-3]

Fibrous or 'hard' plaques are generally thought of as advanced lesions that contain dense fibrous tissue, elastin fibers and proteoglycans. Similar to calcified regions in plaques, dense fibrous plaque components generally reflect ultrasound energy well and thus appear bright and homogeneous on IVUS images.[4] However, one of the major problems with many of the image-based studies performed to date is their dependence on plaque brightness to discriminate fibrous tissue content. As this parameter is highly dependent on the gain setting of the IVUS console and its transmit power, direct comparison of brightness in IVUS images may not be possible. In an attempt to overcome this problem, Hodgson et al suggested comparing the echo reflectance of the plaque with that of the adventitia.[5] Unfortunately, the signal produced by the adventitia may be significantly attenuated by the intervening tissue and consequently produce a dimmer image.

Lipidic or 'soft' plaques have been implicated in acute ischemic syndromes such as plaque rupture. In IVUS images, regions of low echo reflectance are usually labeled soft plaque.[1,5] Echolucent regions believed to be lipid pools were first reported by Mallery et al[6] and expanded upon by Potkin et al.[4] In a similar study comparing IVUS images to histology sections using 40 MHz transducers

329

ex vivo, IVUS detection of lipid deposits was shown to have a sensitivity of 88.9% and a specificity of 100% when compared to clinical interpretation.[7]

In a study by Zhang et al,[8] automated image processing techniques were applied to IVUS images captured from video in an attempt to classify lesions as soft plaque, hard plaque or hard plaque with shadow (calcific). The technique's performance was assessed by comparing the results with those determined by manual image interpretation. Their texture-based approach agreed with the reviewers' interpretation in 89.9% of cases. However, the authors state that: 'expert definition of plaque composition is irreproducible and only quantitative histology can provide an alternative independent standard'.[8] In fact, many of the studies evaluating the efficacy of IVUS in determining plaque composition have also been limited by their reliance on digitizing videotape. This process has major limitations as stated by Vince et al.[3]

Limitations of image analysis methods

Although there are a veritable plethora of studies touting the abilities of image analysis techniques to detect plaque composition in near real-time, there are four major limitations to this approach: (i) digitizing videotapes is time consuming and therefore not feasible for near real-time analysis, (ii) the resolution of the image is reduced to that of videotape, approximately $330\,\mu m$, (3) parameters such as gain, including time gain compensation and intensity can be adjusted by the operator, thereby adding variability to the data set, and (iv) the dynamic range pre and postprocessing of the images depend on the analog-to-digital converters used in the IVUS consoles. Additionally, other system factors like frame averaging and the power level would also induce variability in the data sets.

Signal analysis

More recent studies have realized the importance of gaining access to the raw ultrasound back-scattered signals (Figure 18.3).[9–12] Spectral analysis of the unprocessed ultrasound signal allows a more detailed interrogation of various vessel components than digitization of videotape and studies have shown that differentiation between vessel layers and tissue types is possible ex vivo.[10,13,14] To date, two different approaches have been adopted for characterization of atherosclerotic plaque components by IVUS backscattered signals: time domain analysis,[15] and frequency domain analysis.[9–11,14,16]

Time domain

IVUS A-scans are very 'noisy' signals. Although analysis of this signal in the time domain is possible, it would be inadequate without appropriate calibration techniques, due to the level of noise. Very few studies have been performed with this approach for tissue characterization. Heart and Kitney[15] claimed that they compared the signals to 'predetermined signal parameters' such as amplitude

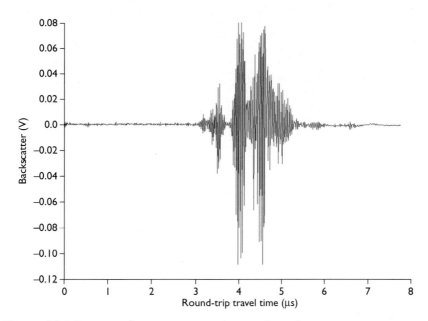

Figure 18.3 *Diagram of one intravenous ultrasound scan line.*

characteristics, peaks or trough level characteristics, variance and phase irregularity to extract information about composition. These predetermined parameters were not calculated from biologic tissue or controls, but from man-made representatives of those tissue types. Extrapolation of these in vitro data to an in vivo environment is questionable.

Frequency domain

More recent studies have realized the importance of spectral analysis to determine tissue composition.[9,11,12,17] Spectral analysis of the RF-signal allows a more detailed analysis of various vessel components than does image analysis of digitized videotape images and can be potentially employed in real-time. Also, the obvious frequency dependence of sound interactions in tissue make this method of analysis an appropriate choice. Early studies by Lizzi et al[18] and O'Donnell and Miller[19] laid out the basis for a theoretical framework pertaining to RF-data analysis. The work performed by Lizzi et al used the power spectrum of RF-data acquired from a perfect reflector to calibrate the tissue data spectrum by subtracting the reflector spectrum from the data spectrum, a technique called inverse filtering. This study was performed with a 10 MHz transducer, and the data were analyzed via the Fast Fourier Transform (FFT). FFT is a method of taking a signal represented in the time domain (i.e. time on the abscissa) and transforming it into frequency data (Figure 18.4). The resulting graph, with power (in dB) on the ordinate and frequency on the abscissa, is known as a power spectrum density

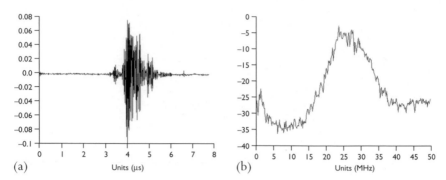

Figure 18.4 *Pulse–echo response (a) and power spectrum (b) from commercial intravenous ultrasound system and catheter.*

plot (PSD). The results from this and other studies of analyzing spectral parameters (Figure 18.5) indicated that the slope and y-intercept of the PSD and a parameter called the mid-band fit are representative of different tissue structures, sizes and intervening attenuation.[18,20] Y-intercept and mid-band fit are also indicative of the ultrasound scatterer concentration.[20] To date, mid-band fit has not been extensively studied for IVUS data, although it has been applied to ultrasonic tissue characterization for other tissues and promises high sensitivity.[20–22] The use of integrated backscatter, the area underneath the PSD, aims to provide an estimation of the backscatter coefficient.[23,24]

Most of the IVUS studies performed to date have adopted the analysis laid out by Lizzi's group, but have utilized clinically available transducers with higher central frequencies (20–40 MHz).[10,14,25] As stated earlier, IVUS transducers are hand-built, single-use devices, and their frequency characteristics vary. Determining the system response of one catheter and then using its spectrum to calibrate RF-data spectra acquired with other catheters would be invalid. In a

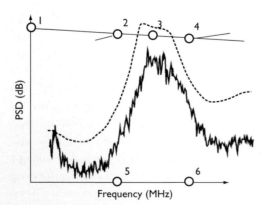

Figure 18.5 *Computation of spectral parameters. A database of parameters is used to compute classification trees for plaque characterization: (1) y-intercept; (2) maximum power; (3) mid-band fit; (4) minimum power; (5) frequency at maximum power; (6) frequency at minimum power.*

recent article by Watson et al,[9] the system response was determined for each catheter before acquiring tissue data, and then utilized for spectral calibration. This group also recognized the importance of accurate correlation between histologic sections and IVUS RF-data. To date, this comparison has been limited to visual assessment via microscopy and visual morphological alignment between histology and the corresponding IVUS image. In fact, Watson et al. state 'at present, no digitized histological image exists, making registration with the ultrasound scan difficult and subject to some uncertainty'.[9] Although methods of digitizing histology images exist, there is no quantitative means of correlating homogeneous histologic regions to corresponding IVUS data. In addition, another recent study by Jeremias et al[25] was directed towards the identification of inflammation around the adventitia of transplant patients. The technique involved selecting a region of interest which encompassed approximately one half of the artery, averaging out the spectral properties of backscatter signals from the vessel wall, plaque and lumen. Although this approach was highly effective in the assessment of transplant vasculopathy, which is a diffuse disease, this method would not be applicable for the identification of plaque constituents as coronary plaques are very heterogeneous. Averaging a large region would be unlikely to produce significant differences between the different plaque components.

Furthermore, many IVUS RF-spectral studies to date have been limited to analysis with the Fourier Transform (FT).[10,16,26] The FT is a mathematical tool for analyzing signals with sinusoidal components. It may not be well suited to decompose short-time, sparse, stochastic biologic signals such as the IVUS backscattered data.[27] As stated earlier, the FFT, which is the algorithm that evaluates the discrete-time Fourier series, has been employed previously and provides limited information about the tissue characteristics of atherosclerotic plaques.[9,10,16] The Welch periodogram, another classic spectral technique, is a modified FFT algorithm that attempts to gain higher resolution in the spectra. The Welch PSD is calculated by windowing a data record in a certain number of segments and overlapping those segments by a specified number of samples.[28] Even though windowing increases stability of the spectral estimates, there are limitations due to trade-offs pertaining to the type of window used and the resolution in the frequency domain. This can result in frequency leakage and side lobes in the spectra.[28]

Autoregressive (AR) modeling of data is yet another way to calculate the spectra. With this method, instead of directly calculating the spectra from the time-based signal, the data are first modeled by mathematical coefficients. Then this model is used to compute the spectra. It has been observed that AR processes result in high resolution of spectral estimates, and no windowing is required with an appropriate model order.[27–29] The model order refers to the number of coefficients used to compute the frequency spectrum.

Clinical application of IVUS backscatter

The analysis of IVUS RF-data is currently undergoing clinical evaluation. A diagram of the overall acquisition system, including the IVUS console and the patient table is shown in Figure 18.6. The ECG-gated RF acquisition system consists of a Pentium computer and a custom-designed ECG-gating box. The PC houses two analog-to-digital converter (ADC) cards, one operating at a sampling frequency of 125 MHz (Gage 8500; Gage Applied, Inc., Montreal, Quebec, Canada) to acquire the IVUS RF-signals, and one sampling at 2.5 KHz (IOTech card, ADAC5500MF, IOTech, Inc., Cleveland, Ohio) per channel to acquire the ECG and trigger signals. These cards are controlled by custom designed software called IVUSLab.

The ECG-gating box has two inputs: an RF input and an ECG input. The RF output provided on the back of the IVUS console is connected to the RF input and the ECG output on the catheterization table is connected to the ECG input. The RF-signal is buffered in the ECG-gating box and fed to the Gage card, which is controlled by the trigger signal, also provided by the ECG-gating box. In addition, the ECG-signal and trigger signal are output from the ECG-gating box and input to the IOTech card. A block diagram illustrating the appropriate connections of the system is shown in Figure 18.7.

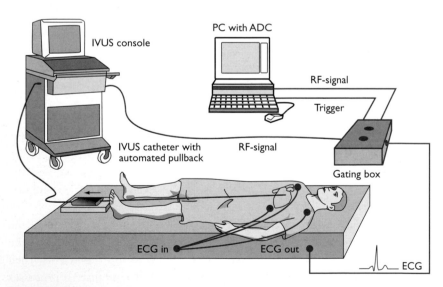

Figure 18.6 *Diagram of the ECG-gated acquisition system setup. The 'RF-signal' from the IVUS console and the 'ECG out' from the catheterization table are input to the ECG-gating box. The ECG, trigger, and RF signals are input to the computer which controls the process with custom-engineered software.*

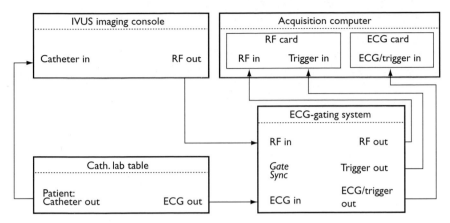

Figure 18.7 *Block diagram of the ECG-gated acquisition system illustrating the connections between all the components. The gating box monitors the ECG signal and outputs trigger pulses for the appropriate scan lines. The instrument computer houses two analog-to-digital converter cards, a Gage card that acquires the RF-signals and an IOTech card that acquires the ECG and trigger signals used for spatial registration of the scan converted intravascular ultrasound images.*

Acquisition of ECG-gated RF-data

Boston Scientific catheters are typically used with this system. These transducers rotate at 1800 rpm and perform 256 pulse–echo acquisitions per revolution. Thirty images are created per second and each scan-converted image contains 256 A-scans. During the pullback, the transducer is continuously firing while the catheter is being slowly withdrawn at a constant rate, typically 0.5 mm/s. The ECG-gating box monitors the ECG signal to determine appropriate image acquisition times during the pullback. Upon detection of the peak R-wave, the ECG-gating box sends 256 consecutive trigger pulses to the Gage card, each corresponding to the firing of the transducer for one A-scan in that image frame. The Gage card receives the trigger pulses and acquires each corresponding scan line. Throughout the pullback, the trigger signal and the ECG signal are continuously acquired with the IOTech card and later used to register IVUS image slices along the arterial segment.

Creation of volume data set

After the pullback acquisition, the IVUS A-scans and the longitudinal spacing information from the trigger signal are used to create the volumetric data set. Each group of 256 A-scans is used to create one IVUS image. The scan lines are processed via typical ultrasonic methods for creating B-mode images. The original, raw RF-data is also stored for later processing. IVUS images are then created, and the images are assimilated into a volume using the inter-slice spacing determined via the trigger signal and pullback speed. An example scan converted image is shown in Figure 18.8a. Also shown is a longitudinal view of a non-gated volume in Figure 18.8b and the same volume resulting from ECG-gating in Figure 18.8c, illustrating the removal of the sawtooth artifact.

Analysis of geometry and composition

Three-dimensional segmentation

After formation of the volumetric data sets, the first step in the analysis is identification of the luminal and medial-adventitial borders in all the images in the volume. The borders are identified using a novel three-dimensional segmentation technique (Figure 18.9).[30,31] In brief, the IVUS images are stacked and control points, approximating the luminal border position, entered on a number of images. The control points entered on one slice are linearly interpolated to generate a closed contour. Initial contours must be placed on the first slice, last slice and several intermediate slices, according to any significant deviations in shape and/or location of the desired borders between adjacent slices. This can be performed manually or automatically. Once the control points are entered the algorithm draws borders through the data set and morphs them in three dimensions to detect the actual border. This process is repeated for the detection of the external elastic membrane. A thorough validation of the technique has been previously described.[32]

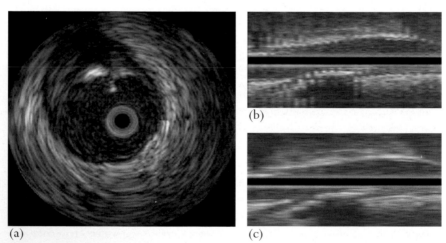

(a) (b) (c)

Figure 18.8 *Example intravascular ultrasound images with (a) scan converted image; (b) longitudinal view without gating; and (c) longitudinal view with ECG-gating.*

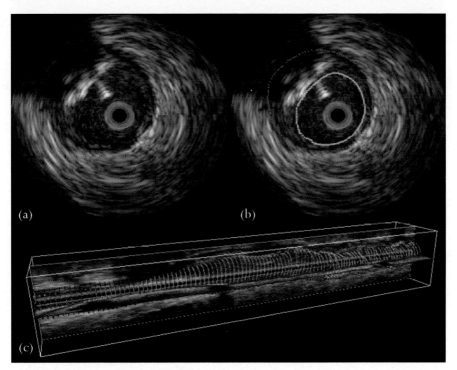

Figure 18.9 *Example intravascular ultrasound images with (a) scan converted image; (b) image with borders detected; and (c) three dimensional reconstruction of the vessel with the luminal (light blue) and medial-adventitial borders (dark blue) identified.*

Spectral analysis

Once the specific areas of plaque have been identified, spectral analysis of the RF-signals backscattered from the plaque provides more detailed analysis of the plaque composition. In previous work by our group, a technique for classification of coronary plaque into one of four categories was developed.[12] Autoregressive models were used to calculate corresponding spectra from RF-signals from within the plaque. These spectra were normalized to remove the catheter/console system response and then several parameters describing the spectra were calculated. These parameters were fed into a statistical classification tree, which is built using a large database of spectral parameters and their corresponding histologic gold standard. Regions of interest, selected from histology, comprised 101 fibrous, 56 fibrolipidic, 50 calcified and 70 calcified-necrotic regions. Classification schemes for model building were computed for autoregressive and classic Fourier spectra by using 75% of the data. The remaining data were used for validation. Autoregressive classification schemes performed well with accuracies of 90.4% for fibrous, 92.8% for fibrolipidic, 90.9% for calcified, and 89.5% for

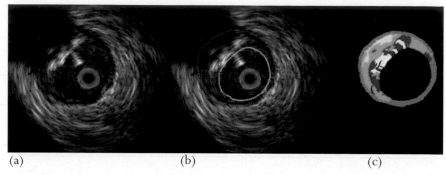

(a)   (b)   (c)

Figure 18.10 Example intravascular ultrasound images with (a) scan converted image; (b) image with borders detected; and (c) reconstructed Virtual Histology™ map. Media, gray; fibrous, green; calcium, white; calcified necrosis, red; fibro-lipid, yellow.

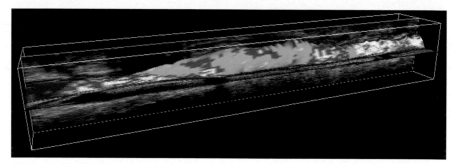

Figure 18.11 Three-dimensional reconstruction of the vessel with plaque components visible. Fibrous, green; calcium, white; calcified necrosis, red; fibro-lipid, yellow.

calcified-necrotic regions in the training data set and 79.7%, 81.2%, 92.8%, and 85.5% in the test data, respectively. Virtual Histology™ images were created using this technique.[11] Figure 18.10 shows the Virtual Histology™ with four histologic categories corresponding to the image with identified plaque regions. These Virtual Histology™ images were created for each frame in the volumetric IVUS RF-data set yielding volumetric composition information (Figure 18.11).

Conclusion

Online acquisition of the RF-data and real-time processing with three-dimensional segmentation and spectral analysis is a potential tool for identification of vulnerable plaque. This system also has unique potential for monitoring progression of atherosclerotic disease in longitudinal studies. The effect of lipid-lowering therapies on atherosclerotic burden has been studied using volumetric

IVUS,[33] and many more studies are under way. ECG-gated acquisition of RF-data, with three-dimensional segmentation and spectral analysis, could not only track the progression of plaque volume over time, it could also identify any changes in composition. Even if the total plaque volume remained constant over time, this system could determine if the relative abundance of the components in that volume of plaque had changed, which is a plausible scenario, according to the theory that lipid-lowering agents remove lipid material from the atherosclerotic wall and stabilize the plaque.[34,35]

Increasing evidence is showing that positive remodeling, along with the composition of the plaque, is an important factor relating to the likelihood of acute coronary syndromes.[36] Positive remodeling and plaque composition, and their impact on plaque vulnerability, have been studied individually, but not until recently has the relationship between these two factors been investigated. Post-mortem studies have shown that positively remodeled plaques have larger lipid content, more inflammation and higher macrophage counts.[37,38] Fusion of three-dimensional segmentation of ECG-gated IVUS image sequences and spectral analysis of the RF-data have provided detailed volumetric assessment of the histologic components of coronary plaques in vivo. The analysis of three-dimensional plaque composition and geometry by IVUS has unique potential for identification of vulnerable plaques, because it can identify two of the main factors involved in the likelihood of plaque rupture – positive remodeling and plaque composition. The tools developed could help elucidate this relationship in vivo, determining the histologic components of positively remodeled plaques, potentially providing insights into plaque rupture that were previously unavailable.

References

1. Gussenhoven EJ, Essed CE, Frietman P et al. Intravascular ultrasonic imaging: histologic and echographic correlation. *Eur J Vasc Surg* 1989; **3**:571–6.

2. Dixon KJ, Vince DG, Cothren RM, Cornhill JF. Characterization of coronary plaque in intravascular ultrasound using histological correlation. *Annu Int Conf IEEE Eng Med Biol Proc* 1997; **2**:530–3.

3. Vince DG, Dixon KJ, Cothren RM, Cornhill JF. Comparison of texture analysis methods for the characterization of coronary plaques in intravascular ultrasound images. *Comput Med Imaging Graph* 2000; **24**:221–9.

4. Potkin BN, Bartorelli AL, Gessert JM et al. Coronary artery imaging with intravascular high-frequency ultrasound. *Circulation* 1990; **81**:1575–85.

5. Hodgson J, Reddy K, Suneja R, Nair R, Lesnefsky E, Sheehan H. Intracoronary ultrasound imaging: correlation of plaque morphology with angiography, clinical syndrome and procedural results in patients undergoing coronary angioplasty. *J Am Coll Cardiol* 1993; **21**:35–44.

6. Mallery JA, Tobis JM, Griffith J et al. Assessment of normal and atherosclerotic arterial wall thickness with an intravascular ultrasound imaging catheter. *Am Heart J* 1990; **119**:1392–400.

7. Di Mario C, The SH, Madretsma S et al. Detection and characterization of vascular lesions by intravascular ultrasound: an in vitro study correlated with histology. *J Am Soc Echocardiogr* 1992; **5**:135–46.

8. Zhang X, McKay C, Sonka M. Tissue characterization in intravascular ultrasound images. *IEEE Trans Med Imaging* 1998; **17**:889–99.

9. Watson RJ, McLean CC, Moore MP et al. Classification of arterial plaque by spectral analysis of in vitro radio frequency intravascular ultrasound data. *Ultrasound Med Biol* 2000; **26**:73–80.

10. Moore MP, Spencer T, Salter DM et al. Characterisation of coronary atherosclerotic morphology by spectral analysis of radiofrequency signal: in vitro intravascular ultrasound study with histological and radiological validation. *Heart* 1998; **79**:459–67.

11. Nair A, Kuban BD, Tuzcu EM et al. Coronary plaque classification with intravascular ultrasound radiofrequency data analysis. *Circulation* 2002; **106**:2200–6.

12. Nair A, Kuban BD, Obuchowski N, Vince DG. Assessing spectral algorithms to predict atherosclerotic plaque composition with normalized and raw intravascular ultrasound data. *Ultrasound Med Biol* 2001; **27**:1319–31.

13. Lockwood GR, Ryan LK, Hunt JW, Foster FS. Measurement of the ultrasonic properties of vascular tissues and blood from 35–65 MHz. *Ultrasound Med Biol* 1991; **17**:653–66.

14. Spencer T, Ramo MP, Salter D, Sutherland G, Fox KA, McDicken WN. Characterisation of atherosclerotic plaque by spectral analysis of 30 MHz intravascular ultrasound radio frequency data. *Proc IEEE Ultrason Symp* 1996; **2**:1073–76.

15. Heart G, Kitney RI. *Ultrasound Scanning*. USA: patient ref. No 98\23210, 1998.

16. Spencer T, Ramo MP, Salter DM, et al. Characterisation of atherosclerotic plaque by spectral analysis of intravascular ultrasound: an in vitro methodology. *Ultrasound Med Biol* 1997; **23**:191–203.

17. Kawasaki M, Takatsu H, Noda T et al. In vivo quantitative tissue characterization of human coronary arterial plaques by use of integrated backscatter intravascular ultrasound and comparison with angioscopic findings. *Circulation* 2002; **105**:2487–92.

18. Lizzi FL, Greenebaum M, Feleppa EJ, Elbaum M. Theoretical framework for spectrum analysis in ultrasonic tissue characterization. *J Acoust Soc Am* 1983; **73**:1366–73.

19. O'Donnell M, Miller JG. Quantitative broad-band ultrasonic backscatter – an approach to non-destructive evaluation in acoustically inhomogeneous materials. *J Appl Phys* 1981; **52**:1056–65.

20. Lizzi FL, Astor M, Feleppa EJ, Shao M, Kalisz A. Statistical framework for ultrasonic spectral parameter imaging. *Ultrasound Med Biol* 1997; **23**:1371–82.

21. van der Steen AFW, Thijssen JM, van der Laak AWM, Ebben GPJ, de Wilde PCM. Correlation of histology and acoustic parameters of liver tissue on a microscopic scale. *Ultrasound Med Biol* 1994; **20**:177–86.

22. van der Steen AFW, Thijssen JM, van der Laak AWM, Ebben GPJ, de Wilde PCM. A new method to correlate acoustic spectroscopic microscopy (30 MHz) and light microscopy. *J Microscopy* 1994; **175**:21–33.

23. Bridal SL, Fornes P, Bruneval P, Berger G. Parametric (integrated backscatter and attenuation) images constructed using backscattered radio frequency signals (25–56 MHz) from human aortae in vitro. *Ultrasound Med Biol* 1997; **23**:215–29.

24. Thomas LJI, Barzilai B, Perez JE et al. Quantitative real-time imaging of myocardium based on ultrasonic integrated backscatter. *IEEE Trans Ultrason Ferroelectr Freq Control* 1989; **36**:466–70.

25. Jeremias A, Kolz ML, Ikonen TS et al. Feasibility of in vivo intravascular ultrasound tissue characterization in the detection of early vascular transplant rejection. *Circulation* 1999; **100**:2127–30.

26. Wilson LS, Neale ML, Talhami HE, Appleberg M. Preliminary results from attenuation-slope mapping of plaque using intravascular ultrasound. *Ultrasound Med Biol* 1994; **20**:529–42.

27. Wear KA, Wagner RF, Garra BS. Comparison of autoregressive spectral estimation algorithms and order determination methods in ultrasonic tissue characterization. *IEEE Trans Ultrason Ferroelectr Freq Control* 1995; **42**:709–16.

28. Marple SL Jr. Digital spectral analysis with applications. In: Oppenheim AV, ed. *Prentice-Hall Signal Processing Series*. New Jersey: Prentice-Hall Inc., 1987.

29. Kay SM. *Modern Spectral Estimation: Theory and Application*. Englewood Cliffs, NJ: Prentice Hall, 1988.

30. Klingensmith JD, Vince DG, Shekhar R et al. Quantification of coronary arterial plaque volume using 3D reconstructions formed by fusing intravascular ultrasound and biplane angiography. *Proc SPIE Int Soc Opt Eng* 1999; **3660**:343–50.

31. Shekhar R, Cothren RM, Vince DG et al. Three dimensional segmentation of luminal and adventitial borders in serial intravascular ultrasound images. *Comput Med Imaging Graph* 1999; **23**:299–309.

32. Klingensmith JD, Shekhar R, Vince DG. Evaluation of three-dimensional segmentation algorithms for the identification of luminal and medial-adventitial borders in intravascular ultrasound images. *IEEE Trans Med Imaging* 2000; **19**:996–1011.

33. Schartl M, Bocksch W, Koschyk DH et al. Use of intravascular ultrasound to compare effects of different strategies of lipid-lowering therapy on plaque volume and composition in patients with coronary artery disease. *Circulation* 2001; **104**:387–92.

34. Amoroso G, Van Boven AJ, Crijns HJ. Drug therapy or coronary angioplasty for the treatment of coronary artery disease: new insights. *Am Heart J* 2001; **141**:S22–S25.

35. Brown BG, Zhao XQ, Sacco DE, Albers JJ. Lipid lowering and plaque regression. New insights into prevention of plaque disruption and clinical events in coronary disease. *Circulation* 1993; **87**:1781–91.

36. Schoenhagen P, Ziada KM, Kapadia SR et al. Extent and direction of arterial remodeling in stable versus unstable coronary syndromes: an intravascular ultrasound study. *Circulation* 2000; **101**:598–603.

37. Burke AP, Kolodgie FD, Farb A, Weber D, Virmani R. Morphological predictors of arterial remodeling in coronary atherosclerosis. *Circulation* 2002; **105**:297–303.

38. Varnava AM, Mills PG, Davies MJ. Relationship between coronary artery remodeling and plaque vulnerability. *Circulation* 2002; **105**:939–43.

19. VULNERABLE PLAQUE DETECTION USING TEMPERATURE HETEROGENEITY MEASURED WITH THE IMETRX THERMOCOIL GUIDEWIRE SYSTEM

Campbell Rogers and Marco Wainstein

In most instances of acute myocardial infarction (MI) or sudden cardiac death, it has been shown that a plaque has ruptured, fissured or ulcerated. Most ruptured plaques contain a dense infiltration of macrophages in a large pool of cholesterol covered by a thin fibrous cap. Hence, plaque inflammation due to activated macrophages very likely plays a crucial role in the pathogenesis of acute coronary syndromes (ACS).

Vulnerable plaques are associated with increased macrophage accumulation as opposed to stable plaques, which lack inflammatory activity. Inflammatory activity has been correlated with increased temperature. Therefore, the determination of temperature heterogeneity due to inflammatory cell activity may have a pivotal role in predicting plaque composition and could differentiate between stable and unstable plaques.

Background

The determination of temperature heterogeneity as a means to differentiate between stable and unstable plaques may prove valuable in treating patients with local invasive treatment and/or medical management.

Techniques for characterizing plaque vulnerability may also contribute to the understanding of how pharmacologic treatments improve clinical outcomes. The techniques are likely to elucidate further the effects of treatment on inflammation, reduction of atheromatous plaque mass, endothelial function or improved geometric remodeling.[1-4]

Ex vivo data

Casscells at al postulated that the acute thrombotic events could be predicted by the heat released by activated macrophages. Measuring the intimal surface temperatures of freshly obtained carotid endarterectomy specimens, they showed

343

a temperature rise up to 2.2 °C in macrophage-rich areas, as well as a significant correlation between macrophage density and local temperature.[5]

Human studies

Recent studies have shown that there is marked thermal heterogeneity within human atherosclerotic coronary arteries. Heterogeneity is larger for unstable angina and AMI than for normal coronary arteries and patients with stable angina.[6]

In addition, there may be a correlation of increasing temperature heterogeneity with increasing risk of an acute event. Stefanadis investigated the relation between the temperature difference between the atherosclerotic plaque and the healthy vessel wall and event-free survival among patients undergoing percutaneous intervention. Local temperature in atherosclerotic plaques was a strong predictor of unfavorable clinical outcomes in patients with coronary artery disease.[7,8]

Animal studies

In studies with hypercholesterolemic rabbits it has been demonstrated that in vivo temperature heterogeneity within arteries is directly linked to atherosclerotic plaque content of macrophages. Furthermore, the temperature heterogeneity disappeared after decreasing macrophage content of plaques via cholesterol lowering.[9]

The device

Thermocoil guidewire

System elements include (Figure 19.1):
- thermocoil guidewire (disposable)
- interface connector, attaching guidewire to handle (disposable)
- motorized pullback handle (reusable)
- data acquisition system (controller box attached to laptop personal computer).

The Imetrx (Mountain View, CA) thermocoil wire is a novel device with the ability to identify temperature fluctuations along the vessel wall and display temperature in real-time on a monitor. The wire is 0.014″ thick, with a tip containing a thermal sensor with temperature resolution of 0.03 °C. The wire is preshaped into a gentle angle, and undergoes motorized rotating pullback. During pullback the tip inscribes a helix touching the inner surface of the artery, interrogating the surface. Its output is via an interface controller box connected to a laptop computer.

The wire is placed into the coronary vasculature through a guide catheter using conventional means. The thermocoil guidewire attaches to the data

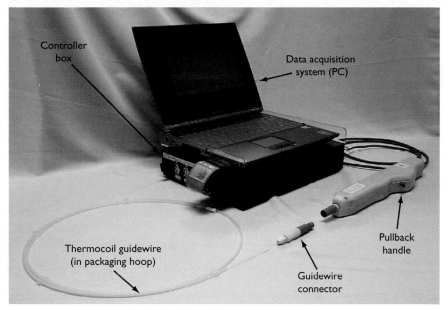

Figure 19.1 *Imetrx thermocoil wire system elements.*

acquisition system via a six-foot integrated cable at the proximal end of the handle. The thermocoil guidewire is advanced approximately 1 cm distal to the arterial segment of interest, then attached to the pullback handle via the interface connector. Thermocoil guidewire sensing is initiated by depressing the actuation button on the pullback handle. Once actuated, the thermocoil guidewire simultaneously rotates at a speed of 30 revolutions per minute and is withdrawn proximally at a rate of 0.5 mm per second. The sensing tip of the wire transmits a signal as it rotates by contacting the vessel wall due to the curvature in the tip. The full automatic cycle of the thermocoil guidewire traverses 5 cm of vessel wall length over approximately 2 minutes. At completion of the cycle the device stops automatically.

The signals are converted to temperature readings displayed as a digital readout and in graphical form on the monitor of the data acquisition system. Once a temperature scan is completed, the clinician may choose to verify results by repeating the process, analyzing a different area by repositioning the thermocoil guidewire, or using the thermocoil guidewire to advance a therapeutic intravascular device, such as an angioplasty balloon or stent delivery catheter, to the lesion.

Interface connector and pullback handle
When the thermocoil guidewire is positioned at the lesion under investigation, it is attached to the pullback handle via the interface connector. The interface

connector is a sterile, disposable component included with the guidewire package. The interface connector is inserted into the pullback handle, which has an actuation button to initiate the temperature scanning. The sensing tip of the guidewire transmits signals to the data acquisition system.

Data acquisition system

Signals from the thermocoil guidewire are converted to temperature readings by the data acquisition system. The signals are displayed both as a digital readout and in graphical form on the monitor.

Preclinical studies using the Imetrx thermocoil guidewire

Preliminary studies used an ex vivo system providing localized and eccentric areas of warming. In this system, temperature rises of 0.13–0.64 °C were reliably detected (Figure 19.2). Tip coordinates were calculated from pullback and rotational information, and temperature variations were then mapped into one and two-dimensional plots by incorporating position coordinates.[10] Animal studies have failed to show any histologic evidence of vascular wall injury caused by the thermocoil guidewire during insertion or pullback.

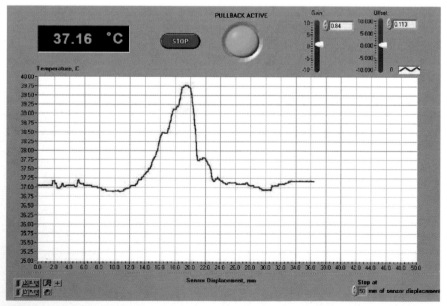

Figure 19.2 *Temperature heterogeneity: temperature data from the thermocoil guidewire tip during rotational pullback through a fluid-filled plastic tube with a short external heat source adjacent to one aspect.*

Clinical studies using the Imetrx thermocoil guidewire

Initial clinical studies were completed in 13 patients in Porto Alegre, Brazil. Patients included those with ACS and those with chronic stable ischemic syndromes. All patients underwent thermography and intravascular ultrasound. No safety issues were identified, and several patients had temperature variations of less that 0.2 °C.

Conclusions and future directions

Published clinical studies have identified localized increases in temperature in areas of the coronary arteries where lesions are present. Some of these lesions do not obstruct the blood flow, but are thought to be associated with ACS. About 60% of acute MI result from previously non-obstructive lesions. Imaging techniques that visualize the plaque locally may provide new insight into the etiology of sudden progression of atherosclerotic disease or acute events. The composition of the atherosclerotic lesion rather than the degree of stenosis is currently considered to be the most important determinant for acute clinical events. Catheter-based visualization modalities can identify components of the atherosclerotic plaque such as local inflammation and predict the occurrence of a clinical event.

Temperature heterogeneity within human atherosclerotic plaque has been shown to be correlated with unfavorable clinical outcome in patients with coronary artery disease. The determination of temperature heterogeneity as a means to differentiate between stable and unstable plaque may prove valuable in treating the patient with ACS by local treatment and/or medical management.

The Imetrx thermocoil guidewire, with a thermal detector at its distal end, functions otherwise in a manner similar to conventional guidewires. Once connected to a data acquisition system, the thermocoil guidewire may be a feasible and atraumatic vulnerable plaque detection tool that safely detects temperature heterogeneity within the atherosclerotic lesion.

References

1. Pasterkamp G, Falk E, Woutman H, Borst C. Techniques characterizing the coronary atherosclerotic plaque: influence on clinical decision making. *J Am Coll Cardiol* 2000; **36**:13–21.

2. Randomised trial of cholesterol lowering in 4444 patients with coronary heart disease: the Scandinavian Simvastatin Survival Study (4S). *Lancet* 1994; **344**:1383–9.

3. Leung WH, Lau CP, Wong CK. Beneficial effect of cholesterol-lowering therapy on coronary endothelium-dependent relaxation in hypercholesterolaemic patients. *Lancet* 1993; **341**:1496–500.

4. Aikawa M, Rabkin E, Okada Y et al. Lipid lowering by diet reduces matrix metalloproteinase activity and increases collagen content of rabbit atheroma: a potential mechanism of lesion stabilization. *Circulation* 1998; **97**:2433-44.

5. Casscells W, Hathorn B, David M et al. Thermal detection of cellular infiltrates in living atherosclerotic plaques: possible implications for plaque rupture and thrombosis. *Lancet* 1996; **347**:1447–51.

6. Stefanadis C, Diamantopoulos L, Vlachopoulos C et al. Thermal heterogeneity within human arterial atherosclerotic coronary arteries detected in vivo. *Circulation* 1999; **99**:1965–71.

7. Stefanadis C, Toutouzas K, Tsiamis E et al. Increased local temperature in human coronary atherosclerotic plaques: an independent predictor of clinical outcome in patients undergoing a percutaneous coronary intervention. *J Am Coll Cardiol* 2001; **37**:1277–83.

8. Stefanadis C, Toutouzas K, Tsiamis E et al. Thermography of human arterial system by means of new thermography catheters. *Catheter Cardiovasc Interv* 2001; **54**:51–8.

9. Verheye S, De Meyer GR, Van Langenhove G et al. In vivo temperature heterogeneity of atherosclerotic plaques is determined by plaque composition. *Circulation* 2002; **105**:1596–601.

10. Courtney et al. In vitro surface temperature images from a guidewire-based thermography system. *Circulation* 2002; [Abstract].

20. INTRAVASCULAR THERMOGRAPHY USING THE THERMOCORE THERMOSENSE™ CATHETER

Stefan Verheye, Glenn van Langenhove, Rob Krams and Patrick W Serruys

Atherosclerosis is an inflammatory process characterized by presence of macrophages and lymphocytes.[1,2] Casscells et al reported increased temperature heterogeneity in ex vivo atherosclerotic specimens of human carotid arteries.[3] Stefanadis et al showed that in vivo temperature heterogeneity was markedly increased in patients presenting with an acute coronary syndrome as opposed to patients having stable angina.[4] We have subsequently shown that by using a dedicated temperature catheter in an animal model of atherosclerosis, in vivo temperature heterogeneity was determined by plaque composition and more specifically by the total macrophage mass.[5] Recently, temperature heterogeneity in the presence of flow appeared to be underestimated in patients with effort angina due to coronary stenosis which was related to cooling of the vessel wall by the blood flow.[6]

Several intravascular thermography catheters have been designed and developed by different people to try to address the relation between inflammation, vulnerability and future ischemic events preferably with a user-friendly and accurate device.[7] The purpose of this chapter is to describe the Thermosense™ Catheter System developed by Thermocore Ltd (Guildford, UK).

Thermosense™ System

The Thermosense™ system consists of three major components: the catheter, the console and the dedicated pullback system.

Thermosense™ catheter

The Thermosense™ catheter is an over-the-wire catheter consisting of several concentric tubings that fit tightly (Figure 20.1). The inner tube is the guidewire tube. This tube can accommodate a 0.014″ guide wire. The over-the-wire system is intended to be compatible with a 7 Fr (0.078″ internal diameter) or larger

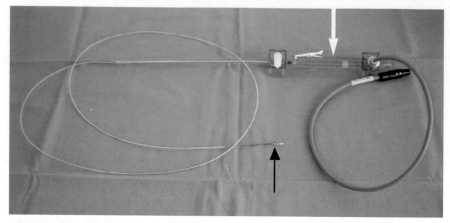

Figure 20.1 *Photograph of the Thermocore Thermosense™ catheter (the white arrow indicates the proximal part, the black arrow indicates the distal tip of the catheter).*

guiding catheter and to be used with a 0.014″ (0.36 mm) or smaller outer diameter long (300 mm) guide wire. The tube can be flushed appropriately using a standard Luer Lock syringe. The tube fits in a second tube that accommodates the temperature sensing electrical leads that are connected to the nitinol branches that contain the thermistors for actual temperature measurement. On the outer side a third tube is present, functioning as covering sheath for the thermistors when in closed position. This tube can also be flushed to ensure the removal of possibly hazardous air bubbles. The distal part has four dedicated thermistors at the distal end of four flexible nitinol strips (each at 90°) that after engagement, with an expansion width of 9 mm, ensure endoluminal surface contact of the vascular wall (Figure 20.2). The thermistors are made of 5k7 bare chips (5 kOhm resistance, curve 7 material), with gold metallization and 40 awg (American wireguage) wires soldered onto the metallization; they can perform up to 25 measurements per second, and are delivered with a certified accuracy of 0.006°C. Retraction of the sheath to engage the thermistors and to obtain actual measurements will be done in an automated fashion, so as to prevent the catheter moving down the coronary artery upon engaging the thermistors. The catheter has a radio-opaque distal tip, and the four thermistor tips are also radio-opaque.

The proximal handheld part of the catheter contains the two flushing valves. It consists of two parts that move in respect to each other, thereby opening and closing the thermistor covering sheath. The proximal part fits exactly on the automated pullback system.

The catheter is connected to the Thermosense™ device through an electrical cable that is mounted upon the catheter, and should be plugged into the device prior to a measuring procedure.

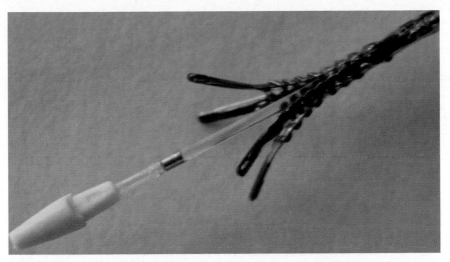

Figure 20.2 *Close-up photograph of a catheter illustrating the four expanded thermistors.*

Thermosense™ console

The Thermosense™ device is a computer-based system with dedicated software to visualize temperature data. Connectors allow for connecting the Thermosense™ catheter as well as the pullback system. After fixing the catheter onto the pullback system the pullback can be started from the Thermosense™ console.

Patient data can be entered into the console by means of a keyboard. The thermistors are measuring resistance changes induced by changes in temperature. The latter changes are transformed into voltage changes via a Wheatstone bridge and recorded by the Thermosense™ console that allows the data to be displayed in real-time (Figure 20.3). Data recorded in the system can be reviewed after finishing the procedure. The system also allows for recording data on a CD-ROM or a diskette in Excel format.

Pullback system

The pullback system is placed on the operating table during the procedure, covered by a sterile sheath (Figure 20.4). Three parts of the pullback system are connected to the catheter system when the catheter is put in place. The first part of the pullback system is connected to the guiding catheter to prevent the nitinol thermistor branches at the distal end of the catheter from moving forward during retraction of the nitinol thermistor branches covering the sheath. The second part of the pullback system is connected to the distal handheld part of the catheter, and the third part of the pullback system to the proximal part of the catheter. Thus these two parts can be moved relative to each other when catheter pullback and

351

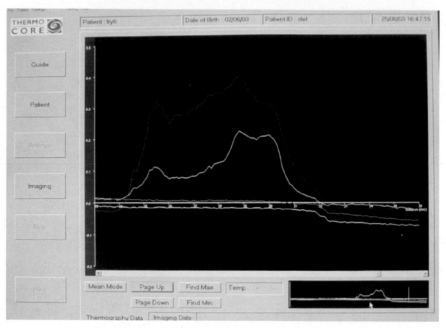

Figure 20.3 *Photograph of the monitor of the Thermosense™ console allowing data to be displayed in real-time.*

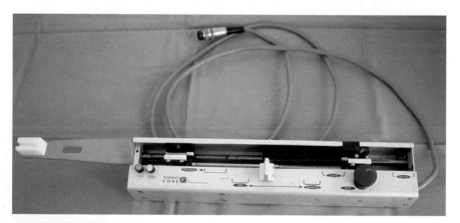

Figure 20.4 *The pullback system is placed on the operating table during the procedure, covered by a sterile sheath.*

engagement of the nitinol thermistor branches is desired. The pullback system is further connected to the console using a dedicated electric connection, to ensure power delivery and pullback system control.

Preclinical data

In vitro experiments

Measurements in a temperature controlled water bath to demonstrate system stability have been made. The measurements recorded with the catheter in a stationary position and with no flow past the sensors showed only 0.01 °C variation. With flow and movement, the maximum temperature variation was 0.03 °C illustrating and confirming the stability of the system in in vitro conditions.

In and ex vivo experiments

Numerous experiments have been performed both in rabbits and pigs to test safety and feasibility. All procedures have been completed successfully, i.e. at no point during or after the procedure did any adverse event (death, stroke, infection, allergic reaction or misbehavior) occur in any of the rabbits or pigs. Intracoronary spasm of pig coronary arteries was noticed in the initial experiments, but the problem was alleviated by administration of intravascular nitrates prior to the investigation. Intra and inter-operator variability testing was performed and found to be very acceptable with no significant differences in the majority of comparisons between measurements. As far as reproducibility is concerned, in an ex vivo setting of a hypercholesterolemic rabbit, a good correlation was found between the repeated measurements (Pearson's coefficient $R^2 = 0.71$; $P<0.0005$).

Recently, we described for the first time that in vivo temperature heterogeneity is determined by plaque composition and more specifically by the total macrophage mass.[5] In a hypercholesterolemic rabbit model, we found that there was marked temperature heterogeneity at sites of thick plaques with a high macrophage content (Figure 20.5). Temperature heterogeneity was not present in

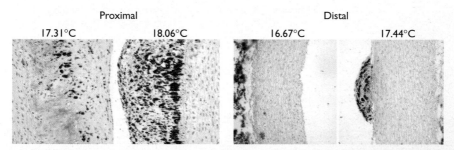

Figure 20.5 *Relation between local temperature measurement and local plaque composition (both thickness and macrophage content) derived from ex vivo experiments. Thick macrophage-rich plaques had a higher temperature than any other plaque. (Adapted with permission from S Verheye et al. Circulation 2002; 105:1061.[5])*

thick plaques with low macrophage content. In addition, this animal study suggested that changes in the macrophage content in the plaque could be detected by in vivo thermography since temperature heterogeneity disappeared when the animals received a lipid-lowering diet for 3 months, which is histopathologically characterized by a marked decrease in macrophage content despite unchanged plaque thickness (Figure 20.6). This also indicates that the effect of cholesterol lowering on at least one parameter of plaque vulnerability (i.e. number of macrophages) can be evaluated in vivo. This study further illustrated that the beneficial effect of cholesterol lowering would have been missed if the results were only based on measurements by intravascular ultrasound (IVUS) or angiography, illustrating the shortcomings of these techniques with respect to mild atherosclerotic plaques. Furthermore, by using this simplified model, a confounding factor such as neovascularization could be excluded since this is not present in this model.

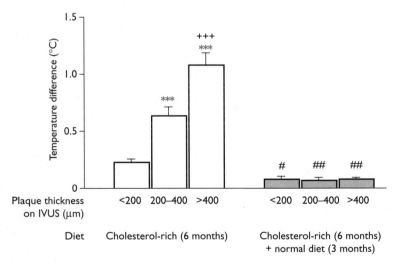

Figure 20.6 *Intravenous ultrasound (IVUS) and temperature data of rabbit aorta with atherosclerotic plaques. After 6 months of cholesterol treatment (open bars), plaques of different thickness were present in the aorta. Temperature differences in the plaques increased with plaque thickness. After 3 months of dietary cholesterol lowering (solid bars), temperature heterogeneity had significantly decreased, although plaque thickness had not changed. Data are given as mean±SEM. ***,P<0.001 vs <200μm; +++,P<0.001 vs 200–400μm; # P = 0.01 vs before cholesterol lowering; ##, P<0.01 vs before cholesterol lowering. (Adapted with permission from S Verheye et al.* Circulation 2002; **105***:1601.[5]*)

Clinical data

Based on the safety and feasibility results obtained in the preclinical setting, a further study was designed to evaluate safety and feasibility of the Thermosense™ catheter in human coronary arteries.

This first-in-man controlled clinical study evaluated 50 control and 50 thermography patients. The primary endpoints of the study were immediate procedural success of coronary temperature assessment (feasibility) and safety of the diagnostic procedure. The secondary endpoints were major adverse cardiac events (MACE) and reoccurrence or occurrence of cardiac events at 15 days, presence of detectable temperature differences within non-stenosed vessels and the potential correlation with clinical syndromes, predictive value of temperature heterogeneity towards the occurrence of any cardiac event (MACE or other), and predictive value of the amount of unstable hot plaques towards the occurrence of any cardiac event. All procedures were successful and there were no differences regarding adverse events between the two groups. Temperature changes over a well defined segment have been recorded in all patients undergoing thermography and mean values for all thermistors including mean maximal temperature difference over the whole analyzed segment were calculated.[8] The results illustrated that intracoronary thermography using the Thermosense™ catheter was safe and feasible. We concluded that intracoronary temperature changes of angiographically normal or mild atherosclerotic coronary artery segments were minimal to absent suggesting absence of inflammatory processes.

Intravascular thermography may well be safe and feasible, but so far, it has not been used to assess occurrence of ischemic coronary events in a prospective manner, at least not in an open natural-history trial. As it is unknown what the prognostic value is of non-obstructive atherosclerotic plaques showing temperature heterogeneity, we designed the PARACHUTE (Percutaneous Assessment of Regional Acute Coronary Hot Unstable plaques by Thermographic Evaluation) trial, a prospective, open, non-randomized reproducibility and prognostic trial using thermography. The PARACHUTE trial is a multicenter trial and will run from Spring 2004.

The primary endpoint of the trial is the predictive value of temperature heterogeneity toward the occurrence of ischemic coronary events and hospitalization for ischemia and/or angina. The secondary endpoints are the predictive value of amount of unstable hot plaques towards the occurrence of any cardiac event, assessment of safety of the procedure, assessment of temperature reproducibility and heterogeneity in coronary arteries, as defined by the total thermal burden towards the occurrence of any cardiac event. Results are expected in early 2005.

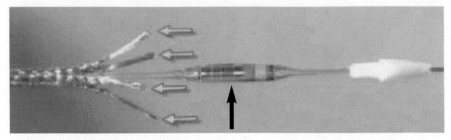

Figure 20.7 *Thermosound catheter combining intravascular ultrasound (IVUS) (distal probe, indicated by black arrow) with intravascular thermography (ultrasensitive thermistors proximal to the IVUS probe, indicated by horizontal arrows).*

Perspectives

Temperature measurement is a functional technique in the approach of detecting vulnerable plaques. There is widespread agreement that optimal assessment of a vulnerable plaque, at least invasively, perhaps should be done by combining both functional and morphologic parameters. Developing such a catheter is a challenge, however, Thermocore Ltd. has recently designed and developed a catheter combining IVUS with intravascular thermography, enabling assessment of the atherosclerotic coronary tree using morphologic information in combination with functional measurements (Figure 20.7). Future plans are to incorporate intravascular elastography in a similar way.

Conclusion

Intracoronary thermography using the Thermosense™ catheter is a safe and feasible technique with reproducible results. Applying this technique in an atherosclerotic model, we have been able to demonstrate a link between increased temperature heterogeneity and inflammation as represented by macrophages. Intracoronary thermography may therefore be proposed as a valuable tool for assessing the degree of temperature heterogeneity in human arteries with macrophage-rich plaques.

References

1. Davies MJ, Woolf N. Atherosclerosis: what is it and why does it occur? *Br Heart J* 1993; **69**:S3–11.

2. Ross R. Atherosclerosis – an inflammatory disease. *N Engl J Med* 1999; **340**:115–26.

3. Casscells W, Hathorn B, David M et al. Thermal detection of cellular infiltrates in living atherosclerotic plaques: possible implications for plaque rupture and thrombosis. *Lancet* 1996; **347**:1447–51.

4. Stefanadis C, Diamantopoulos L, Vlachopoulos C et al. Thermal heterogeneity within human atherosclerotic coronary arteries detected in vivo: a new method of detection by application of a special thermography catheter. *Circulation* 1999; **99**:1965–71.

5. Verheye S, De Meyer GRY, Van Langenhove G, Knaapen MW, Kockx MM. In vivo temperature heterogeneity of atherosclerotic plaques is determined by plaque composition. *Circulation* 2002; **105**:1601.

6. Stefanadis C, Toutouzas K, Tsiamis E et al. Thermal heterogeneity in stable human coronary atherosclerotic plaques is underestimated in vivo: the 'cooling effect' of blood flow. *J Am Coll Cardiol* 2003; **41**:403–8.

7. Verheye S, Diamantopoulos L, Serruys PW, Van Langenhove G. Intravascular imaging of the vulnerable atherosclerotic plaque: spotlight on temperature measurement. *J Cardiovasc Risk* 2002; **5**:247–54.

8. Verheye S, Van Langenhove G, Diamantopoulos L et al. Temperature heterogeneity is nearly absent in angiographically normal or mild-atherosclerotic coronary segments: interim results from a safety study. *Am J Cardiol* 2002; **105**:1596–601.

21. LIGHTLAB™ IMAGING OPTICAL COHERENCE TOMOGRAPHY

Paul Magnin

Optical coherence tomography (OCT) is a light-based imaging modality utilizing newly developed fiberoptic technologies for medical imaging applications. It was initially developed by researchers at the Massachusetts Institute of Technology in the early 1990s and the first report was published in *Science* in 1991.[1] OCT technology uses a broadband light source to create images in a manner analogous to pulse-echo ultrasound. Since the speed of light is five orders of magnitude faster than the speed of sound, an 'interferometric' technique must be used to 'range gate' the returning reflections. The major difference in the image is that the resolution of OCT is an order of magnitude higher that commercially available intravascular ultrasound (IVUS) imaging systems, however, the penetration is significantly worse.

The second dimension of the two-dimensional image is created by a physical translation or rotation of a fiberoptic probe. In this dimension the resolution is limited by diffraction and is also an order of magnitude higher than IVUS. Figure 21.1 shows an in vivo comparison of a swine coronary artery image from a

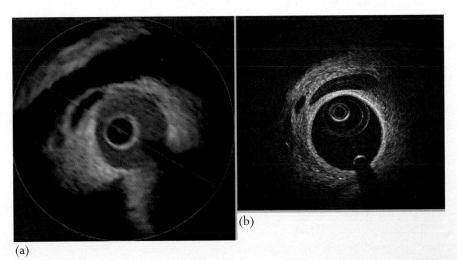

(a)

(b)

Figure 21.1 (a) an intravascular ultrasound (IVUS) image of in vivo swine coronary artery made with a commercially available IVUS imaging system. (b) Optical coherence tomography image of the same section of the artery. The scale applies to both images.

commercially available IVUS system and the same section imaged with the LightLab™ OCT system. One can clearly see the increased resolution of the OCT image.

Description of the device

Technological background

OCT, like ultrasound, produces images from backscattered reflections but uses infrared light, rather than sound to create the image. Typically a wavelength of around 1300 nm is used since it minimizes the absorption of the energy in the light beam caused by proteins, water, hemoglobin and lipids. It is important to remember, however, that while the dominant mode of signal attenuation in ultrasound is absorption, the dominant mode in OCT is multiple scattering. It is the multiple scattering caused by the red blood cells that causes the very large signal loss when trying to image through blood. It is for this reason that the blood must be displaced by saline or a contrast medium while imaging.

Internal microstructures within biologic tissues reflect the light waves back to the catheter as a result of their differing optical indices and backscattering cross-sections. While standard electronic techniques are adequate for processing ultrasonic echoes that travel at the speed of sound, interferometric techniques are required to extract the reflected optical signals from the infrared light used in OCT. It was in fact an interferometer, used to make an accurate measurement of the speed of light by Albert Michelson and Edward Morley in 1887, that verified a central conclusion of Einstein's theory of relativity. An interferometer operates by comparing two light beams with each other. This can be done most simply by letting the two light beams impinge on different faces of a half-silvered mirror. The first signal is sent down a 'reference arm' and the second is sent down the 'sample arm.' The sample arm includes the fiberoptics that carry the light to the catheter, the catheter itself and the range in depth of the tissue being examined. The reference arm is completely internal to the OCT system and its length can be changed very rapidly over about 4 mm with the use of either a moving mirror or some other optical device that has the ability to rapidly vary the length of an optical path. When the length of the reference arm and sample arm are exactly the same, they sum coherently. The scattered light that returns from all other distances in the tissue sums incoherently and gets 'washed out'. Using the interferometer, only the depth that corresponds exactly to the reference arm length will be recorded in the image.

The output, measured by an interferometer, is converted to an electrical signal then processed by a computer in real-time to produce high-resolution, cross-sectional, or three-dimensional images of the tissue. This powerful technology provides in situ images of tissues at near histologic resolution without the need for excision or processing of the specimen.

Light from a broadband infrared light source is sent down a fiber waveguide and then split into the two arms of the interferometer: the sample arm and the reference arm. This is not a conventional laser light source since such a source would have no range resolution but rather a wide bandwidth source such as a super luminescent diode or a pulsed laser. The transmitted light travels through the sample arm into a rotary optical coupler and then into the catheter and out into the tissue. In the distal tip of the catheter, the light passes through a tiny microscope consisting of three optical components as shown in Figure 21.2. The first is a diverging lens which expands the light from the fiber optic core where it travels most of the length of the catheter. The second is the focusing, or objective lens, that creates the focus in the tissue and the third is a prism that steers the light at an angle of 90° to the axis of the catheter. After the light passes through the microscope it passes into the tissue. In the body the light is reflected from the microstructures in the tissue and returns through the microscope into the optical fiber core, through the rotary coupler and back into the half silvered mirror. At this point the light returning from the sample combines with the light from the reference arm. In the OCT system shown in Figure 21.3, the length of the reference arm is rapidly changed by reflecting off a rotating cam-like disk. The distance from the fiber to the cam and back varies, linearly in time, over 4.7 mm. This is effectively the variable part of the reference arm that allows range gating of the returning sample arm reflections from 0 to 3.6 mm in the depth dimension in the tissue. The difference between the 4.7 mm reflecting cam movement and the 3.6 mm radial range is a result of the optical index of the tissue being different than the index of air. The cam spins at a rate sufficient to create up to 4000 image lines per second. The interference pattern that is created contains information regarding the physical qualities of the sample.

The optical core, inside the catheter, is rotated through 360° to provide the second dimension in the two-dimensional image in a manner identical to

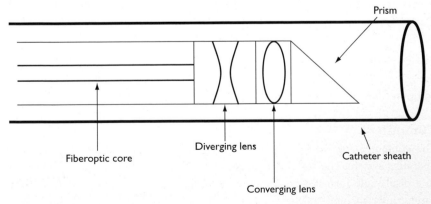

Figure 21.2 Catheter tip microscope.

361

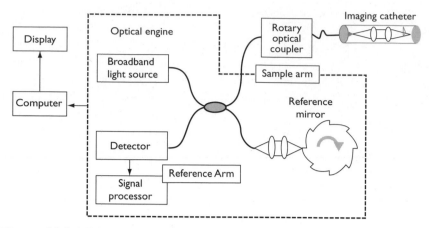

Figure 21.3 *OCT system schematic.*

mechanically scanned IVUS systems. The information from each line is then combined into a two-dimensional representation of the tissue and displayed on the computer screen.

Summary of the OCT system

The LightLab™ OCT system (Figure 21.4) uses advanced fiberoptic interferometers coupled with a mid infrared (1320 nm), low power, broad bandwidth and a light source. It is capable of imaging in real-time using video scanning rates of up to 30 frames per second. The range resolution is 12 μm and the lateral and out of plane resolution is 20 μm at the focus. The OCT imaging system is a portable tool for use in the cardiac catheterization laboratory. The system hardware is divided into four major components: the OCT imaging engine, the computer, patient interface unit and the catheters.

OCT imaging engine

The imaging engine is responsible for emitting and receiving the infrared signals. The broadband light source is housed in the engine, along with interferometer, the reference arm and the detection circuitry. The detected signal is sent to the computer for processing into an image.

Computer

The computer consists of a computer processor system running an embedded operating system. The computer processes the OCT information and converts it to a displayable format. The computer also controls the optical engine and the patient interface unit and serves as the image storage device for both still frame and video images.

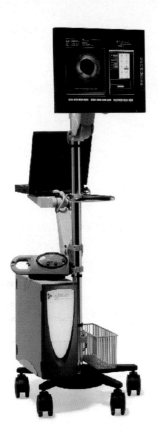

Figure 21.4 LightLab™ OCT imaging system.

Patient interface unit

The patient interface unit (PIU) (Figure 21.5) serves as the human interface for the interventional cardiologist and the location where the imaging catheter plugs into the system. It starts and stops the imaging, and selects whether the catheter is to be automatically pulled back inside the catheter sheath or moved manually. The PIU provides the motor drive that spins the imaging core to create the circular image and performs the automated pullback to collect the third dimension of image information if that mode is selected by the human interface. Inside the PIU is a rotary coupler that connects the stationary optical fiber to the rotating catheter imaging core. There is also a foot switch that mirrors the two buttons on the PIU to make operation more convenient for the interventionalist.

Catheter system

The catheter system consists of the two catheters: the 'balloon delivery catheter' and the 'imagewire catheter' (Figure 21.6). The imagewire catheter directs the infrared light into the tissue and returns the reflected light transmitting it back through the PIU to the optical engine. It is delivered to the imaging site through

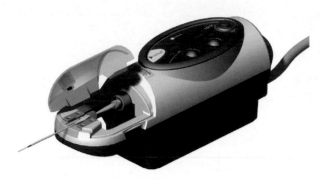

Figure 21.5 Patient interface unit.

the lumen of the balloon delivery catheter. The balloon delivery catheter is used to decrease the blood flow and deliver a modest amount of saline flush to the imaging location during the period of time that the image is being collected. The balloon delivery catheter consists of a soft balloon and a guidewire lumen. In the current design the guidewire is exchanged for the imagewire when the balloon delivery catheter is in a location proximal to the imaging site. The inflation pressure in the balloon can be kept low so as not to unnecessarily stretch the artery wall or it can be undersized to avoid stretching the artery at all.

The LightLab™ imaging catheter or 'imagewire' is a single lumen catheter. The small lumen holds the imaging fiber that consists of the optical fiber, the lenses and the turning prism. The imaging core is made of glass with a polymer coating on the outside to strengthen it both in torsion and in flexion. The proximal end of the catheter has a chamber that captures the imaging core and allows it to move along the catheter axis to perform an 'automated pullback' while spinning.

The outside of the imaging catheter is stationary with respect to the vessel wall. The imaging core is rotated and translated inside of the external catheter sheath. The distal end of the imagewire has an atraumatic spring tip to prevent

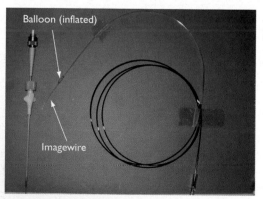

Balloon (inflated)

Imagewire

Figure 21.6 Imagewire inside the balloon occlusion catheter.

injury when this catheter exits the balloon delivery catheter. The proximal end of the catheter is designed to allow for both rotational and translational movement of the probe tip.

Future prospect

The LightLab™ OCT system incorporates two separate signal processing channels to allow for additional information to be extracted from the returning signal in the future. Since the infrared light is a transverse wave, it can be polarized and the polarization axis can be determined from two transversely polarized receiving channels. This allows one to determine the degree of birefringence in the tissue being examined. Such information may be helpful in determining the structure of the tissue since highly oriented tissue fibers are birefringent while randomly oriented cells are not. It is also possible to use the second signal processing channel to create a Doppler image simultaneous with the reflection (or anatomical) image. This will permit color flow mapping in real-time in a manner analogous to Doppler flow mapping on echocardiology systems. Finally, the second channel can be used to create a spectroscopic image simultaneously with the reflection image. In this case, the various parts of the infrared spectrum can be detected separately and color coded to provide insight into the size, orientation and even chemical content of the structures scattering the light back to the probe. While to date there is no OCT available and approved for use in the coronary arteries, this new modality has the potential to provide a new level of anatomical detail and a new dimension of information for the diagnosis of coronary artery disease (Figures 21.7–21.10).

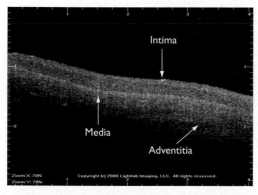

Figure 21.7 *Normal human coronary artery showing intimal, medial, and adventitial layers using OCT microscope format.*

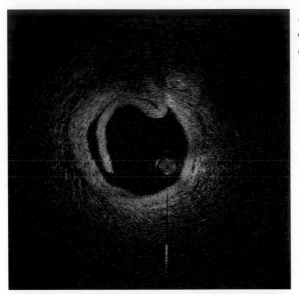

Figure 21.8 OCT image of *an intimal dissection in a human cadaver.*

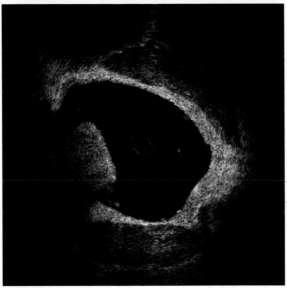

Figure 21.9 OCT image of *thrombus and calcified lesions in a human cadaver.*

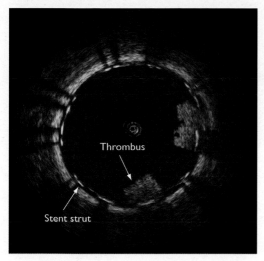

Figure 21.10 *In vivo OCT image of a stent with two large thrombi.*

References

1. Huang D, Swanson E, Lin CP et al. Optical coherence tomography. *Science* 1991; **254**:1178–81.

22. MASSACHUSETTS GENERAL HOSPITAL OPTICAL COHERENCE TOMOGRAPHY SYSTEM

Masamichi Takano, Brett Bouma, Guillermo J Tearney and Ik-Kyung Jang

Every year approximately 1.5 million patients in the United States suffer acute coronary syndromes (ACS), such as sudden cardiac death, acute myocardial infarction (MI), and unstable angina. Spontaneous rupture or erosion of atherosclerotic plaques with subsequent thrombosis is the most frequent underlying cause of ACS. Autopsy studies have identified several histologic characteristics of plaques that are prone to disruption, the so-called vulnerable plaques. Pathologic characteristics of these vulnerable plaques are (i) a thin fibrous cap (<65 µm), (ii) a large lipid pool, and (iii) activated inflammatory cells, such as monocytes, macrophages, foam cells, lymphocytes and neutrophils near the fibrous cap.[1–5]

To date, a variety of diagnostic tools to detect structural abnormalities in vulnerable plaques have been developed. Intravascular optical coherence tomography (OCT) is a recently developed optical imaging tool that provides high-resolution, cross-sectional images of tissues in situ. In this chapter, an outline of the Massachusetts General Hospital (MGH) OCT system and the results of studies using this system are presented.

MGH OCT system overview

The optical source power is 5 mW, centered at 1300 nm, with a bandwidth of 70 nm, giving an axial resolution of 10 µm. A high-speed phase control delay line is used for coherence gating and is capable of performing 2000 axial scans per second. Images are acquired at either eight frames per second (500 angular pixels × 250 radial pixels) or four frames per second (250 angular pixels × 250 radial pixels). OCT images are displayed in real time using an inverse gray-scale lookup table and are digitally stored.

The commercially available 3.2 Fr intravascular ultrasound (IVUS) catheter was modified by replacing a core with an optical fiber. This catheter consisted of a single-mode optical fiber within a wound stainless steel cable.[6] At the distal tip of fiber, a gradient index lens and a microprism are used to produce a focused output beam that propagates transversely to the catheter axis.[6] The transverse resolution provided by the distal optics was 25 µm. The mechanical properties of this catheter were tested in the porcine experiments and were found to be comparable to those of the 3.2 Fr IVUS catheter.[7] The proximal end design was similar to those described in previous publications.[6,8] The stainless steel cable that carried the fiber and the focusing optics were cemented to an FC fiberoptic connector that could be attached to and detached from the rotating end of the rotational coupler (Figure 22.1). The coupler consisted of two gradient index lens collimators separated by an air gap precisely aligned to ensure maximal throughput. A stabilized electric motor is used to spin the rotating end of the coupler (4–8 Hz) with the catheter through a belt drive. The rotating coupler, the motor, and the drive are enclosed in a compact (12 cm × 5 cm) handheld unit compatible with the requirements of the cardiology suite (see Figure 22.1).

In vitro optical coherence tomography imaging of human arteries

Plaque types and thickness of fibrous cap

OCT criteria based on previous comparison studies between OCT and histology are shown in Table 22.1[7,9–11] OCT images of 357 atherosclerotic arterial segments, including 162 aortas, 105 carotid bulbs and 90 coronary arteries from 90 cadavers (48 male and 42 female, mean age 74.5±13.2 years) were correlated with histology in order to assess accuracy of objective OCT image criteria for atherosclerotic plaque characterization in vitro. The degree of agreement between histopathologic diagnosis and the results obtained by OCT readers and the OCT interobserver and intraobserver variability were quantified by the k test of concordance.[12] OCT image criteria for three types of plaque, the fibrous, fibrocalcific, and lipid-rich plaque were formulated by analysis of a subset (n = 50) of arterial segments. In non-atheromatous artery segments, differentiation of intima, media and adventitia was possible due to differences in signal intensity from these layers (Figure 22.2). In non-atheromatous segments, the media was

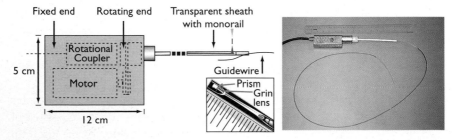

Figure 22.1 Schematic of the optical coherence tomography catheter.

Table 22.1 OCT image features of vessel wall structure by histopathologic finding

Histopathologic finding	OCT finding
Internal hyperplasia	Signal-rich layer nearest lumen
Media	Signal-poor middle layer
Adventitia	Signal-rich, heterogeneous outer layer
Internal elastic lamina	Signal-rich band (~20 µm) between the intima and media
External elastic lamina	Signal-rich band (~20 µm) between the media and adventitia
Plaque	Loss of layered appearance, narrowing of lumen
Fibrous plaque	Homogeneous, signal-rich region
Macrocalcification	Large, heterogeneous, sharply delineated, signal-poor or signal-rich region or alternating signal-poor and signal-rich region
Lipid pool	Large, homogeneous, poorly delineated, signal-poor region
Fibrous cap	Signal-rich band overlying signal-poor region

OCT, optical coherence tomography.

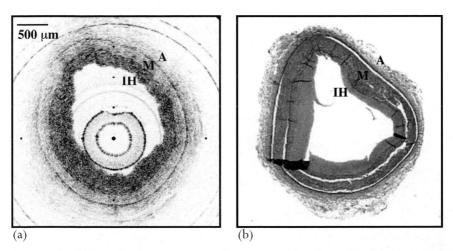

(a)   (b)

Figure 22.2 *Optical coherence tomography image and histology of a coronary artery with intimal hyperplasia. (a) The intimal hyperplasia (IH), media (M), and adventitia (A) are clearly seen. (b) Corresponding histology (Movat's pentachrome stain).*

low signal than either the intima or the adventitia, and then intimal hyperplasia was clearly identified (Figure 22.2). Calcification within the plaques was identified by the presence of well delineated, signal-poor regions with sharp borders (Figures 22.3 and 22.4). Lipid pools were identified by the presence of signal-poor regions with diffuse borders (Figures 22.3 and 22.5). Fibrous tissue was identified by the presence of homogeneous, signal-rich regions (Figures 22.3 and 22.6).

Independent validation of OCT image criteria by two OCT readers for the remaining segments ($n = 307$) demonstrated a sensitivity and specificity ranging from 71% to 79% and 97% to 98% for fibrous plaques, 95% to 96% and 97% for fibrocalcific plaques, and 90% to 94% and 90% to 92% for lipid-rich plaques, respectively (overall agreement, $k = 0.83–0.84$). The interobserver and intraobserver reliabilities of OCT assessment were high (k values of 0.88 and 0.91, respectively).

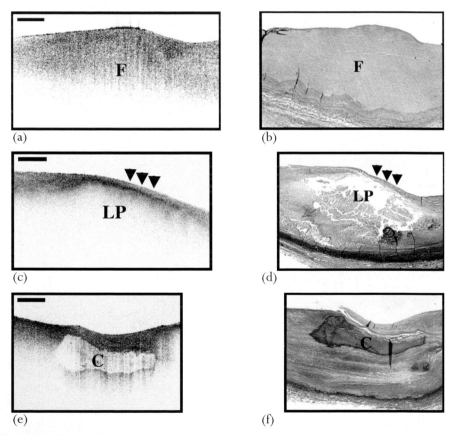

(a) (b) (c) (d) (e) (f)

Figure 22.3 *Optical coherence tomography image and histology of aortic plaques. (a,b) Fibrous plaque. Dense fibrous tissue (F) was seen. (c,d) Lipid-rich plaque. Lipid pool (LP) and overlying thin fibrous cap (arrows) were seen. (e,f) Calcified plaque. Calcification (C) was seen. (Scale bars, 500 μm.)*

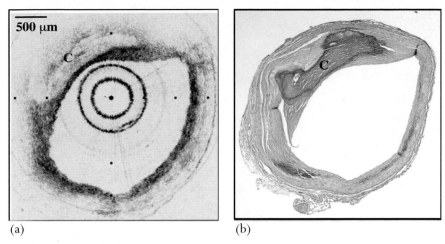

(a) (b)

Figure 22.4 *Optical coherence tomography image and histology of a calcified coronary plaque. (a) The OCT image showing intimal and medial calcifications (C). (b) Corresponding histology (hematoxylin and eosin stain).*

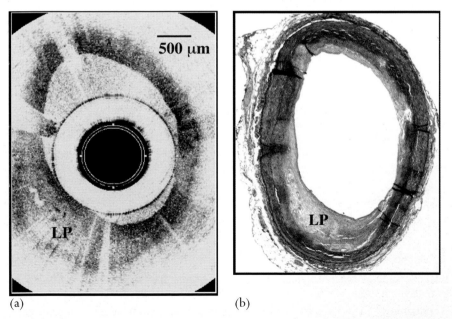

(a) (b)

Figure 22.5 *Optical coherence tomography image and histology of a coronary plaque with lipid pool. (a) The OCT image showing lipid pool (LP). (b) Corresponding histology (Movat's pentachrome stain).*

373

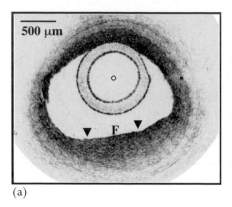
(a)

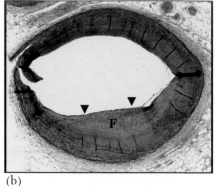
(b)

Figure 22.6 *Optical coherence tomography (OCT) image and histology of a fibrous coronary plaque. (a) The OCT image showing dense fibrous tissue (F). (b) Corresponding histology (Movat's pentachrome stain).*

Fibrous caps were measured by OCT (30–450 μm), and cap thickness correlated well with histology in the 10 specimens. There was a high degree of correlation between the two measurements (R = 0.98).

The results of this study showed that atherosclerotic plaque could be discriminated in vitro with a high degree of sensitivity and specificity by using objective OCT image criteria, and this technique may hold promise for identifying morphologic features of coronary plaques at risk for rupture.

Quantification of macrophage content in atherosclerotic plaques

OCT images of 26 lipid-rich atherosclerotic arterial segments (19 aortas and seven carotid bulbs) obtained at autopsy were correlated with histology in order to evaluate the potential of OCT for identifying macrophages in fibrous caps.[13] Cap macrophage density was quantified morphometrically by immunoperoxidase staining with CD68 and smooth muscle actin and compared with the standard deviation of the OCT signal intensity at corresponding locations. There was a high degree of positive correlation between OCT and histologic measurements of fibrous cap macrophage density (R = 0.84, P<0.0001) and a negative correlation between OCT and histologic measurements of smooth muscle actin density (r = –0.56, P<0.005). A range of OCT signal standard deviation thresholds (6.15%–6.35%) yielded 100% sensitivity and specificity for identifying caps containing >10% CD68 staining. The results of this study suggest that the high contrast and resolution of OCT enables the quantification of macrophages within fibrous caps and this technology may be suited for identifying vulnerable plaques in living patients.

In vivo OCT imaging of swine coronary arteries

Normal coronary arteries, intimal dissections, and stents were imaged in five swine with OCT and compared with IVUS.[7] In the normal coronary arteries, visualization of all the layers of the vessel wall was achieved with a saline flush, including the intima which was not identified by IVUS. Following dissections, detailed layered structures including intimal flaps, intimal defects and disruption of the medial wall were visualized by OCT. IVUS failed to show clear evidence of intimal and medial disruption. The microanatomic relationships between stents and the vessel walls were clearly identified only by IVUS. This study demonstrated that in vivo OCT imaging of normal coronary arteries, intimal dissections and deployed stents is feasible, and identification of clinically relevant coronary artery morphology with high-resolution and contrast. In this preclinical study the mechanical properties of the OCT catheter were found to be almost identical to those of the IVUS catheter.

In vivo OCT imaging of human coronary arteries

The first OCT study in living patients was reported in 2002.[11] In this study, a total of 17 IVUS and OCT image pairs in 10 patients were compared and the feasibility and the ability of intravascular OCT were evaluated. In order to remove blood from the field of view and allow clear visualization of the vessel wall, OCT images were recorded during intermittent 8–10 ml saline flushes through the guide catheter. Axial resolution measured $13.3\pm3\,\mu m$ with OCT and $98\pm19\,\mu m$ with IVUS. All OCT procedures were performed without complications. All fibrous plaques, macrocalcifications and echolucent regions identified by IVUS were visualized in corresponding OCT images. Intimal hyperplasia and echolucent regions, which may correspond to lipid pools, were identified more frequently by OCT than by IVUS (Table 22.2). This study result demonstrated that intracoronary OCT was feasible and safe. Moreover, this modality identified most architectural features detected by IVUS and may provide additional detailed structural information for detection of vulnerable plaques.

Another report revealed that plaque prolapse after stent deployment was clearly identified not by IVUS but by OCT (Figure 22.7).[14] This report demonstrated OCT might be useful in improving the outcome of coronary intervention.

Recent clinical studies using intracoronary OCT have revealed several characteristics in the culprit lesion of ACS. In 17 patients with ST-elevation acute MI (57.6 ± 10.6 years, 13 male), lipid-rich plaque was found in 13 patients (76%), fibrous plaque in 4 patients (24%), and calcification in 3 patients (18%). Disrupted fibrous caps were observed in 10 patients (59%) and thrombus in 15 patients (88%) (Figure 22.8).[15] The high incidence of lipid-rich plaque in

Table 22.2 IVUS and OCT findings for corresponding image pairs (n = 17)

Feature	Identified by both OCT and IVUS	Identified by OCT alone
Intimal hyperplasia	3 (3 patients)	8 (7 patients)
Internal elastic lamina	Not evaluated	11 (8 patients)
External elastic lamina	Not evaluated	10 (7 patients)
Plaque	17 (10 patients)	0
Fibrous plaque	13 (10 patients)	0
Calcific plaque	4 (4 patients)	0
Echolucent region	2 (2 patients)	2 (2 patients)

IVUS, intravenous ultrasound; OCT, optical coherence tomography.

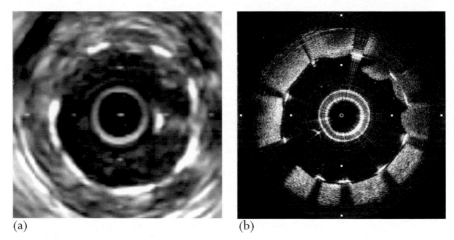

(a) (b)

Figure 22.7 *IVUS and OCT images after stenting. Due to strong sigal from stent struts adjacent tissue between the struts is not well seen on the IVUS image, whereas vessel wall between the struts is well visualized on the OCT image. Tissue prolapse (one o'clock) is more evident on OCT.*

association with thrombus observed in this study, was consistent with prior autopsy studies.

In 20 patients with non-ST-elevation MI or unstable angina (58.5±9.8 years, 15 male), lipid-rich plaque was found in 13 patients (65%), fibrous plaque in 7 patients (35%), and calcification in 5 patients (25%). Disrupted fibrous caps were observed in 8 patients (40%), erosion in 2 (10%), and thrombus in 11 patients (55%).[16]

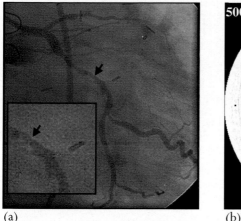
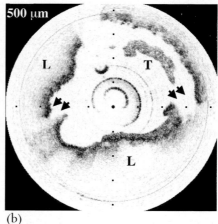

(a)   (b)

Figure 22.8 Disrupted plaque in patient with an acute coronary syndrome. (a) Coronary angiogram showing mild irregularity of the contour in the mid portion of the left circumflex artery (arrow). (b) The optical coherence tomography image this lesion. Disruption (arrows) of lipid-rich plaque (L) and thrombus (T) were clearly seen.

In the combination study with OCT and IVUS, the relation between the plaque characterization and distensibility, index of mechanical property in vessel wall, were investigated.[17] ECG-gated IVUS images, the 29 non-culprit lesions with 30–50% stenosis on coronary angiogram, were obtained to calculate systolic and diastolic external elastic membrane (EEM) area and lumen cross-sectional area (CSA). Distensibility index was calculated as Δ lumen CSA / (lumen CSA in diastole $\times$ Δ P) $\times$ 10^3 (mmHg^{-1}), where Δ lumen CSA is the difference between systolic and diastolic lumen CSA and Δ P is the difference between systolic and diastolic intracoronary pressure. Plaque morphology was classified as lipid-rich plaque (n = 7), mixed plaque (n = 6), or fibrous plaque (n = 16) according to OCT criteria. Distensibility index was significantly higher in lipid-rich plaques compared to other plaque types (P<0.005). The results of this study suggested that plaques with high distensibility might be one of the mechanical characteristics in the vulnerable plaques.

Future role of optical coherence tomography

Identification of vulnerable plaques might lead to a therapeutic strategy specifically designed for a given patient to prevent ACS including sudden cardiac death. In addition, OCT could be used to monitor structural changes in response to genetic, pharmacologic, or other forms of intervention. Finally, with its high resolution, this imaging modality may help us to optimize percutaneous coronary intervention.

Conclusion

We have demonstrated that the MGH OCT system is capable of identifying all architectural features of vulnerable coronary plaques. First, the capability of the MGH OCT system to identify the different components of atherosclerotic plaque was tested in vitro study using arterial specimens. The feasibility and evaluation of the intravascular catheter system were performed in the porcine experiments. Finally, this novel imaging modality was applied for the first time in humans undergoing cardiac catheterization by our group. All of this work provided the basic work for the next step to identify vulnerable coronary plaque.

References

1. Falk E, Shah PK, Fuster V. Coronary plaque disruption. *Circulation* 1995; **92**:657–71.

2. Davies MJ. Detecting vulnerable coronary plaques. *Lancet* 1996; **347**:1422–3.

3. Lee RT, Libby P. The unstable atheroma. *Arterioscler Thromb Vasc Biol* 1997; **17**:1859–67.

4. Virmani R, Kolodgie FD, Burke AP et al. Lesions from sudden death: a comprehensive morphological classification scheme for atherosclerotic lesions. *Arterioscler Thromb Vasc Biol* 2000; **20**:1262–75.

5. Naruko T, Ueda M, Haze K et al. Neutrophil infiltration of culprit lesion in acute coronary syndromes. *Circulation* 2002; **106**:2894–900.

6. Tearney GJ, Boppart SA, Tearney GJ et al. Scanning single-mode fiber optic catheter-endoscope for optical coherence tomography. *Opt Lett* 1996; **21**:1–3.

7. Tearney GJ, Jang IK, Kang DH et al. Porcine coronary imaging in vivo by optical coherence tomography. *Acta Cardiol* 2000; **55**:233–7.

8. Tearney GJ, Bouma BE, Brezinski ME et al. In vivo endoscopic optical biopsy with optical coherence tomography. *Science* 1997; **276**:2037–9.

9. Brezinski ME, Tearney GJ, Bouma BE et al. Imaging of coronary artery microstructure (in vitro) with optical coherence tomography. *Am J Cardiol* 1996; **77**:92–3.

10. Brezinski ME, Tearney GJ, Bouma BE et al. Optical coherence tomography for optical biopsy: properties and demonstration of vascular pathology. *Circulation* 1996; **93**:1206–13.

11. Jang IK, Bouma BE, Kang DH et al. Visualization of coronary atherosclerotic plaques in patients using optical coherence tomography: comparison with intravascular ultrasound. *J Am Coll Cardiol* 2002; **39**:604–9.

12. Yabushita H, Bouma BE, Houser SL et al. Characterization of human atherosclerosis by optical coherence tomography. *Circulation* 2002; **106**:1640–5.

13. Tearney GJ, Yabushita H, Houser SL et al. Quantification of macrophage content in atherosclerotic plaques by optical coherence tomography. *Circulation* 2003; **107**:113–19.

14. Jang IK, Tearney GJ, Bouma BE. Visualization of tissue prolapse between coronary stent struts by optical coherence tomography: comparison with intravascular ultrasound. *Circulation* 2001; **104**:2754.

15. Jang IK, MacNeill BD, Yabushita H et al. In-vivo characterization of coronary plaques in patients with ST elevation acute myocardial infarction using optical coherence tomography (OCT). *Circulation* 2002; **106**:3440 [abstract].

16. Jang IK, MacNeill BD, Yabushita H et al. In-vivo visualization of coronary plaques in patients with non-ST elevation myocardial infarction/unstable angina using optical coherence tomography. *Circulation* 2002; **106**:3239 [abstract].

17. MacNeill BD, Shaw JA, Yabushita H et al. Lipid rich plaques display greater vessel distensibility than fibrous plaques: a combined optical coherence tomography and intravascular ultrasound study. *Circulation* 2002; **106**:3237 [abstract].

23. pH AS A MARKER OF PLAQUE ACTIVITY: A POSSIBLE TECHNIQUE FOR pH BASED DETECTION OF VULNERABLE PLAQUE

Tania Khan, Babs Soller, S Ward Casscells,
James Willerson and Morteza Naghavi

A recent consensus statement by word leaders in cardiovascular medicine has described the vulnerable plaque as the precursor lesion prone to thrombosis or rapid progress in the near future.[1] Structural classification of the relative sizes of the fibrous cap and lipid cores have historically been used to characterize plaques after surgical intervention and histology, or with several promising new minimally or non-invasive techniques such as intravascular ultrasound (IVUS),[2,3] magnetic resonance imaging (MRI)[4,5] and optical coherence tomography.[6] It is widely accepted that plaque rupture or erosion depends more on the plaque composition than on the degree of stenosis. However, lipid accumulation may not be the only precondition for plaque rupture.

A functional classification, based on physiologic and inflammatory processes, was proposed earlier by Naghavi et al[7] as an adjunct to structural information. Macrophages and inflammatory cells, found preferentially in vulnerable plaque, might contribute to plaque rupture through the release of proteases.[8] Thermal sensors have been employed to study the relation between functional and structural heterogeneity, and may be a useful functional measure of vulnerability.[9,10] Temperature change correlated with the cell density and proximity of cells to the fibrous cap.[9] Lower pH in lipid-rich plaques and considerable pH heterogeneity has been also demonstrated in human atherosclerotic lesions, and Wantanabe cholesterol fed rabbits.[11]

Near-infrared spectroscopy (NIRS) is one of many techniques available for non-destructive analysis of tissues. The determination of tissue pH using NIRS has been reported in the muscle during ischemia[12] and in the intestines during hemorrhagic shock.[13] It is relatively inexpensive compared to other modalities such as nuclear magnetic resonance spectroscopy, ultrasound, and nuclear (x-ray) radiography. Spectroscopic methods have been proposed by several researchers to characterize the relatively static, structural or chemical properties of atherosclerotic plaques in ex-vivo tissue.[14] This chapter focuses on the feasibility of using NIRS to measure tissue pH in an oxygenated media bath preparation that maintains the plaque in as close to in vivo status as possible.

Materials and methods

Fresh carotid plaque tissue was collected from UMass Memorial Healthcare's Vascular Surgery operations at the university campus over a period of three months under approval by the Institutional Review Board for human studies (Docket #10041). The plaque was immediately placed in a tissue culture medium (Minimum Essential Medium (MEM), Invitrogen, MD) which had a pH of 7.4, and contained 5.6 mM glucose, 26.2 mM sodium bicarbonate, and non-essential amino acids supplement. The plaque was maintained at $37°C$ in a heated porcelain bath and bubbled continuously with a 75% O_2/20% N_2/5% CO_2 gas mixture. The media bath was equilibrated with the gas mixture for half an hour prior to tissue addition. The entire tissue bath apparatus was enclosed in a humidified $37°C$ incubator. The MEM was chosen because it was the only available prepared sterile liquid medium with high glucose concentration that did not contain phenol red, a pH-sensitive, colored dye that is used to indicate gross pH changes in the liquid medium. Phenol red interferes with the spectral data collection in the visible (500–700 nm) regions and therefore was avoided. This procedure was used for five plaques and all spectral, tissue pH, and temperature measurements were made while the plaque was immersed in the oxygenated media.

The fiber optic, diffuse reflectance sensor used had a forward-viewing design with an optical window. The 1 mm thick quartz optical window was mounted on the face of the sensor. A center bundle of seven fibers were separated from an outer ring of 12 fibers by 0.005 cm, which provided a minimum optical depth penetration of 450 μm in aortic tissue for wavelengths 500–2250 nm.

Spectra from 667 to 2436 nm (15 000–4097 cm^{-1}), were collected using a Nicolet Nexus 670 Fourier Transform NIRS (75 W tungsten–halogen lamp/quartz beamsplitter) employing a room temperature InGaAs detector and a fiberoptic probe module connected to the fiberoptic sensor as described above. The acquisition time was ~42 seconds for each spectrum; 128 interferogram scans were collected and averaged at a spectral resolution of 32 cm^{-1} (~2.5 nm). A reference spectrum was collected using a 50% reflectance standard (Labsphere, NH) prior to each tissue spectrum. The software automatically calculates the absorbance spectrum for each tissue measurement. Additional spectral data from 400 to 1100 nm were taken with the same fiberoptic sensor using a Control Development (South Bend, IN) 512 element photodiode array (PDA) spectrometer with a room temperature silicon detector, and converted to absorbance using a dark current-corrected, reference spectrum. The spectral resolution of the PDA spectrometer was 0.5 nm. The light source used was a separate unmodulated, ~7.5 W tungsten–halogen lamp (Ocean Optics,

FL). The integration time was set to be 3.6 seconds, and sample averaging 15, resulting in an acquisition time of 54 seconds on the PDA spectrometer. The visible tissue spectrum from the PDA spectrometer was offset to the peak value at 970 nm for the same tissue spectrum collected on the FT-NIR spectrometer, and the data were spliced together to form a full range spectrum (400–2400 nm).

Micro-pH electrodes in a sharp, beveled 21-gauge needle (~750 μm diameter, MI-407 Microelectrodes Inc., NH) were used to make the reference tissue pH measurements. The reference junction electrode was placed in the media bath and both electrodes are connected to a Thermo Orion 720A pH meter. The electrodes were calibrated prior to each experiment using five NIST-traceable buffers (Fisher Scientific, 4.00, 6.00, 7.00, 7.40, and 10.00 at 25 °C). The pH meter readout was automatically temperature corrected to the in-vitro media temperature. The tissue pH measurements were recorded after spectral acquisition from the same plaque location used for spectral assessment. Tissue temperature measurements were also made in the same location using a T-type needle thermistor probe (Omega Engineering, CT). After each tissue pH measurement, the electrodes were rinsed in warm Tergazyme solution and distilled water, then checked for drift in a 4.00 buffer at 37 °C. This was done to avoid protein buildup and electrode drift from location to location. An average of four points were collected from each of the five plaques. A total of 20 points were used initially. Statistical methods were used to remove points that were significantly different.

The quantitative determination of NIRS tissue pH was performed using multivariate calibration or chemometric techniques. Partial least squares data analysis (PLS)[15,16] and leave one sample out cross-validation was performed. Briefly, the spectral data are compressed and a linear regression is made against the known reference tissue pH values (or other desired analyte) and a mathematical model is created. Statistical methods, based on an F-ratio test, are used to remove points that are extreme outliers from the rest of the data set.[16] The optimal number of vectors to which the spectral data are compressed is determined by the cross-validation procedure such that the error in the NIRS predicted values is minimized. These vectors can be qualitatively reviewed after calibration to determine if the model is appropriate for the system studied.[15] The ability of the NIRS model to predict trends in pH is assessed by calculating the coefficient of determination (R^2) and the accuracy of the pH measurement is assessed by calculating the cross-validated standard error of prediction (CVSEP).[16] All calculations were performed using Grams32/PLSIQ software (Galactic Industries, NH).

Results of the study

The reference pH values measured with the microelectrodes and the tissue temperatures were analyzed prior to developing PLS models. No correlation was observed in the points used for the PLS tissue pH model. The correlation coefficient between tissue pH and tissue temperature data was 0.002.

The spectra from five plaques (a total of 17 distinct data points) are shown in Figure 23.1. Three pH values were removed from the 20 collected based on statistical outlier detection (F-ratio >3). The most accurate PLS models were developed using three distinct spectral regions, rather than the entire spectral range. The spectral regions are marked in Figure 23.1 (Region 1: 400–615 nm, Region 2: 924–1889 nm, and Region 3: 2043–2341 nm). The correlation of the NIRS pH values to the reference values is shown in Figure 23.2. The coefficient of determination was 0.75 and estimated accuracy was 0.09 pH units. The range of the reference tissue pH was 6.99–7.55. The optimal number of vectors in the model was three. This calibration model has acceptable results using 17 points.

The chemical peaks for the spectra (see Figure 23.1) are assigned and listed in Table 23.1. Between 500–600 nm, the spectral features are varied. Not all the spectra exhibit hemoglobin bands, and in some spectra, the signal is fairly flat and featureless. There is an anomaly observed at 633 nm in all spectra. This was investigated and found to be unrelated to the tissue characteristics and the spectral data from 615 to 920 nm was not used in the model. The top most spectrum was taken from an area of plaque that contained a large amount of blood. Below ~515 nm of this spectrum, strong hemoglobin absorption occurs (~×10 or an order of

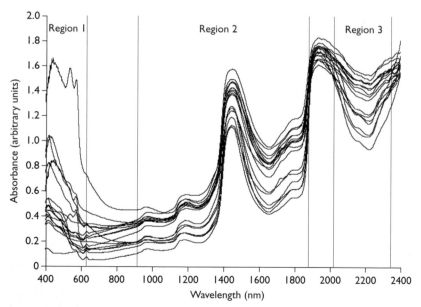

Figure 23.1 *Seventeen spectra from five living human carotid plaques measured in vitro oxygenated tissue culture at 37°C. The three spectral regions used solely for the partial least squares data analysis models are marked. Region 1: 400–615 nm, Region 2: 924–1889 nm, and Region 3: 2043–2341 nm.*

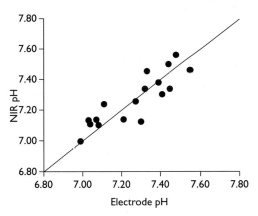

Figure 23.2 *Correlation between the tissue pH measured with microelectrodes in five human carotid plaques in vitro tissue culture media and the NIRS pH determination. Solid line is unity line. Coefficient of determination, $R^2 = 0.75$. Estimated accuracy of NIRS pH was 0.09 pH units. NIRS, near-infrared spectroscopy.*

Table 23.1. Peak assignments for spectra shown in Figure 23.1.

Peak wavelength (nm)	Chemical species	References
417	OxyHb	20
540	OxyHb, OxyMb	20, 21
574	OxyHb	20
633	Optical anomaly	Removed before models built
970	Water	22
1196	Water	23
1449	Water	24
1650	OxyHb	17
1730 (weak, broad)	Cholesterol, lipids, alkyl CH groups, proteins	24, 25
1780 (weak, broad)	Cholesterol, lipids, alkyl CH groups, proteins	24, 25
1943	Water (lipids)	23, 25
2168 (weak)	Non-specific proteins	24
2318 (weak, broad, shoulder)	C-H combinations from lipids	18, 19

Hb, hemoglobin; Mb, myoglobin.

magnitude higher than the amount at 575 nm). The observed muted signal is a result of the spectrometer's decreased efficiency below 515 nm. Region 2 is dominated by the water peak at ~1450 nm. Various proteins and lipids absorb in Regions 2 and 3.

The percent variance captured is summarized in Table 23.2. For each additional vector used, the more variance is explained in both the spectral (X) and reference pH (Y) data. The percent variance captured by each vector is calculated by taking the difference between the sum of squares (variance) of the reconstructed spectra using n vectors and the variance of the reconstructed spectra using $n-1$ vectors, over the total variance of the original spectra. This is calculated in a similar fashion for the pH values. The total, or cumulative, % variance describes how much improvement the successive vector has in capturing the total variability in the original spectra (X) or measured pH values (Y) in an additive fashion. More vectors would capture more variability, and eventually describe the original system. However, too many vectors can also lead to overfit of the model, and lead to erroneous prediction of NIR pH values if not monitored. Incremental variability could be due to spectral noise and not real variability of the tissue pH. Table 23.2 shows that using three vectors to reconstruct and model the data, 98% of the original spectral variance (X) is captured. The corresponding ability of the three vectors used in the model to predict NIR pH values shows that 84.3% of the original tissue pH variance (Y) is captured.

Figure 23.3 depicts the three model vectors used and their contribution to the tissue pH calibration in each wavelength region used. Figure 23.3a shows the three vectors in spectral Region 1 (400–615 nm). The second vector (dashed) clearly shows the oxyhemoglobin doublet at 540 and 574 nm. The first vector (solid line) shows the doublet albeit with a lesser magnitude. Figure 22.3b shows the three model vectors in spectral Region 2 (924–1889 nm). The water band at ~1450 nm is a strong contributor and is apparent in all three vectors in this region. A small oxyhemoglobin band at 1650 nm is also apparent in all three

Table 23.2 Percent variance captured by PLS (partial least squares data analysis) tissue pH model shown in Figure 23.2. Variance of original data captured by reconstructed spectra (X) and pH values (Y) from each successive vector in a linear additive fashion

Factor #	Spectral variance (X)		Reference tissue pH variance (Y)	
	% Variance captured	Total %	% Variance captured	Total %
1	48.9	48.9	57.8	57.8
2	45.1	94	7.3	65.1
3	4.0	98	19.2	84.3

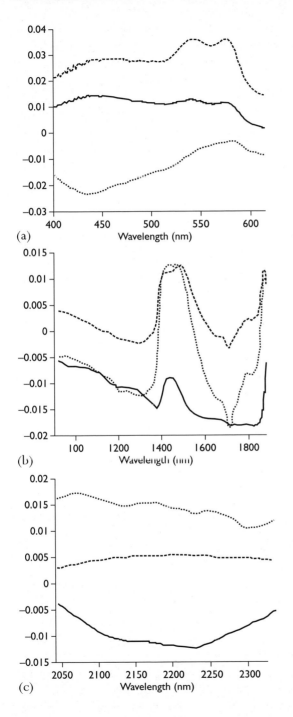

Figure 22.3 *Tissue pH vectors in each wavelength region of the model. (a) Region 1, 400–615 nm, (b) Region 2, 924–1889 nm and (c) Region 3, 2043–2341 nm. Hemoglobin bands at ~540 and 575, and also at 1650 nm, are apparent in vector 2 and vector 1 in (a) and (b), respectively. The water band at ~1450 nm is also a strong contributor to the model (b), all three vectors. Solid line = vector 1, Dashed line = vector 2, Dotted line = vector 3.*

vectors. Figure 23.3c shows the three vectors in spectral Region 3 (2043–2341 nm). Many non-specific proteins and lipids absorb in this region. Using the Region 3 model vectors did not significantly improve or degrade the overall model in terms of correlation and accuracy of the NIRS pH values.

Discussion

The quantitative model results showed that tissue pH determination in atherosclerotic plaque is feasible. Qualitatively, this model has vectors that resemble hemoglobin and water absorption. The cumulative percent variation captured by the three vectors, in each wavelength region contributing to the model, showed positive correlation peaks at the wavelengths where oxyhemoglobin absorb in both the visible (Figure 23.3a, vectors 2 and 3) and near-infrared (Figure 23.3b, vector 1). Alam et al demonstrated in lysed blood experiments,[17] that the 1650 nm peak is a pH-inducible shift in the absorption spectrum of the histidine residue of the hemoglobin molecule, further corroborating the validity of the tissue pH model in atherosclerotic plaques. The other dominant feature contributing to the NIRS pH model is water at 1450 nm (Figure 22.3b, vector 3). This may be related to hydrogen bonding effects from pH-induced changes in water. Most of the spectral variation is captured by the third factor (98%), however, only 84% of the variation in the reference tissue pH was explained. This unmodeled variability could account for the limited accuracy of the model. Additional vectors could be used, however, this both increases model complexity and unwanted noise correlation. An optimal model using the three-vector model is acceptable for the 17 points used for the tissue pH determination and does not indicate over or underfit of the data.[25] Therefore, quantitatively and qualitatively, the model is appropriate for the in-vitro tissue pH measurement of atherosclerotic plaque studied.

The reference pH values were consistent with the values observed in prior studies of plaque pH.[7,11] The electrodes have a reported measurement error of 0.03 pH units. However, the volume of tissue measured optically may be too large compared to the approximate volume measured by the electrode measurement (2 mm working optical diameter versus a ~750 μm working diameter of electrode). This difference in volume may affect the calibration accuracy and prediction.

In a previous work describing optical tissue pH calibration and real tissue pH heterogeneity in vivo in the myocardium,[19] similar challenges of matching the optical volume and reference measurement volume were outlined. However, when ischemic changes occur in the intact myocardium, the direction of pH change is homogeneous and may be more optically predictable compared to the atherosclerotic plaque. Improvement of the optical depth resolution that was required in the myocardium was on the order of 3–5 mm. The spatial distribution of tissue pH in the atherosclerotic plaque is more heterogeneous, in the order of micrometers. In addition, due to the histological variability of necrotic and living tissue in the order of micrometers, the direction of pH change due to ischemic, hypoxic or anaerobic conditions in the in vitro situation may not be as optically predictable. The averaging effect of the optical probe volume in this research may be a large contribution to the limited accuracy of the optical calibration.

Correlation analysis demonstrated that the measured tissue temperature was uncorrelated to the tissue pH reference measurements in this data set. This is an important finding because the PLS method employed here could inadvertently model some other variable if it is related to the desired calibration variable of tissue pH. Therefore, spurious correlation to temperature can be ruled out in assessing the calibration models interpretability. The fact that PLS models could be created with real temperature variation is another indicator that the NIRS pH determined values in this in vitro setting is robust with respect to temperature changes that can affect near-infrared measurements.

Both Casscells[9] and Stefanadis[10] have demonstrated thermal heterogeneity associated with inflammation in atherosclerotic plaques. In this study, no attempt was made to correlate measured tissue temperature with inflammation. It was observed that the tissue temperatures were different in different locations of the plaque and were stable throughout the experiment because of the in vitro temperature control. Stefanadis et al[10] described in vivo human coronary artery studies that showed significant thermal heterogeneity with a novel thermistor-based catheter in stable and unstable angina, and acute myocardial infarction. It should be possible then to determine vulnerability based on metabolic processes of inflammatory cells in the atherosclerotic plaque, whether temperature or pH based.

The study discussed here demonstrates feasibility of the NIRS measurement of tissue pH in atherosclerotic plaque in vitro. Significant challenges still exist to bring this technique in vivo such as the fiberoptic sensor size, signal-to-noise ratios that can be achieved, and improving the PLS models with more in vitro data. Minimally invasive measurements of metabolic derangements such as tissue pH, in combination with one of the localization or structural techniques, could be superior to cholesterol concentration determinations alone. NIRS tissue pH measurement would indicate macrophage activity and acidic plaque, as well as the influence of hypoxic cells on their way to necrosis or apoptosis. A catheter-based fiberoptic, NIRS system is ultimately envisioned to determine the pH of atherosclerotic plaques. The use of a tissue pH value as a determinant of vulnerability is yet to be evaluated, but a non-destructive NIRS tissue pH measurement could be potentially valuable for deciding between different interventional therapies to treat the vulnerable plaque.

References

1. Naghavi M, Libby P, Falk E et al. From vulnerable plaque to vulnerable patient: a call for new definitions and risk assessment strategies: Part I. *Circulation* 2003; **108**:1664–72.

2. Nissen S, Yock P. Intravascular ultrasound: novel pathophysiological insights and current clinical applications. *Circulation* 2001; **103**:604–16.

3. Takano M, Mizuno K, Okamatsu K et al. Mechanical and structural characteristics of vulnerable plaques: analysis by coronary angioscopy and intravascular ultrasound. *J Am Coll Cardiol* 2001; **38**:99–104.

4. Flacke S, Fischer S, Scott M et al. Novel MRI contrast agent for molecular imaging of fibrin: implications for detecting vulnerable plaques. *Circulation* 2001; **104**:1280–5.

5. Fayad Z, Fuster V. Clinical imaging of the high-risk or vulnerable atherosclerotic plaque. *Circ Res* 2001; **89**:305–16.

6. Patwari P, Weissman N, Boppart S et al. Assessment of coronary plaque with optical coherence tomography and high-frequency ultrasound. *Am J Cardiol* 2000; **85**:641–4.

7. Naghavi M, John R, Nakatani S et al. pH heterogeneity of human and rabbit atherosclerotic plaques; a new insight into detection of vulnerable plaque. *Atherosclerosis* 2002; **164**:27–35.

8. Sukhova G, Shi G, Simon D, Chapman H, Libby P. Expression of the elastolytic cathepsins S and K in human atheroma and regulation of their production in smooth muscle cells. *J Clin Invest* 1998; **102**:576–83.

9. Casscells W, Hathorn B, David M et al. Thermal detection of cellular infiltrates in living atherosclerotic plaques: possible implications for plaque rupture and thrombosis. *Lancet* 1996; **347**:1447–9.

10. Stefanadis C, Diamantopoulos L, Vlachopoulos C et al. Thermal heterogeneity within human atherosclerotic coronary arteries detected in vivo: a new method of detection by application of a special thermography catheter. *Circulation* 1999; **99**:1965–71.

11. Grasu R, Kurian KC, van Winkle B et al. pH heterogeneity of human and rabbit atherosclerotic plaques. *Circulation* 1999; **100**:I-542–I-542.

12. Zhang S, Soller BR, Micheels R. Partial least-squares modeling of near infrared reflectance data for noninvasive in-vivo determination of deep tissue pH. *Appl Spectroscopy* 1998; **52**:400–6.

13. Puyana JC, Soller BR, Zhang S, Heard SO. Continuous measurement of gut pH with near infrared spectroscopy during hemorrhagic shock. *J Trauma* 1999; **46**:9–15.

14. Cassis LA, Lodder RA. Near-IR imaging of atheromas in living tissue. *Anal Chem* 1993; **65**:1247–56.

15. Martens H, Naes T. *Multivariate Calibration*. New York: John Wiley & Sons, 1989.

16. Haaland DM, Thomas EV. Partial least-squares methods for spectral analyses. 1. Relation to other quantitative calibration methods and the extraction of qualitative information. *Anal Chem* 1988; **60**:1193–1202.

17. Alam KM, Franke JE, Niemczyk TM et al. Characterization of pH variation in lysed blood by near-infrared spectroscopy. *Appl Spectroscopy* 1998; **52**:393–9.

18. Jaross W, Neumeister V, Lattke P, Schuh D. Determination of cholesterol in atherosclerotic plaques using near infrared diffuse reflectance spectroscopy. *Atherosclerosis* 1999; **147**:327–37.

19. Wang J, Geng YJ, Guo B et al. Near-infrared spectroscopic characterization of human advanced atherosclerotic plaques. *J Am Coll Cardiol* 2002; **39**:1305–13.

20. Di Iorio E. Proteolytic enzymes. *Methods Enzymol*. 1981; **80**:57,76.

21. Rothgeb TM and Gurd FRN. *Methods Enzymol*. 1978; **52**:473.

22. Palmer KF, Williams D. Optical properties of water in the near infrared. *J Opt Soc Am* 1974; **64**:1107–10.

23. Hale GM, Querry MR. Optical constants of water in the 200 nm to 200 μm wavelength region. *Appl Opt* 1973; **12**:555–63.

24. Martin K. In vivo measurements of water in skin by near-infrared reflectance. *Appl Spectroscopy* 1998; **52**:1001–7.

25. American Society for Testing and Materials. *Standard Practices for Infrared, Multivariate, Quantitative Analysis; Annual Book of ASTM Standards*. 3.06(E 1655), 1995; 1–24.

26. Zhang S, Soller BR. In-vivo determination of myocardial pH during regional ischemia using near-infrared spectroscopy. *SPIE* 1998; **3257**:110–17.

24. INTRAVASCULAR ELASTOGRAPHY: FROM IDEA TO TECHNIQUE

Chris L de Korte, Johannes A Schaar, Frits Mastik,
Patrick W Serruys and Anton FW van der Steen

Intravascular ultrasound (IVUS) is the only commercially available clinical technique providing real-time cross-sectional images of the coronary artery in patients.[1] IVUS provides information on the severity of the stenosis and the remaining free luminal area. Furthermore, calcified and non-calcified plaque components can be identified. Although many investigators studied the value of IVUS to identify the plaque composition, identification of fibrous and fatty plaque components remains limited. The sensitivity to identify fatty material remains in the order of 60–70%.[2,3] Recent radiofrequency (RF)-based tissue identification strategies appear to have better performance.[3,4] Using these techniques, sensitivities and specificities in the order of 90% were found. However, since these techniques require a substantial window-length, the resolution of these approaches is in the order of 200 μm or worse. As a consequence, identification of a thin fibrous cap is difficult.

Identification of different plaque components is of crucial importance to detect the vulnerable plaque since these are characterized by an eccentric plaque with a large lipid pool shielded from the lumen by a thin fibrous cap.[5,6] Inflammation of the cap by macrophages further increases the vulnerability of these plaques.[7] The mechanical properties of fibrous and fatty plaque components are different.[8–10] Furthermore, inflamed fibrous caps with macrophages are weaker than caps without inflammation.[11] Because the lipid pool is unable to withstand forces, all the stress that is applied on the plaque by the pulsating blood is concentrated in the cap.[12,13] The cap will rupture if it is unable to withstand the stress applied on it. This increased circumferential stress will result in an increased radial deformation (strain) of the tissue due to the incompressibility of the material. Therefore, methods that are capable of measuring the radial strain provide information that may influence clinical decision making.

In 1991, Ophir et al proposed a method to measure the strain in tissue using ultrasound.[14] The tissue was strained by applying an external force on it. Different strain values were found in tissues with different mechanical properties. Implementing this method for intravascular purposes has potential to identify the vulnerable plaque by (i) identification of different plaque components and

(ii) detection of high strain regions. In this chapter, the technique behind, the method for, and the validation of intravascular palpography are discussed.

Principle

Ophir and colleagues[14,15] have developed an imaging technique called elastography, which is based on (quasi-)static deformation of a linear isotropic elastic material. The tissue under inspection is deformed by the force and the amount of deformation (strain) is directly related to its mechanical properties. The strain of the tissue is determined directly or indirectly using displacement with ultrasound using pairs of ultrasound signals.[16] The method was developed for tumor detection and characterization in breast. Nowadays, this principle is applied in many other fields including tumor detection in prostate, detection of kidney failure and assessment of myocardial viability. Although Ophir et al never explored the quasi-static approach for intravascular purposes this approach seems to be the most fruitful concept. In this application, besides knowledge of the mechanical properties of the different plaque components, the strain in itself may be an excellent diagnostic parameter. Furthermore, the compression can be obtained from the systemic pressure difference that is already available in intravascular applications. Eventually, user-controlled deformation is possible by using a compliant intravascular balloon.[17]

The principle of intravascular elastography is illustrated in Figure 24.1. An ultrasound image of a vessel-phantom with a hard vessel wall and a soft eccentric plaque is acquired at a low pressure. In this case, there is no difference in echogenicity between the vessel wall and the plaque resulting in a homogeneous IVUS echogram. A second acquisition at a higher intraluminal pressure (pressure differential is approximately 5 mmHg) is performed. The elastogram (image of the radial strain) is plotted as a complementary image to the IVUS echogram. The elastogram reveals the presence of an eccentric region with increased strain values thus identifying the soft eccentric plaque. The different strategies to perform intravascular elastography (i.e. assess the local deformation of the tissue) are in the way of detecting the strain and the source of deforming the vascular tissue.

Implementation of the technique

Typically in intravascular elastography, intraluminal pressure differences in the order of 5 mmHg are used. The strain induced by this pressure differential in vascular tissue is in the order of 1%. This means that a block of tissue with an initial size of 100 μm will be deformed to 99 μm. To differentiate between strain levels, sub-micron estimation of the deformation is required.

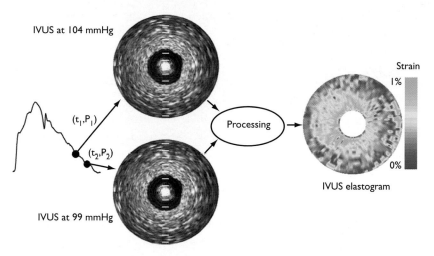

Figure 24.1 *Principle of intravascular elastography measurement procedure. An intravenous ultrasound (IVUS) echogram is acquired with a low (P_2) and a high (P_1) intraluminal pressure during the heart cycle (t_2 and t_1 respectively). Using cross-correlation analysis on the high frequency radiofrequency data, the radial strain in the tissue is determined. This information is plotted as an additional image to the IVUS echogram. In this example an eccentric soft lesion is visible between 6 and 12 o'clock in the elastogram where this lesion cannot be identified from the IVUS echogram.*

Envelope-based methods

Two groups worked on intravascular elastography using the envelope of the ultrasound signal. Talhami et al introduced a technique to assess the strain that is based on the Fourier scaling property of the signals and uses the chirp Z-transform.[18] The scaling property is a direct estimator of the strain in the tissue. The chirp-Z transform was determined from the envelope signal to overcome decorrelation of the RF-signal due to deformation of the tissue. The result is displayed as a colour-coded ring around the image of the vessel. Initial results on vascular tissue in vitro and in vivo are described. Although the technique seems relatively easy to implement, it was not further developed and validated. Ryan and Foster developed a technique based on speckle tracking in video signals.[19] The strain can be determined from these displacement estimates. The technique was tested using vessel-mimicking phantoms. It was shown that in a phantom that was partly made of soft and partly made of hard material the displacement in soft material was larger than the displacement in hard material.

An advantage of envelope-based methods is the fact that the correlation function is smoother than the RF-based correlation function. This prevents 'peak hopping', meaning that the correlation function is maximized around the wrong peak. This makes the method less noise sensitive. Furthermore, the video signal is commonly available from any commercial echo system. A disadvantage is the limited resolution and the low sensitivity of the method for low strain values. Since small tissue strains are expected for intravascular applications, and the arterial wall is relatively thin, it is expected that the use of the high frequency RF-signal will greatly improve the resolution. Based on work of Varghese and Ophir, a smaller variance of the strain estimate is expected using RF-data instead of envelope data.[20]

RF-based methods

Shapo et al developed a technique based on cross-correlation of A-lines.[21,22] The group proposes a large deformation to maximize the signal-to-noise ratio of the displacement and strain estimation. Since the deformation that is needed is larger than the deformation that occurs in arteries in vivo, the tissue is deformed using a non-compliant balloon that is inflated up to 8 atm. Large displacement will decorrelate the ultrasound signals to such an extent that correlation detection is unreliable. For this reason, the cross-correlation is calculated in several intermediate steps of intraluminal pressure. For detection, they use a phase-sensitive speckle tracking technique. The technique was demonstrated in simulations and tissue-mimicking phantoms. Recently this group presented data on a compliant balloon containing an intravascular catheter.[23,24] The compliant balloon is inflated to 2 atm to obtain strain values up to 40%. This method was tested in phantoms and in vitro. The phantom (with one half soft and one half hard material) revealed strains from 20–40% in the soft part and strains lower than 20% in the hard part. These results were corroborated by finite element analysis. In vitro, low strain values (7%) were found for fibrous tissue in the human femoral artery and high strain values (35%) were found in thrombus in a rabbit aorta.

de Korte et al[25,26] incorporated 'correlation-based' elastography[14] for intravascular purposes. The vascular tissue is strained by different levels of the intraluminal pressure. The local displacement of the tissue is determined using cross-correlation analysis of the gated RF-signals (Figure 24.2). A cross-correlation function between two signals will have its maximum if the signals are not shifted with respect to each other. If a shift between the signals is present, the peak of the cross-correlation function is found at the position representing the displacement of the tissue. For each angle, the displacement of the tissue at the lumen–vessel wall boundary is determined. Next, the displacement of the tissue in the plaque (350 µm from the lumen–vessel wall boundary) is determined. The strain of the tissue can be calculated by dividing the differential displacement (displacement of tissue at boundary – displacement of tissue in plaque) by the distance between these two regions (350 µm) The strain for each

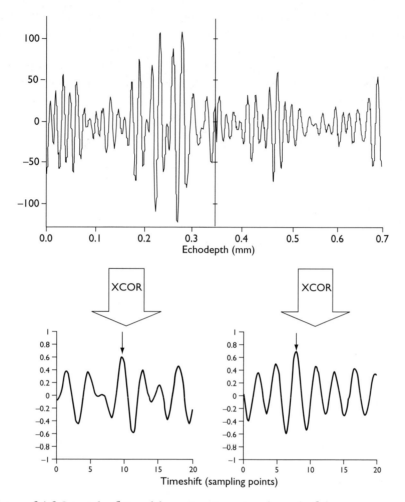

Figure 24.2 Principle of time delay estimation using the peak of the cross-correlation coefficient function. In the upper part, both the radiofrequency traces (the trace acquired at increased intraluminal pressure is preshifted for better visual comparison) are shown for the two windows (at the vessel wall boundary and in the plaque). In the lower part, the corresponding cross-correlation functions for both the windows are plotted, showing a decreasing position of the peak with increasing echodepth. The difference in peak position represents the differential displacement.

angle is color-coded and plotted as a ring (palpogram) at the lumen–vessel wall boundary.[27–29] If the strain is determined for multiple regions per angle, a two-dimensional image of the strain can be constructed. This additional image to the IVUS echogram is called elastogram. The method was validated using vessel phantoms with the morphology of an artery with an eccentric soft or hard

397

plaque.[30] The plaque could be clearly identified from the vessel wall using the elastogram, independently of the echogenicity contrast between vessel wall and plaque. The technique was validated in vitro and tested in atherosclerotic animal models and during interventions in patients (as discussed later in this chapter).

This cross-correlation based technique is especially suited for strain values smaller than 2.5%. These strain values are present during in vivo acquisitions when only a part of the heart cycle is used to strain the tissue.[31] The maximum strain that will be present between the systolic and diastolic pressure is in the order of 10%. For these strain rates, another approach that takes into account the change in shape of the signals can be applied. This 'local scaling factor estimation' technique[32] has been recently described for intravascular purposes[33] and has proven to be more robust to large deformations. The signal after compression is processed as a delayed and scaled replica of the signal before deformation. An adaptive strain estimation method based on the computation of local scaling factors has been applied to compute elastograms of cryogel phantoms mimicking vessels and of a freshly excised human carotid artery using a 30 MHz mechanical rotating single element ultrasound scanner (ClearView, CVIS, Boston Scientific Corp, San Jose, CA).[34]

In vitro validation

de Korte et al performed a validation study on excised human coronary ($n = 4$) and femoral ($n = 9$) arteries (Figure 24.3). Data were acquired at room temperature at intraluminal pressures of 80 and 100 mmHg. Coronary arteries were measured using a solid state 20 MHz array catheter (EndoSonics, Rancho Cordova, CA, USA). Femoral arteries were investigated using a single element 30 MHz catheter (DuMed/EndoSonics, Rijswijk, The Netherlands) that was connected to a modified motor unit (containing the pulser and receiver and a stepper-motor to rotate the catheter). The RF-data was stored and processed off-line. The visualized segments were stained on the presence of collagen, smooth muscle cells and macrophages. Matching of elastographic data and histology was performed using the IVUS echogram. The cross-sections were segmented in regions ($n = 125$) based on the strain value on the elastogram. The dominant plaque types in these regions (fibrous, fibro-fatty or fatty) were obtained from histology and correlated with the average strain and echointensity.

IVUS echograms and elastograms of 45 cross-sections were acquired (see Figure 24.3). Mean strain values of 0.27, 0.45 and 0.60% were found for fibrous, fibro-fatty and fatty plaque components, respectively. The strain for the three plaque types as determined by histology differed significantly ($P = 0.0002$). This difference was independent on the type of artery (coronary or femoral) and was mainly evident between fibrous and fatty tissue ($P = 0.0004$). The plaque types did not reveal echointensity differences in the IVUS echogram ($P = 0.992$).

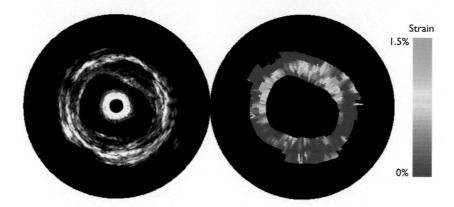

Figure 24.3 *In vitro intravascular echogram and elastogram of a human femoral artery. The elastogram reveals that the plaque at 12 o'clock contains a soft core that is covered from the lumen by a stiff cap. At 9 o'clock soft tissue is present at the lumen–vessel wall boundary. A different strain was found at 9 and 3 o'clock and this difference was not present in the echogram.*

Conversion of the strain into Young's modulus values was performed by the relation $E = \Delta P / 2\varepsilon$. Because the pressure differential and thus the stress are only known at the boundary between lumen and vessel wall and due to non-linearity of this parameter this gives only a first order approximation of the modulus. Conversion of strain in modulus resulted in values of 493, 296 and 222 kPa for fibrous, fibro-fatty and fatty plaques, respectively. Although these values are higher than values measured by Lee et al,[10] the ratio between fibrous and fatty material is similar. Since fibrous and fatty tissue demonstrated a different strain value and high strain values were often co-localized with increased concentrations of macrophages, these results reveal the potential of identification of the vulnerable plaque.

Although plaque vulnerability is associated with the plaque composition, detection of a lipid or fibrous composition does not directly warrant identification of the vulnerable plaque. Therefore, a study to evaluate the predictive power of elastography to identify the vulnerable plaque was performed. In histology, a vulnerable plaque was defined as a lesion with a large atheroma (>40%), a thin fibrous cap with moderate to heavy infiltration of macrophages. A plaque was considered vulnerable in elastography when a high strain region was present at the lumen–plaque boundary that was surrounded by low strain values. This in vitro study in 54 diseased coronary arteries revealed that elastography has a high sensitivity and specificity to identify plaques with a typical rupture-prone morphology (see Chapter 5).

399

In vivo validation

IVUS elastography was validated in vivo using an atherosclerotic Yucatan mini-pig.[36,37] External iliac and femoral arteries were made atherosclerotic by endothelial Fogarty denudation and subsequent atherosclerotic diet for the duration of 7 months. Balloon dilation was performed in the femoral arteries and the diet was discontinued. Before termination, 6 weeks after balloon dilation and discontinuation of the diet, data were acquired in the external iliac and femoral arteries in six Yucatan pigs. In total, 20 cross-sections were investigated with a 20 MHz Visions® catheter (JOMED, Rancho Cordova, CA). The tissue was strained by the pulsatile blood pressure. Two frames acquired at end-diastole with a pressure differential of ~4 mmHg were taken to determine the elastograms.

After the ultrasound experiments and before dissection, x-ray was used to identify the arterial segments that had been investigated by ultrasound. The specimens were frozen in liquid nitrogen. The cross-sections (7 μm) were stained for collagen (picrosirius red and polarized light), fat (oil red O) and macrophages (alcalic phosphatase). Plaques were classified as absent, as early fibrous lesion, as early fatty lesion or as advanced fibrous plaque. The mean strain in these plaques and normal cross-sections was determined.

Strains were similar in the plaque free arterial wall and the early and advanced fibrous plaques (Table 24.1). Univariate analysis of variance revealed significantly higher strain values in cross-sections with early fatty lesions than in fibrous plaques ($P = 0.02$). Although a higher strain value was found in plaques with macrophages than in plaques without macrophages, this difference was not significant after correction for fatty components. The presence of a high strain spot had a high predictive value to identify the presence of macrophages (a sensitivity and specificity of 92%). In cases where there was no high strain spot present, no fatty plaque was found (Table 24.2).

Table 24.1 Mean strain value in plaque types and normal artery in Yucatan pig

Plaque	Strain (%)	
	Mean	Range
Absent ($n = 6$)	0.21	0.13–0.33
Early fatty lesions ($n = 9$)	0.46	0.28–0.80
Early fibrous lesions ($n = 3$)	0.24	0.21–0.27
Advanced fibrous plaque ($n = 6$)	0.22	0.17–0.28

Table 24.2 Relation between a high strain spot and fat or macrophages in Yucatan pig

High strain spot	Fat		Macrophages	
	Present	Absent	Present	Absent
Present	9	3	11	1
Absent	0	12	1	11

Initial patient results

Preliminary acquisitions were performed in patients during percutaneous transluminal coronary angioplasty (PTCA) procedures.[31,38] Data were acquired in patients ($n = 12$) with an EndoSonics InVision echo apparatus equipped with an RF-output. For obtaining the RF-data, the machine was working in ChromaFlo mode resulting in images of 64 angles with unfocused ultrasound data. The systemic pressure was used to strain the tissue. This strain was determined using cross-correlation analysis of sequential frames. A likelihood function was determined to obtain the frames with minimal motion of the catheter in the lumen, since motion of the catheter prevents reliable strain estimation. Minimal motion was observed near end-diastole. Reproducible strain estimates were obtained within one pressure cycle and over several pressure cycles. Validation of the results was limited to the information provided by the echogram. Strain in calcified material (0.20%) was lower ($P<0.001$) than in non-calcified tissue (0.51%).

Recently, high-resolution elastograms were acquired using an EndoSonics InVision echo apparatus.[39] The beam-formed image mode (512 angles) ultrasound data ($f_c = 20$ MHz) was acquired with a PC-based acquisition system. Frames acquired at end-diastole with a pressure difference of ~5 mmHg were taken to determine the elastograms. An elastogram of an eccentric plaque with calcification in the central part, revealed low strain values in this part of the plaque. However, increased strain values were found at the shoulders of this plaque (Figure 24.4).

Discussion

Identification of plaque components and the proneness of a lesion to rupture is a major issue in interventional cardiology. IVUS echography is a real-time, clinical available technique capable of providing cross-sectional images and identifying calcified plaque components. Since elastography only requires ultrasound data sets that are acquired at different levels of intraluminal pressure, it can be realized

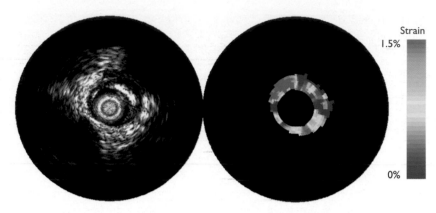

Strain
1.5%

0%

Figure 24.4 Intravascular echogram and elastogram of a coronary artery obtained in vivo in a patient. The echogram suggests a calcified region between 12 and 3 o'clock. The elastogram reveals low strain values in this region corroborating this finding. High strain values were found at the shoulders of this eccentric plaque.

using conventional catheters. It has been shown by several groups that elastograms of vessel-like phantoms and arteries in vitro can be produced. Furthermore, the feasibility of IVUS elastography in vivo in animals and patients was demonstrated.

The question still not answered is the relevance of the information given by the elastogram. An elastogram is an image of the strain and is therefore an artifactual representation of the Young's modulus. Using finite element analysis, an image of the Young's modulus can be reconstructed using the strain and/or displacement information (also known as solving the inverse problem).[40,41] Analysis of more complex geometries has to be performed to identify the differences between and the similarities of strain and modulus images. Currently, the inverse problem is being solved for strain images acquired from human artery specimen in vitro. The resulting Young's modulus images and the strain images will be related to the histology.[42]

Currently, there is no clinical available technique capable of identifying the rupture-prone plaque. Identification of these plaques is of paramount importance to investigate the underlying principle of plaque rupture, the effectiveness of pharmaceutical treatments and on the long-term prevention of sudden cardiac deaths. IVUS elastography has proven to be able to identify the rupture-prone plaque in vitro with high sensitivity and specificity and in vivo experiments demonstrate the power to identify fibrous and fatty plaque components. Therefore, IVUS elastography may be one of the first techniques that can be applied in patients to assess the vulnerability of plaques. Since IVUS palpography is a faster and more robust technique, introduction of this technique in the catheterization laboratory may be easier. Although palpography reveals no information on the composition of material deeper in the plaque, it may be a powerful technique to identify the weak spots in an artery. If a plaque will rupture, this rupture will start at the lumen–vessel wall boundary and this region is imaged with palpography. A natural history study is a prerequisite to assess the predictive value of intravascular palpography to identify the rupture-prone plaque.

Conclusion

Intravascular elastography has proved to be a technique capable of providing information on the plaque composition. IVUS elastography was tested in vitro in several institutes using different IVUS systems, different sources of mechanical stimulus and different processing techniques. Experiments in vivo in animals and patients demonstrate that IVUS palpography may develop into a clinical available tool to identify the rupture-prone plaque.

Acknowledgment

The research that resulted in this chapter had been funded by grants from the Dutch Technology Foundation (STW) (NWO), Deutsche Herzstiftung (DHS), Dutch Heart foundation (NHS) and JOMED.

References

1. Mintz GS, Nissen SE, Anderson WD et al. ACC Clinical Expert Consensus Document on Standards for Acquisition, Measurement and Reporting of Intravascular Ultrasound Studies (IVUS). A report of the American College of Cardiology Task Force on Clinical Expert Consensus Documents. *J Am Coll Cardiol* 2001; **37**:1478–92.

2. Prati F, Arbustini E, Labellarte A et al. Correlation between high frequency intravascular ultrasound and histomorphology in human coronary arteries. *Heart* 2001; **85**:567–70.

3. Komiyama N, Berry G, Kolz M et al. Tissue characterization of atherosclerotic plaques by intravascular ultrasound radiofrequency signal analysis: an in vitro study of human coronary arteries. *Am Heart J* 2000; **140**:565–74.

4. Hiro T, Fujii T, Yasumoto K et al. Detection of fibrous cap in atherosclerotic plaque by intravascular ultrasound by use of color mapping of angle-dependent echo-intensity variation. *Circulation* 2001; **103**:1206–11.

5. Falk E, Shah P, Fuster V. Coronary plaque disruption. *Circulation* 1995; **92**:657–71.

6. Fuster V, Stein B, Ambrose J et al. Atherosclerotic plaque rupture and thrombosis. Evolving concepts. *Circulation* 1990; **82**:II.47–II.59.

7. Moreno PR, Falk E, Palacios IF et al. Macrophage infiltration in acute coronary syndromes: implications for plaque rupture. *Circulation* 1994; **90**:775–8.

8. Loree HM, Tobias BJ, Gibson LJ et al. Mechanical properties of model atherosclerotic lesion lipid pools. *Arterioscler Thromb* 1994; **14**:230–4.

9. Loree HM, Grodzinsky AJ, Park SY, Gibson LJ, Lee RT. Static circumferential tangential modulus of human atherosclerotic tissue. *J Biomech* 1994; **27**:195–204.

10. Lee RT, Richardson G, Loree HM et al. Prediction of mechanical properties of human atherosclerotic tissue by high-frequency intravascular ultrasound imaging. *Arterioscler Thromb* 1992; **12**:1–5.

11. Lendon CL, Davies MJ, Born GVR, Richardson PD. Atherosclerotic plaque caps are locally weakened when macrophage density is increased. *Atherosclerosis* 1991; **87**:87–90.

12. Loree HM, Kamm RD, Stringfellow RG, Lee RT. Effects of fibrous cap thickness on peak circumferential stress in model atherosclerotic vessels. *Circ Res* 1992; **71**:850–8.

13. Richardson PD, Davies MJ, Born GVR. Influence of plaque configuration and stress distribution on fissuring of coronary atherosclerotic plaques. *Lancet* 1989; **21**:941–4.

14. Ophir J, Céspedes EI, Ponnekanti H, Yazdi Y, Li X. Elastography: a method for imaging the elasticity in biological tissues. *Ultrason Imag* 1991; **13**:111–34.

15. Céspedes EI, Ophir J, Ponnekanti H, Maklad N. Elastography: elasticity imaging using ultrasound with application to muscle and breast in vivo. *Ultrason Imag* 1993; **17**:73–88.

16. Céspedes EI, Huang Y, Ophir J, Spratt S. Methods for estimation of subsample time delays of digitized echo signals. *Ultrason Imag* 1995; **17**:142–71.

17. Sarvazyan AP, Emelianov SY, Skovorada AR. Intracavity device for elasticity imaging. US patent, 1993.

18. Talhami HE, Wilson LS, Neale ML. Spectral tissue strain: a new technique for imaging tissue strain using intravascular ultrasound. *Ultrasound Med Biol* 1994; **20**:759–72.

19. Ryan LK, Foster FS. Ultrasonic measurement of differential displacement and strain in a vascular model. *Ultrason Imag* 1997; **19**:19–38.

20. Varghese T, Ophir J. Characterization of elastographic noise using the envelope of echo signals. *Ultrasound Med Biol* 1998; **24**:543–55.

21. Shapo BM, Crowe JR, Erkamp R et al. Strain imaging of coronary arteries with intraluminal ultrasound: experiments on an inhomogeneous phantom. *Ultrason Imag* 1996; **18**:173–91.

22. Shapo BM, Crowe JR, Skovoroda AR et al. Displacement and strain imaging of coronary arteries with intraluminal ultrasound. *IEEE Trans Ultrason Ferroelectr Freq Control* 1996; **43**:234–46.

23. Choi CD, Skovoroda A, Emelianov S, O'Donnell M. Strain imaging of vascular pathologies using a compliant balloon catheter. IEEE Ultrasonics Symposium, Puerto Rico, USA, 2000.

24. Choi CD, Skovoroda AR, Emelianov SY, O'Donnell M. An integrated compliant balloon ultrasound catheter for intravascular strain imaging. *IEEE Trans Ultrason Ferroelectr Freq Control* 2002; **49**:1552–60

25. de Korte CL, Céspedes EI, van der Steen AFW, Pasterkamp G, Bom N. Intravascular ultrasound elastography: Assessment and imaging of elastic properties of diseased arteries and vulnerable plaque. *Eur J Ultrasound* 1998; **7**:219–24.

26. de Korte CL, van der Steen A, Céspedes EI et al. Characterisation of plaque components and vulnerability with intravascular ultrasound elastography. *Phys Med Biol* 2000; **45**:1465–75.

27. Doyley MM, Mastik F, de Korte CL et al. Advancing intravascular ultrasonic palpation towards clinical applications. *Ultrasound Med Biol* 2001; **27**:1471–80.

28. Doyley MM, de Korte CL, Mastik F, Carlier S, van der Steen AFW. Advancing intravascular palpography towards clinical applications. In: Wells PNT and Halliwell M (eds), *Acoustical Imaging*, Bristol, 2000, Vol. 25. New York: Plenum Press.

29. Céspedes EI, de Korte CL, van der Steen AFW. Intraluminal ultrasonic palpation: assessment of local and cross-sectional tissue stiffness. *Ultrasound Med Biol* 2000; **26**:385–96.

30. de Korte CL, Céspedes EI, van der Steen AFW, Lancée CT. Intravascular elasticity imaging using ultrasound: feasibility studies in phantoms. *Ultrasound Med Biol* 1997; **23**:735–46.

31. de Korte CL, Carlier SG, Mastik F et al. Intracoronary elastography in the catheterisation laboratory: preliminary patient results. IEEE Ultrasonics Symposium, Lake Tahoe, CA, USA, 1999.

32. Alam S, Ophir J, Konofagou E. An adaptive strain estimator for elastography. IEEE Trans Ultrason Ferroelectr Freq Control 1998; **45**:461–72.

33. Brusseau E, Perrey C, Delachartre P et al. Axial strain imaging using a local estimation of the scaling factor from RF ultrasound signals. *Ultrason Imag* 2000; **22**:95–107.

34. Brusseau E, Fromageau J, Finet G, Delachartre P, Vray D. Axial strain imaging of intravascular data: results on polyvinyl alcohol cryogel phantoms and carotid artery. *Ultrasound Med Biol* 2001; **27**:1631–42.

35. de Korte CL, Pasterkamp G, van der Steen AFW, Woutman HA, Bom N. Characterization of plaque components using intravascular ultrasound elastography in human femoral and coronary arteries in vitro. *Circulation* 2000; **102**:617–23.

36. de Korte CL, Sierevogel M, Mastik F et al. Intravascular elastography in Yucatan pigs: validation in vivo. *Euro Heart J* 2001; **22**:251.

37. de Korte CL, Sierevogel M, Mastik F et al. Identification of atherosclerotic plaque components with intravascular ultrasound elastography in vivo: a Yucatan pig study. *Circulation* 2002; **105**:1627–30.

38. de Korte CL, Carlier SG, Mastik F et al. Morphological and mechanical information of coronary arteries obtained with intravascular elastography: a feasibility study in vivo. *Eur Heart J* 2002; **23**:405–13.

39. de Korte CL, Doyley MM, Carlier SG et al. High resolution IVUS elastography in patients, IEEE Ultrasonics Symposium, Puerto Rico, USA, 2000.

40. de Korte CL, Céspedes EI, van der Steen AFW, Lancée CT. Image artifacts in intravascular elastography, IEEE EMBS, Amsterdam, The Netherlands, 1996.

41. Soualmi L, Bertrand M, Mongrain R, Tardif JC. Forward and inverse problems in endovascular elastography. In: Lees S, Ferrari LA, eds. *Acoustical Imaging*, Vol. 23. New York: Plenum Press, 1997:203–9.

42. Baldewsing R, de Korte CL, Schaar J, Mastik F, van der Steen AFW. Comparison of finite elements model elastograms and IVUS elastograms acquired from phantoms and arteries. IEEE Ultrasonics Symposium Proceedings, Munich, Germany, 2002: 1873–6.

INDEX

417